MEASUREMENT AND ANALYSIS IN PSYCHOSOCIAL RESEARCH

Measurement and Analysis in Psychosocial Research

The Failing and Saving of Theory

SHEYING CHEN
Department of Psychology, Sociology and Anthropology
The College of Staten Island
The City University of New York

Avebury

Aldershot • Brookfield USA • Hong Kong • Singapore • Sydney

Published by
Avebury
Ashgate Publishing Limited
Gower House
Croft Road
Aldershot
Hants GU11 3HR
England

Ashgate Publishing Company
Old Post Road
Brookfield
Vermont 05036
USA

British Library Cataloguing in Publication Data

Chen, Sheying
    Measurement and analysis in psychosocial research : the
    failing and saving of theory
    1. Developmental psychology 2. Psychological tests
    3. Psychology - Research
    I. Title
    155'.072

ISBN 1 85972 571 6

Library of Congress Catalog Card Number: 96-86721

Printed in Great Britain by the Ipswich Book Company, Suffolk

Contents

Tables and diagrams   ix
Acknowledgments   xv

Introduction: Psychosocial research and the failing of theory
    - Measurement and analysis issues   1

 Psychosocial research and the failing of theory   1
 Measurement and analysis issues and objectives of the book   3
 The chronic crisis in validation and the overlooked issue
  of relation   5
 The Chen Approaches to Unidimensionalized Scaling (CAUS)   7
 Psychosocial mechanism of affective functioning: Social
  support, stress, and depression   8

1 Theories on psychosocial mechanism of affective
   functioning   12

 Affective functioning and depression: An overview   13
 Causative outlook   13
 The psychosocial aspects   19
 Social support theory   21
 Stress and disease   22
 The stress buffering hypothesis   24

2   Issues in measurement and analysis   26

Elements and dimensions of social support   27
The state of the art of scale development   29
Psychosocial determinants of depression: A critique of
    current practice in measurement and analysis   32
Research objectives   36

**3   Social well-being, mental health, and quality of life:
        A research framework**   38

Dimensions of well-being, health and functioning and
    problems of confounding   39
The logic of relational analysis and the requirement for
    construct validity   41
Definition of depression, social support, stress, and
    related concepts   42
Culture and mental health   52
Aging and affective functioning   57

**4   Modeling psychosocial mechanism of affective
        functioning**   61

Social support, stress, coping, and depression   61
Subjective aspects of social support and cognitive
    processes in depression   73
Cultural differentiation: A new perspective   76
Affective disorders in old age: The gerontological
    approach   77
Gender comparison: A feminist viewpoint   79
Psychosocial determinants of depression among elderly
    Chinese and Chinese Americans   80

5   Multifactorial scaling methods   84

Statistical reduction and beyond: A perspective on
    psychosocial measurement   84
Theoretical approach to unidimensionalization: Learning
    from science   88
Weighting and multiple regression: A practical strategy   92

6 Empirical data and analysis plan   96

The data sets   97
Variables and original scales   99
Some consideration of measures and operationalization
    of the path model   104
Scale development and hypothesis testing: An integral
    and optimal approach to data analysis   106
Analysis procedures and a caveat about causation   108

7 Scale development   113

Item selection and content and construct validity   113
The domain of social support   115
The measurement of life stress   118
Symptoms of depression   124
Personal coping: Health behaviors and social attitudes   126

8 Factor analysis: Dimensionality and subscales   127

Descriptive statistics and factor analysis procedures   127
The Social Support Scale (SSS)   130
The Life Stress Scale (LSS)   141
The Depression Scale (DS)   154
The personal coping proxy scales   160

9 The CAUS and the falsification of measurement models   164

Theory-guided unidimensionalization   165
Practice-oriented unidimensionalization   172
Examination of scaling hypotheses by comparing derived
    scales: Criterion-related validity   181
Conclusion on scaling effectiveness   203

10 Substantive analysis and model testing   206

Depression among Chinese and Chinese-American elderly   207
Social network support   210
Stress and coping   211
Correlates of depression   214
Social support, life stress, and personal coping   225
Statistical control via multiple regression   230

Path analysis   233

11   Conclusion   246

Psychosocial research and the saving of theory: Toward
    unidimensionalized scaling   247
Validity, relation, and unconfounded logic   249
Multiple measurement, scaling effectiveness, and standardi-
    zation of research results   252
Social support, stress, and depression in a context of aging
    and Chinese culture   254
The limitation of research   257
Relevance to practice and policy making   261
Suggestions to future research   262

Appendix

1a Lubben Social Network Scale (LSNS) items and
        scaling methods   265

1b Items used for the Social Support Scale (SSS) development   269

2   Items used for the Life Stress Scale (LSS) development   279

3a Modified CES-D (17 items)   290

3b Items used for the Depression Scale (DS) development   291

4a Items used in personal coping proxy measure 1:
        Health Behaviors and Beliefs (HBB)   297

4b Items used in personal coping proxy measure 2:
        Attitudes Toward Social Support (ATSS)   300

4c Items used in personal coping proxy measure 3:
        Attitudes Toward Elderly (ATE)   302

Bibliography   303

Tables and diagrams

Table 4.1   Summary of individual hypotheses involved in the
theoretical model   83

Table 6.1   Summary of the loosened individual hypotheses to be
tested   106

Table 8.1   Descriptive statistics of the items for major scales
development   128

Table 8.2   Correlation matrix of the Social Support Scale (SSS) items   131

Table 8.3a SSS: Final statistics for factors extracted by principal
axis factoring (PA)   132

Table 8.3b SSS: Final statistics for factors extracted by principal
components analysis (PC)   133

Table 8.4a SSS: Factor matrix extracted by principle components
analysis (PC)   134

Table 8.4b SSS: Rotated factor matrix (varimax)   135

Table 8.4c SSS: Pattern matrix (oblimin rotation)   136

Table 8.4d SSS: Structure matrix (oblimin rotation)   137

Table 8.4e SSS: Factor correlation matrix (oblimin rotation)   139

Table 8.5a SSS: Factor score coefficient matrix (oblimin rotation)   139

Table 8.5b   SSS: Factor score coefficient matrix (varimax rotation)   140

Table 8.6   LSS: Final statistics for factors extracted by principal
              components analysis (PC)   142

Table 8.7a   LSS: Rotated factor matrix (varimax)   143

Table 8.7b   LSS: Pattern matrix (oblimin rotation)   146

Table 8.7c   LSS: Factor correlation matrix (oblimin rotation)   149

Table 8.8a   LSS: Factor score coefficient matrix (oblimin rotation)   150

Table 8.8b   LSS: Factor score coefficient matrix (varimax rotation)   152

Table 8.9   DS: Final statistics for factors extracted by principal
              components analysis (PC)   155

Table 8.10a   DS: Rotated factor matrix (varimax)   156

Table 8.10b   DS: Pattern matrix (oblimin rotation)   157

Table 8.10c   DS: Factor correlation matrix (oblimin rotation)   157

Table 8.11a   DS: Factor score coefficient matrix (oblimin rotation)   158

Table 8.11b   DS: Factor score coefficient matrix (varimax rotation)   159

Table 8.12a   HBB: Final statistics for factors extracted by principal
              components analysis (PC)   160

Table 8.12b   HBB: Rotated factor matrix (varimax)   161

Table 8.12c   HBB: Factor score coefficient matrix (varimax rotation)   161

Table 8.13a   ATSS: Final statistics for factors extracted by principal
              components analysis (PC)   161

Table 8.13b   ATSS: Rotated factor matrix (varimax)   162

Table 8.13c   ATSS: Factor score coefficient matrix (varimax rotation)   162

Table 8.14a ATE: Final statistics for factors extracted by principal
            components analysis (PC)   162

Table 8.14b ATE: Rotated factor matrix (varimax)   163

Table 8.14c ATE: Factor score coefficient matrix (varimax rotation)   163

Table 9.1a   Regression of the SSS with the DS (RDSCESD)   176

Table 9.1b   Regression of the SSS with the LSS (RLSRDSC)   177

Table 9.1c   Regression of the SSS with the HBB (RHBRDSC)   178

Table 9.1d   Regression of the SSS with the ATSS (RASRDSC)   179

Table 9.1e   Regression of the SSS with the ATE (RAERDSC)   180

Table 9.2a   List of the Depression Scales (DS) and basic statistics   182

Table 9.2b   List of the Life Stress Scales (LSS) and basic statistics 183

Table 9.2c   List of the Social Support Scales (SSS) and basic statistics 184

Table 9.2d   List of the Health Behaviors and Beliefs (HBB) measures
            and basic statistics   185

Table 9.2e   List of the Attitudes Toward Social Support (ATSS)
            measures and basic statistics   186

Table 9.2f   List of the Attitudes Toward Elderly (ATE) measures
            and basic statistics   187

Table 9.3   Correlation coefficients of the Depression Scales (DS)
            with criterion variables   189

Table 9.4   Correlation coefficients of the Life Stress Scales (LSS)
            with criterion variables   192

Table 9.5a   Correlation coefficients of the Health Behaviors and
            Beliefs (HBB) measure with criterion variables   194

Table 9.5b   Correlation coefficients of the Attitudes Toward Social
             Support (ATSS) measure with criterion variables   195

Table 9.5c   Correlation coefficients of the Attitudes Toward Elderly
             (ATE) measure with criterion variables   196

Table 9.6a   Correlation coefficients of the Social Support Scales (SSS)
             with Depression Scales (DS)   198

Table 9.6b   Correlation coefficients of the Social Support Scales (SSS)
             with Life Stress Scales (LSS)   199

Table 9.6c   Correlation coefficients of the Social Support Scales (SSS)
             with personal coping proxies   200

Table 10.1   Depression measured by multiple selected scales and
             suggested cutoff points   209

Table 10.2   Social support measured by multiple selected scales and
             suggested cutoff points   212

Table 10.3   Correlations between depression and life stress using
             multiple scales   215

Table 10.4   Correlations between depression and social support using
             multiple scales   215

Table 10.5a Correlations between depression and health behaviors and
             beliefs using multiple scales   217

Table 10.5b Correlations between depression and attitudes toward
             social support using multiple scales   217

Table 10.5c Correlations between depression and attitudes toward
             elderly using multiple scales   218

Table 10.6   Aging and affective functioning: Correlations   218

Table 10.7   Gender difference in affective functioning: T-Tests   220

Table 10.8a Cultural differentiation in affective functioning (measured
             by 17-item CES-D): One-Way ANOVA   222

Table 10.8b Cultural differentiation in affective functioning (measured
by DSS): One-Way ANOVA   222

Table 10.8c Cultural differentiation in affective functioning (measured
by DSSD): One-Way ANOVA   223

Table 10.8d Cultural differentiation in affective functioning (measured
by DSS1A): One-Way ANOVA   223

Table 10.8e Cultural differentiation in affective functioning (measured
by DSSD1A): One-Way ANOVA   224

Table 10.8f Cultural differentiation in affective functioning (measured
by DSH2): One-Way ANOVA   224

Table 10.9 Correlations between life stress and social support using
multiple scales   226

Table 10.10a Correlations between life stress and health behaviors and
beliefs using multiple scales   226

Table 10.10b Correlations between life stress and attitudes toward
social support using multiple scales   227

Table 10.10c Correlations between life stress and attitudes toward
elderly using multiple scales   227

Table 10.11a Correlations between social support and health behaviors
and beliefs using multiple scales   229

Table 10.11b Correlations between social support and attitude toward
social support using multiple scales   229

Table 10.11c Correlations between social support and attitude toward
elderly using multiple scales   229

Table 10.12 Psychosocial mechanism of affective functioning:
Multiple regression   234

Table 10.13 Correlation matrix input in path analysis   235

Table 10.14 Residual covariance matrices (LS solution)   238

Table 10.15   Measurement equations with standard errors and test
statistics   239

Table 10.16   Standardized solutions of path analysis   240

Table 10.17a Total effects with nonstandardized values   243

Table 10.17b Indirect effects with standard errors and test statistics   244

Table 10.18   Total and direct effects with standardized values   245

Diagram 4.1   The relationship between social support and depression   62

Diagram 4.2   The relationship between stress and depression   63

Diagram 4.3   A general diathesis-stress model   64

Diagram 4.4   Social support as stress buffer (combined with its direct
effect)   67

Diagram 4.5   Personality and coping as stress buffers   70

Diagram 4.6   An integrated model   72

Diagram 4.7   Psychosocial determinants of depression: A theoretical
model   82

Diagram 6.1   Psychosocial determinants of depression: The working
model   106

Diagram 10.1 A path diagram plotted by EQS   236

Diagram 10.2 Psychosocial determinants of depression: A modified
and tested model   242

Acknowledgments

I owe many people to whom this volume is dedicated. I am grateful to those who have prepared me to undertake the writing of the book. The unique mix of qualifications they gave me for the project includes my training in social welfare, mental health, social epidemiology, gerontology, sociology, behavioral and social research methodology, statistics, engineering mechanics, scientific methods, epistemology, and philosophy. The writing of the book has been so demanding a task that lack of preparation in any of the above areas would prevent it from the achievements. Brought to the project are also my interdisciplinary perspectives, cross-cultural insights, and years of research experience. It is hard to imagine that I could have survived all the challenges without the people that stood behind me. I need not name all of them, but many have been essential to my support and will thus be memorized. I must record, however, that this book has benefitted from the comments and encouragement of experts in the fields of social support (Dr James Lubben, Chair of the Department of Social Welfare, University of California, Los Angeles), mental health (Dr Stanley Sue, Director of the National Research Center on Asian American Mental Health), and cultural studies (Dr Harry Kitano, Professor of Social Welfare and Sociology, and Dr Mitchell Maki). Drs Harry Kitano and James Lubben, along with Dr Iris Chi at the University of Hong Kong, are also thanked for permitting me to use their survey data for empirical analysis. I am grateful to Ms Anne Keirby, Ms Sarah Markham, and Ms Valerie Polding at Avebury, whose effort finally made the book possible.

Introduction: Psychosocial research and the failing of theory - Measurement and analysis issues

Psychosocial research and the failing of theory

Psychosocial research in this book refers to any behavioral and social science pursuit, especially in such professional fields as health and human services where the behavioral and the social aspects can hardly be distinguished from each other.

Inspired by the speculative spirit of science, behavioral and social investigators tend to understand the psychosocial aspects of physical diseases, mental disorders and interpersonal problems in terms of some general theoretical constructs. Among these, stress and social support are two leading approaches to contemporary psychosocial studies dealing with health issues in general and mental problems in particular. Striving to demonstrate the usefulness of such theoretical products, researchers have labored to work out their conceptual details with a variety of elaborate schemes on one hand, and develop some refined analytic procedures using advanced computer technology on the other. With the flourish of literature stemming from such work, there seems no reason for one not to be satisfied with the progress that the sciences have made or have been making.

A potential gap between research and theory, however, has developed while psychosocial research has headed toward details, i.e., components, items, or fractions of the theoretical constructs. Since such parts and portions tend to point to very different dimensions, theorists cannot help but give up their original (often innovative), general ideas and turn to some lower-level, specific conceptions, which are only various facets of the original constructs and need be specifically defined before they can be used on behalf of the original thoughts and notions. Methodologists, on the other side, cater to this tendency and go farther in their own way with hypothesized latent structures, which essentially deny the significance or feasibility of any kind of general theoretical constructs. It is surprising indeed when one finds out that meaningful constructs could be generated (generalized) but cannot be scaled, and that theories that make perfect sense could be logically derived but cannot be empirically (at least, directly) tested. In this regard, theory seems to have largely failed research in psychosocial studies.

Some may argue that the current way of scaling and testing *is* a way for psychosocial research to address theoretical concerns and apply abstract ideas (we will examine the current research practice in more specific terms in the succeeding chapters). However, few, if any, would be a hundred percent confident that breaking the constructs down into pieces is always better than keeping them as-is (if possible at all) in representing, testing, and applying the original thoughts and theories. It is more likely that unless a theorist is interested in showing off her/his knowing of the "advanced technology," s/he would not like to see her/his relatively simple ideas be bogged down in an often excessively complicated research model represented by, for example, a FASEM (Factor Analytic Simultaneous Equation Model) diagram (Bentler, 1986). Indeed, the theorist would be confused because what s/he expects is but some simple quantitative indication of the actual relationship between her/his theoretical constructs. Yet almost for certain s/he will be told by senior research workers that they cannot help with the apparently too broad or general concepts unless s/he is going to be fooled by some dull treatments. The hopeless theorist, however, has a right to complain and to appeal to more relevant research. After all, scientific tenets instruct that pertinence, accuracy, and simplicity are the essence of good research approaches.

This book is about these stated principles as embodied in research measurement and analysis in relation to theory development in behavioral and social sciences including applied psychosocial studies. Although it confines its scope to psychosocial research, the issues it raises and the solutions it proposes may apply to a broader field and add to the whole and integrated body of "biopsychosocial" knowledge.

Measurement and analysis issues
and objectives of the book

In real terms, it is research that has largely failed theory in psychosocial studies. Two major problems can be identified in empirical research: a) lack of a guideline in conceptualization and operationalization, and b) poor treatment in scaling. With regard to the first problem, many research commentators have cited the problem of theoretical confounding. No one, however, has actually articulated a way out, while most research workers are not even certain whether or not this problem is avoidable. As for the other problem, modern psychometrics deserves great recognition for clarifying the issue of dimensionality and introducing powerful statistical tools for dimensional analysis, especially the popular factor analysis. Nevertheless, despite its sophistication with the use of advanced analytic procedures such as the LISREL technique (Jöreskog & Sörbom, 1989), the incompetence or negligence of psychometrics in dealing with extracted, especially uncorrelated, factors/components has left scaling methods largely incomplete. Since factor analysis is intimately related to issues concerning scientific generalization (Nunnally, 1978), this has set an invisible limit for psychosocial research. Indeed, if factor hypotheses set the extent to which one can generalize results across variables that are given the same name, dimensional analysis would in effect become an insurmountable barrier to the advancement of knowledge in terms of generalization finally up to the original theoretical levels. This would certainly lead to a gap between theory and research.

With the consequence that practice has been poorly directed, psychosocial researchers have been largely left unguided in dealing with extracted factors/ components. There are many people who have endeavored in developing various scales and scaling procedures around important psychosocial constructs. Yet few, if any, have fully proved the utility of the invented devices and explained why. Although an original theoretical idea could be considered extremely important and insightful, it would rarely be deemed as scalable unless it breaks up theoretically or empirically, which, however, would at once wipe out the original idea itself as a general theoretical construct.

Unsatisfied with the way theoretical ideas have been represented in psychosocial research, this book aims at advancing "the state of the art" by providing a comprehensive conceptual scheme to guide analysis, and articulating some theoretical and practical approaches to unidimensionalization to improve measurement. In the first place I want to show, on one hand, that confounding is unavoidable by conventional understanding, while on the other, that clear boundaries are possible by tracing the roots of the problem and stressing the role of purpose in understanding the specific meaning of a theoretical formulation and mastering the particular design of a research investigation. I shall endeavor to clarify the general relationship among social well-being, mental health, and quality of life by focusing on a few major theoretical constructs in contemporary psychosocial research (i.e., life stress, coping, social support, affective functioning and depression).

In the second place, I will not only develop some scales using specific data sets to tackle the technical issues in measurement, but aim more fundamentally at illuminating the way in which psychosocial scaling could be done more orderly, reasonably, systematically, and effectively. I will demonstrate that theoretical constructs in psychosocial studies, such as stress, social support, and mental symptomatology, tend to be multidimensional in nature,[1] and blind unidimensional treatments are unreasonable indeed. Showing the results of factor (principal component) analysis by using specific data sets, I will not only stress the significance of dimensional analysis but focus on an unresolved and even overlooked issue of how to deal with the extracted components, regardless of how well a latent factor structure could be constructed and confirmed. The arbitrary manner of using factor(component)-based scales will be exposed and castigated as much as the blind unidimensional treatments in current practice. At the heart of the study, the book sets forth a central theme of unidimensionalization and articulates the Chen Approaches to Unidimensionalized Scaling (CAUS). The primary purpose is to provide some guidelines with the advancement of certain scientific standards to promote and direct exploration in scaling practice.

The book involves a number of important topics: social support, social networks, social well-being, well-being, health, mental health, functioning, affective functioning, depression, life satisfaction, quality of life, stress, coping, health beliefs and behaviors, attitudes toward social support and the elderly, culture and mental health, mental health and aging, the logic of causal modeling, the analysis of psychosocial mechanism, psychosocial measurement, dimensional analysis, scaling, and unidimensionalization. The audience of the book includes students and professionals in psychology, mental health, behavioral/social epidemiology, community health science and other public health fields, nursing, social work/welfare, sociology, gerontology, medical anthropology,

4

Asian American studies, and Chinese studies. In general, any one who engages in theoretical thinking and/or empirical research, especially who deals with conceptualization, modeling, operationalization, measurement and instrumentation, application of statistics, data analysis, scaling, and proposal and report writing may find something useful or suggestive, which s/he is unlikely to find elsewhere.

Because of the wide coverage and multiple purposes of the book, a combination of different approaches are used. First, the book is both theory and practice oriented. In the theory part, a thorough review of the research literature and a pertinent theoretical analysis are provided in a "broad brush" manner to allow the reader to grasp the essence of the all too complicated subject matter without too much pain. As a guide for research practice, the book contains detailed illustrations of the research procedures that the reader should be able to replicate with their own study programs without missing anything substantial. Second, the book is both a comprehensive reading for instructional use and a specific report of my own research program. It is an in-depth study but would also serve as a general text/reference book explicating how research could be done in a desirable manner in psychosocial studies.

The chronic crisis in validation and the overlooked issue of relation

Validity is a (if not *the*) most important and ingrained concept in measurement and scaling theory. Although the term is somehow overused to imply "all things good about a measuring instrument" (Nunnally, 1978:86), psychometricians do attempt to make it explicitly indicate "the standards by which measuring instruments must be judged" (ibid.). The special effort they have made is to distinguish the different meanings of the idea, which has resulted in different types of validity employed in scaling practice. Preoccupied with "what is supposed to measure" in terms of a certain universe of content or a psychological attribute, psychometricians have focused on scaling individual constructs. Their embeddedness in construct validity has been accompanied by an attention mainly paid to unidimensional constructs plus a consideration of the method factor or some general measurement conditions. To maintain the underlying assumptions and validate various scales, analytic procedures such as confirmatory factor analysis (CFA) are valued.

A "chronic crisis" in psychological measurement and assessment, however, is observed in terms of the problems in validation (Meier, 1994). Meier (ibid.) attributes the problems to a considerable ambiguity in the application of Campbell and Fiske's (1959) criteria to demonstrate convergent and discriminant validity. As Meier (1994) complains, "No specific level exists for determining when differences between correlations are sufficient to proclaim a test-construct as possessing adequate convergent or discriminant validity (e.g., Jackson, 1975)."

The real issue, however, is with the limitation of the notion of validity itself. The idea of validity focuses on individual constructs yet overlooks the relationship among the constructs as well as the necessary conditions to validate such relations. In real terms, the idea of construct validity even tends to deny or preclude any significant relationship among different constructs, since if such relationship does exist, it would easily be interpreted as an indication of low discriminant validity in measurement (e.g., Meier, 1991). On the other hand, the achievement of convergence, content, construct or any other kind of validity does not necessarily mean a good measuring instrument as required by a relational analysis. Indeed, psychometric studies of validity contributes little to theory development with regard to the increasing appeal to better measurement tools as a solution to theoretical confounding in empirical research. Not only is validity unable to resolve the confounding problem, but is the pursuit of validity more likely to contribute to it, especially when people pursue validity without purpose, or try to establish universal or all-purpose validity (e.g., Cohen, Kessler & Gordon, 1995). In this regard, the logic of relational analysis needs to be stressed, which will help redress the role of validity in scale development and address the paradoxical needs for both conceptually valid and theoretically useful measurement.

Judging whether a scale could be a good one in a relational analysis needs to take into consideration the conceptual boundaries between different constructs. This book will articulate some principles and provide a masterful understanding of the scaling issues for a discerning and meaningful relational analysis. With a sound, prerequisite logical basis, our scaling efforts could center on vigorous exploration and systematic development of multiple measurement tools rather than simply fall on compliant tests. Aiming at the power of unconfounded measurement or the effectiveness of scaling methods, the use of criteria will be part of an aggressive scaling process in order to achieve the fullest theoretical results.

Owing to the impact of the interrelations among theoretical constructs on their respective content areas and structures, theoretical formulations in empirical research will always be considered as flexible and specific. The price for avoiding confounding will be the modification of the definitions of various constructs. It seems unlikely that one must possess a theory valid enough to predict how test data should appear (Meier, 1994), but that the theory is to be finally specified in the validation process in which data could also be predicted. The viewpoint of relativity is important, and the role of research purpose will be stressed.

The Chen Approaches to Unidimensionalized Scaling (CAUS)

It is ironical that although theoretical constructs like stress and social support are fervently hailed for their significance to psychosocial studies, it is not well recognized that they have to suffer from being torn to pieces or reduced to some mere events in empirical research, or they would be declared unscalable at all. Dimensional analysis seems to have provided a return only to kill the original ideas. Theorists did so by content analysis; methodologists did so by using advanced techniques such as the LISREL approach which borrows ideas like the FASEM that emphasizes on elaborate confirmatory factor analysis. In this book I will attempt to reestablish the integrity of those important theoretical products by proving them scalable "as-is" (at the generalized levels). I do not intend to deny the value of confirmatory factor analysis or the FASEM approach. But I do hope to bring the discussion a step beyond, with an alternative approach to empirical testing and research, to directly or eventually address the need of theory development. I believe when structural equations modeling and the LISREL or the EQS package are used for simple path analysis using good global measures of the psychosocial constructs, they would contribute more directly to behavioral and social theories. The theme of unidimensionalization I set forth indicates the need to move from extracted factors and readily available subscales to the global level. Specifying only one latent variable in the LISREL or FASEM model, however, does not necessarily mean a good or the best measure. The Chen Approaches to Unidimensionalized Scaling (CAUS) tries to accomplish this in a general and desirable manner without resorting to the abstract and in-effective psychometric thinking about factoring at higher levels (especially in light of uncorrelated components). This will help bridge over the gap between

7

the theoretical psychometricians and the practical scale developers.

It is cynical indeed that even psychometricians would allow tremendous variation in practical scale constructions. But now, at least some sort of standardization is possible. In this book I intend to shape some principles in scaling process starting from the very first step. These include the clarification of specific research objectives, basic logical requirements in conceptualization and operationalization for a meaningful relational analysis, item sampling adequacy, good item characteristics, the clarification of dimensionality of the items pool at different extraction levels, the articulation of various scaling assumptions guided by the CAUS, the systematic construction of multiple scales, the falsification or validation of the developed scales and scaling programs according to their measurement power or scaling effectiveness for the specific research purpose (emphasizing relational authenticity of the theory rather than absolute validity of individual constructs), and the multiple trials of selected scales in substantive analysis. Results from different studies can thus be compared against these universal criteria and standards.

In terms of the state of the art of scale development, the CAUS has some fundamental implications with standardized scaling methods formulated to establish comparability among various measures. In contrast to the variety of elaborate schemes of theorists in content analysis and the advanced techniques of methodologists for confirmatory factor analysis, the new approach represents a significant step toward the standardization of research results.

Psychosocial mechanism of affective functioning:
Social support, stress, and depression

Stress and social support are two leading approaches to contemporary psychosocial studies of affective functioning and depression. The genuine effects of stress and social support, however, are not made very clear in empirical research because of various confusions among theoretical constructs as well as serious limitations in multidimensional scaling methods. This book aims at shedding light on these specific topics by providing a comprehensive conceptual scheme to guide operationalization and analysis, and articulating some theoretical and practical approaches to unidimensionalization to improve measurement.

In terms of substantive analysis, the book stresses the importance of statistical control, but not in abstract terms that would call for the awesome complexity of available techniques. Many students, and professionals as well, are actually prevented from studying such complicated subjects as the multilateral relations among psychosocial constructs, including the prominent triad topic of social support, stress, and depression. Research has produced so overwhelming a literature in each field involved that few are able to wade through and arrive at a thorough understanding of all of the domains. With regard to the procedures of analysis, many folks have to stay with simple cross-tabulations and/or zero-order correlations, or at most a single multiple regression model although more advanced techniques such as structural equations modeling are now available. This book will give a step-by-step illustration so that the novice reader can easily follow the logic of causal analysis and replicate it for his/her own research programs. The book tries to present the subject matter in a more masterly manner to help people on campus as well as in the research community at large who have only limited time and resources while urgently need such readings. Beyond the instructional purpose, the results of substantive analysis using specific data sets as well as the particularly developed measures will inform and interest people in related fields. The substantive results have a place in their own right since the significance and pathways of the interrelations among those constructs are not yet made very clear. In addition, no one seems to have successfully applied the popular research paradigms to the Chinese, especially the elderly population. Therefore, the results of the relational analyses as well as the obtained specific measures will make up a special contribution to cross-national and cross-cultural studies.

A causal model is created in the book by integrating the main research assumptions in the literature as well as by taking into account the potential impacts of aging, gender, and cultural differentiation. A reduced working model as well as some major individual hypotheses are tested against data on 1,504 elderly Chinese living in Beijing, Shanghai and Guangzhou and 204 elderly Chinese Americans living in Los Angeles, which were collected in cross-national surveys conducted during 1990-1992. The outcome is remarkable for an integral and optimal approach to data analysis incorporating both emphases on scale development and hypothesis testing. For each construct, different results obtained with different scale instruments are compared, and those proven more powerful or effective in detecting the relationships among the theoretical constructs are recommended. Holding a multiple and systematic measurement approach to psychosocial research, the study opens up some important topics for inquiry and debate. It reveals some unique opportunities for promoting the leading research hypotheses via the Chen Approaches to Unidimensionalized Scaling (CAUS). On the whole, the findings reconfirm significant associations among affective functioning (depression), life stress and social support, with an appropriate understanding of the relationships among mental health, social well-being, and quality of life. The role of personal coping in assuaging stress and depression is also betokened. The hypothetical impact of aging, however, gains only marginal support from the empirical data. Gender difference, on the other hand, is relatively noticeable. Evidence is also obtained for the difference between elderly Chinese and Chinese Americans, though the results do not lend themselves to the myth that Chinese culture is associated with extremely low rates of depression.

The content of the book falls into eleven chapters, including chapter eleven, a concluding one. Chapters one and two provide a review of the perspectives on psychosocial mechanism of affective functioning and identify the major issues in psychosocial scaling and theory building. Chapter three articulates the logic of relational analysis by providing a comprehensive theoretical framework, based on which a specific theoretical causal modeling is carried out in chapter four. Chapter five explains multifactorial scaling methods by setting out a central theme of unidimensionalization. Chapter six introduces the specific data sets used in the study and clarifies some general methodological concerns about the research. The following four chapters, namely chapters seven through ten, are the presentation of the empirical findings on scale development and substantive hypothesis testing. The scaling item pools used in the study are listed in the appendices to allow a smooth flow in the text. Other components in the book to augment the textual discussions include ten modeling diagrams and eighty-three tables (numeric results).

This book breaks new ground in scale and theory development and puts forth a new approach to carrying out behavioral and social research. The book is intended to fill in some major gaps in psychosocial studies. My thoughts about the volume are, in sum, for it to be an in-depth study as well as a general text/reference book explicating how research should be done in a variety of fields of scientific inquiry.

Note

1. In psychometrics the issue of dimensionality is often related to Coombs' (1964) data theory, which is represented by a three-dimensional data matrix for H responses of N persons to K stimuli. Traditional Multidimensional Scaling (MDS) or factor analysis, however, is concerned with the scaling of stimuli or people, and the notion of multi-dimensionality refers to the groupings of elements along either of the two dimensions of the data matrix. This book focuses on the issue of grouping variables in scaling people, and therefore refers multi-dimensional scaling technique primarily to factor analysis rather than MDS as a special procedure mainly concerned with scaling stimuli.

1 Theories on psychosocial mechanism of affective functioning

This chapter sets off by introducing and distinguishing between such core concepts as depression, emotion, affective functioning, affective disorders, mood disorders, and negative and positive mental health. An epidemiological description follows presenting a picture of depressive disorders as the most common mental health problems in industrialized countries as well as other regions including Chinese communities. A causative outlook is depicted by highlighting the role of such basic variables as age, gender, race/ethnicity, geographic location, socioeconomic status, and family history. Noting the fact that "psychosocial factors" have been widely believed to significantly influence depressive disorders, the chapter introduces different groupings of depression according to different etiological theories. Stressing the distinction between etiological taxonomy and clinical nosology, the chapter raises several questions for further literature examination. The purpose is to clarify the general body of knowledge in order to apply the major theoretical perspectives and research insights to the study of some fundamental measurement and analysis issues. It will also help to locate the most significant theoretical and empirical concerns in the exploration into a specific population residing in a particular cultural setting.

Affective functioning and depression:
An overview

Depression has to do with a range of emotional states. "'Emotion' usually refers to the total range of cognitive, bodily, and behavioral changes that fluctuate in psychic life" (Klerman, 1987:3). It is observed that "mood" and "affect" are terms that are often used interchangeably with "emotion." Yet, as Klerman writes, "'Mood' usually refers to a sustained emotional state, and 'affect' refers to the minute-to-minute fluctuations of emotion" (ibid.). In psychopathological studies, "mood disorders" is now considered a more precise term than "affective disorders" in designating certain clinical conditions, in which the emotional changes are pervasive and sustained. However, since "historical continuity and clinical usage have preferred 'affective disorders'" (ibid.), that term is still frequently used in the literature, and accordingly also in this book. With such understanding, mood disturbance is considered as the central feature of affective disorders (Paykel, 1992).

Generally speaking, the evaluation of emotional states is a matter of assessing affective functioning in the study and practice of mental health. "Although human experience includes a variety of emotions, such as fear, anger, pleasure, and surprise, the clinical conditions considered within the affective disorders usually involve depression and mania" (Klerman, 1987:3). Depression is characterized by depressed mood, sadness, as well as a number of other accompanying symptoms, whereas mania is featured by elevated mood in contrast to depression. The focus on such psychopathological states reflects a traditional negative perspective of mental health, that is, the study of affective functioning only when it goes "wrong." Recent trend, nevertheless, has rendered an emphasis on positive mental health (Herzog et al., 1982). This provides ground not only for the inclusion of "normal depression" in the general study of affective disorders (Klerman, 1987), but for the extension of the interest of this book to the conditions of optimal or successful affective functioning.

Causative outlook

Affective disorders are probably the most common mental health problems. With the narrow meaning of the term, the prevalence of affective disorders in industrialized countries and regions may range up to 20% of the population or more (Weissman & Myers, 1978), depending on criterion. Depression has the greatest prominence, whereas mania is less common. In clinical practice, affective disorders fall into two major diagnostic categories, that is, unipolar and bipolar depressions. Here "bipolar" refers to the occurrence of both depressive and manic phases or, in other words, to a state of depression implicating manic episodes. The term "major depression" is used for most unipolar depressions, whereas unipolar mania is seldom considered a separate entity of affective disorders (American Psychiatric Association, 1987). Epidemiological data from industrialized countries and regions show a general rate of about 1% lifetime prevalence for bipolar disorder and a rough range of 2.9% to 12.6% lifetime prevalence for major depression (Smith & Weissman, 1992). There is another milder but more chronic form of depression, dysthymia (previously called depressive neurosis), which adds to the prevalence rates while is somewhat less widespread than major depression (ibid.).

An important approach to the factors associated with the depressive disorders is epidemiological investigation. In its extensive search for the demographic distributions of the disorders, all significant person characteristics as well as time and place variables are examined in relation to specific diagnoses so that their causes can be distinguished. In terms of potential risk factors, investigators tend to firstly look into an epidemic for its gender and age differences. There is no sex difference found in bipolar illness. On the other hand, there is increased risk of unipolar depressions in women, with the sex ratios of females to males being about 2:1 (ibid.). This is seen remarkably consistent across cultures and persistent over time. However, as Perris (1992) summarizes, none of the single variables explored so far (e.g. methodological, endocrine, psychosocial, and genetic factors) is enough to account for the increased rates of depression among women.

Cross-national data suggest that bipolar disorder, when compared with unipolar depression, has an earlier onset and narrower period of risk. For major depression, until recently the conventional wisdom has been that it increases with age (Smith & Weissman, 1992). Studies throughout the 1970s, however, began to show that persons 18-44 years of age were at highest risk for all forms of depression (ibid.). It seems that older age turns out to be more protective. Nonetheless, when even a decrease was found in lifetime prevalence with age, this hypothesis on the simple age effect became not only counter-intuitive but logically uninterpretable. That is because lifetime risks are cumulative and should increase with age, or at least flatten if older age is completely protective

14

(ibid.). A number of additional hypotheses have been made to account for potential artifacts operating in the relationship between age and depression. These include a memory loss effect with increasing age, selective mortality and/or institutionalization, selective migration, changing diagnostic criteria, threshold changes in reporting among mental health professionals and/or society at large, and reporting bias of interviewees (Klerman & Weissman, 1989). Moreover, a period effect is hypothesized to illuminate the time or historical dimension. And a birth-cohort effect is articulated to recapitulate the differences in the lifetime experience of different cohort groups (Smith & Weissman, 1992).

Racial/ethnic differences are issues important to investigators from multi-racial/ethnic and/or multiculturalist countries as well as to all researchers interested in cross-cultural studies. In the United States, there is no convincing evidence showing significant differences in rates for depression by race independent of socioeconomic status (Smith & Weissman, 1992). Cross-national studies, however, indicate the possible influence of some cultural factors. Asian, especially Chinese, communities demonstrated the lowest prevalence for depressive disorders. However, since there were possibly artifacts in translation and cultural interpretation, whether or not such a difference represents true diagnostic racial variability is yet open to inquiry (ibid.).

The geographic factor, i.e., the rural-urban distinction, may have an impact on the distribution of depressive disorders. Although its role in effecting depression is yet hard to decide, it has been hypothesized that the greater instability in the more transitional small-town areas would result from the conflict in values between the industrialized metropolitan area and traditional rural areas. And this would have an effect on the rates of depressive disorders by increasing the psychological stress on their residents (ibid.).

Socioeconomic status is generally accepted as a significant factor in social and health surveys. Epidemiological data, however, seem to be far from validating its complicated relationship with depressive disorders. Results of community surveys variously indicated higher rates of bipolar illness for higher social class (Dunham, 1967; Weissman & Myers, 1978; Krauthammer & Klerman, 1979), particularly for professional and/or highly educated people (Welner et al., 1979; Woodruff et al., 1971), and lower rates of major depression for the employed and/or financially independent. Studies also tried to connect major depression to education (Smith & Weissman, 1992). However, research studies have not produced consistent findings regarding the relationships between socioeconomic status variables and depressive disorders. And the causal directions of those ever hypothesized associations are generally unclear.

Conventional epidemiological inquiry into family ties of the sufferers of depressive disorders attaches most interest to the hereditary or genetic aspect. Although epidemiologists usually do not assess family history, suggestions from clinical studies on the familial nature of major depression and bipolar illness are held in high regard. It is hypothesized that genes play a role in the etiology of major depression, although their role is not as great as in bipolar disorder (ibid.). On the other hand, marital status is often considered a risk factor, and divorced persons are identified most likely to have major depressive and bipolar disorders. Differentiating between marital history and current status, however, Smith and Weissman (1992) underscore the quality of marital relationship by pointing to the change of marriage and divorce system in the past decades.

It seems that the current system of scientific knowledge dealing with depressive disorders has included different approaches to the issues involved, ranging from biological-physiological and psychodynamic studies to epidemiological and social investigations. Particularly, "psychosocial factors" have been believed to significantly influence depressive disorders. Researchers seem to agree that such variables play a significant role in the predisposition, onset, lifetime course, and systems impact of depression (Becker & Kleinman, 1991).

However, there are different groupings of depression. Tremendous efforts have been made in clinical practice and research to classify depressive disorders (e.g. World Health Organization, 1978; American Psychiatric Association, 1987), which provide various nosological categories aiming primarily at effective diagnosis and treatment of depressive disorders. On the other hand, in the study of pathogenesis of depressive disorders, it is noted that research findings on their psychosocial determinants have not proven to be as consistently replicable or predictive as expected. And much of the mixed results obtained is attributed to the heterogeneity of depressive diagnoses (Becker & Kleinman, 1991).

Etiological theorists have tried to provide different models to account for affective disorders. Especially, there have been two major conceptions of depression, namely, the endogenous and the reactive. Endogenous depression refers to a hereditary disorder characterized either by a bipolar course of episodes (i.e., depressive and manic episodes are alternating) or by recurrent depressive episodes (unipolar depression), whereas reactive depression is a depressive episode provoked by a single major life event or by enduring psychosocial circumstances (Bech, 1992). Interesting enough, the classical works on endogenous depression (e.g. Kraepelin, 1921) and the classical studies on reactive depression (e.g.

Freud, 1959) give rather similar clinical descriptions of depression in spite of their etiological differences (Bech, 1992). The potential differences in their determinants other than symptoms are therefore important aspects of diagnostic scales for the endogenous-reactive distinction. Such scales take into consideration a) psychosocial stressors, b) personality, c) onset, duration and persistence of clinical picture, d) previous episodes of depression, e) diurnal variation, f) reactivity of symptoms, g) biological symptoms (quality of depression, early awakening, weight loss), and h) psychological symptoms (anxiety, phobias, aggression) (ibid.).

Generally, however, the endogenous-reactive distinction is not confirmed, and we seem to be yet far from an etiological classification of the depressive disorders. In real terms, even deciding whether or not a particular depression has been precipitated by some outside factor can be quite difficult (Grove & Andreasen, 1992). Here it is important not to confuse etiological taxonomy with clinical nosology; the latter is based primarily on symptoms or the phenomenology of depression. However, the identification of disorders, if it is to be of full use, must lead to their effective treatment and prevention. And that will eventually demand elucidations of their determinants including psychosocial factors with some specificity.

In the following, I will seek to lay some theoretical groundwork for an empirical research into a specific population residing in a particular cultural setting in order to illuminate some important measurement and analysis issues. The psychosocial aspects of depressive disorders, especially the relationship between social support and depression in the context of aging and Chinese culture, are specified as the domain to be addressed in the literature exploration. However, behavioral/social science theory rooted in the Chinese society, especially that derived from studies of its older people, is yet hardly available on the selected topic. For the purpose of the book which is intended to draw on a wide range of behavioral/social science knowledge, an approach will be taken to start from the most commonly accepted core of worldwide research literature. The commitment is, therefore, in the clarification of the general body of knowledge and application of the major theoretical perspectives and research insights to the study of social well-being and mental health of the Chinese/Chinese-American elderly.

The task of the inquiry is fourfold. First, the boundaries of the general body of knowledge and the scope of current research should be specified and, based on such information, the topic for discussion should be narrowed down to find out some significant but manageable theoretical and empirical issues for further examination. Second, a thorough analysis of the contributions to knowledge and limitations of various theoretical approaches and empirical studies is crucial to subsequent research that entails a proper theoretical framework. Third, as this body of knowledge is mainly a product of Western, especially English-speaking, industrialized societies (though enriched with some cross-cultural study and international research), the issues and perspectives discerned from current theory and research should be perused with an appropriate understanding of the cultural issues involved. And finally, the characteristics of the aging population should especially be heeded. The applicability of such knowledge to the advancement of aging research in Chinese cultural settings, in the last analysis, lies at the center of the empirical inquiry.

In spotting the boundaries of the field by recapitulating its major themes and narrowing down to the present topic, this body of knowledge has been evidenced to be sufficiently broad. A thorough review of both theoretical and empirical research writings, however, is possible only after a clear statement of the questions to be examined is made. The selection of the questions is based on both their theoretical significance and the need to guide the specific empirical research to be performed afterward. In the first place, efforts invested in the psychosocial studies of depressive disorders have yielded a few very important perspectives. Each of them has formed an affluent body of knowledge on its own and we should trace the main ideas therein. In the second, the interplay among different approaches and perspectives have resulted in some prevailing research paradigms in the field. We need to examine their utility by summing up the empirical results. Age- and culture-related issues will be discussed in greater detail to illuminate their relevance to the research of Chinese and Chinese-American elderly. The applicability of the body of knowledge will also be considered in light of some general issues remaining to be resolved. To be specific, answers to the following questions are to be sought in the theoretical discussions:

1)   What are the major approaches and perspectives in contemporary psychosocial studies of affective mental health in general and depressive disorders in particular?

2)   What are the main themes of each of these approaches and perspectives, especially of the social support theory?

3)   How the themes and theses, especially the stress-buffering hypothesis,

are maintained and advanced by empirical research findings?

4) What are the major issues in pursuing the correlations among social support, stress, and affective functioning (depression)?

5) What are the characteristics of depressive disorders among elderly population?

6) What is the influence of Chinese culture?

7) How would the theoretical approaches and empirical findings inform research design on Chinese and Chinese-American elderly?

The literature review will first look at various psychosocial aspects of depression by examining the meaning of "psychosocial" in some representative writings of the field. It is underscored that this dimension of affective functioning and depression has become more and more evident, with both its social precipitators and social moderators attracting wider and wider research attention. Specifically, social support, life events, and depression have become a hot triadic topic in pursuing the social process of mental health. With a research interest in thus constructed psychosocial mechanism, the rest of the chapter will make brief yet effective visits to the research fields of social support, stress and disease, and finally arrive at the "stress buffering" hypothesis. In view of the overwhelming information in these fields, the material presented in this chapter is highly refined to ensure the reader to get the essence of each subject as well as the sense of significance of linking these topics together.

The psychosocial aspects

Recent progress made in genetic, neurochemical, and neuroendocrinological studies considerably illuminated biological aspects of the etiology of depressive disorders. Efforts aimed at gaining understanding of their pathogenesis or patho-physiology also contributed to rather effective medication and physical treatment. On the other hand, along with the surge of behavioral/social epidemiology, there has been a rapid growth in the literature on psychosocial aspects of depressive disorders. The study of depression is now so diversified that it seems one can hardly master all of its domains ranging from the mechanism of action of antidepressant drugs to the mediating or moderating role of social support networks. Whereas an all-sided view of the major variables contributing to the disorders should serve as an indispensable basis, the inquiry here is intended to focus on some major psychosocial factors associated with depressive disorders.

The meaning of "psychosocial," however, appears to be somewhat too broad, or too loosely defined. Under the rubric of "Psychosocial Aspects of Depression," Becker and Kleinman (1991) included the following topics: a) epidemiological studies of depression, b) theoretical and empirical issues in differentiating depression from anxiety, c) cross-cultural studies of depression, d) life stress and depression, e) interpersonal aspects of depression from psychodynamic and attachment perspectives, f) empirical studies of the interpersonal relations of adult depressives, g) life stressors, social resources, and the treatment of depression, and h) the mediating role of personality in recurrent mood disorders. There were still many other interpersonal domains that were precluded because of space limitations but were relevant in the view of the two U.S. editors, such as social cognition, impression management, circumflex models or the impacts of immigration, unemployment, political upheaval, and the drug culture on depressive phenomena. In a book published earlier in 1982 while entitled the same as above, Freden, a Swedish author, used a different set of headings for his contents. With a sociological perspective and claiming an interest in social psychiatry as well as a comprehensive strategy, the author made comparison between the psychodynamic approach, the behavioral approach, and Ernest Becker's multidimensional approach. Characteristics of the depressed were reviewed in terms of childhood background, education, social class, personality, sex, and the social antecedents of depression. The author paid much attention to the role of stressful events in terms of loss of close relative, loss of work, problems at work, somatic illness, separation, problems in the partner relationship, family problems, "nothing special," and other problems. It is worth noting that even more regard was given to social ties such as parental, marital, and friend relations as means of social support (Freden, 1982).

It seems that a psychosocial dimension of affective functioning in general and depression in particular has become more and more evident, with both its social precipitators and social moderators attracting wider and wider research attention. Specifically, social support, life events, and depression have become a hot triadic topic in pursuing the social process of mental health (Lin, Dean, & Ensel, 1986). The research here is particularly interested in the social approach to affective functioning and depressive disorders. We may well proceed with the recent trend to clarify the current "state of the art" of the field and identify the major issues for further inquiry.

Social support theory

Social support became a heated term when a branch of learning of "psychosocial epidemiology" recently achieved its phenomenal existence (Lin, Dean, & Ensel, 1986). Its being a research subject, nevertheless, can be pursued far back in the modern history. The roots of interest in social support are now often traced to early sociologist Durkheim's classic work (Vaux, 1988). Especially, his study of suicide in 1897 has been directly related to the formation of a social psychiatry (Dean, 1986). Based on sociological studies thereafter, there has been a belief that morale and well-being are sustained through primary group ties, the absence of which may result in psychological disorder and social problem. On the other hand, psychodynamic thinking such as Freudian theory also provided a precedent for the study of social relationships and well-being by highlighting the importance of early attachment and the needs served by later social relationships that in some views harken back to childhood issues (Vaux, 1988).

With all such theoretical tradition setting the stage for social support study, however, it did not automatically become an outspoken subject for either sociological or psychological pursuit. Rather, the research interest of social support over the past two decades has largely grown out of the practice of some helping professions, especially the health sciences. Epidemiologists John Cassel (1974) and Sidney Cobb (1976) laid much of the groundwork for the discussion of the psychosocial processes implicated in disease etiology. In particular, Cassel argued that social support plays a key role in stress-related disorders. Both animal and human studies had provided evidence supporting this point of view (Cassel, 1976). Therefore, he advocated the mobilization of social support as a more feasible direction for intervention than attempting to reduce exposure to environmental stressors. This is a viewpoint that has underlaid much of the interest in social support (Vaux, 1988). Another influential figure responsible for current interest in social support, Gerald Caplan (1974), incorporated the role of social support in preventive psychiatry and community mental health. Later, Gottlieb (1983) examined the direct and indirect ways that social support may affect health, and outlined directions for mental health practice that involve the mobilization and strengthening of social support. Through the work of these pioneers and their followers, the role of social support in maintaining good mental health in general and normal and successful affective functioning in particular has been gradually recognized.

It is noticeable that the social pathogenesis of affective disorders is now frequently expressed in terms of life events and social stress (Paykel & Cooper, 1992). And the role of social support tends to be understood as a "moderator" or "buffer" of their negative mental and physical health effects (Cassel, 1976; Cobb, 1976; Cohen & Wills, 1985). The enhancement of social support networks, therefore, is advocated along with the modification of stressful environments and the development of individual coping skills as social approaches to the treatment and prevention of affective disorders (Scott, 1992).

Stress and disease

It is hard indeed to imagine the elevation of social support dialogue without a knowledge of the mighty achievement of stress study. The term is so fashionable nowadays that it seems that human beings have entered an "age of stress." Hans Selye, the founding father of stress research, defines stress as the *nonspecific* or *common* result of any demand upon the body, be the effect mental or somatic (Selye, 1982). The formulation of the definition is based on objective indicators such as bodily and chemical changes that appear after any demand. In Selye's view, it is this conceptualization that has brought the subject up from the level of cocktail party chitchat into the domain of science, which is now so trendy that it is often referred to as "stressology" (ibid.).

Selye's major contribution is the identification of the general adaptation syndrome (GAS) in his original, biologic research, which serves as the basis of the stress conception (Selye, 1936). The syndrome, in his words, consists of several stages starting from alarm reaction, through adaptation or resistance, then ending with exhaustion. Yet, according to Selye, the stage of exhaustion does not always need to be irreversible and complete, as long as it affects only parts of the body. Since he articulated the nonspecific stress syndrome, discoveries in science have linked it with numerous biochemical and structural changes of previously unknown origin. Functions of the nervous and vascular-hormonal systems in stress response have been remarkably illustrated by animal studies. The mediation of stress reactions via biological mechanisms of the organism is also part of the major research efforts, which involve countless hormonal and chemical changes that check and balance the body's functioning and stability during stress. In general, the nervous and hormonal stress responses aid adaptation to environmental change or stimuli.

The significance of Selye's finding, however, would not be so great should the stress concept not be connected with all kinds of diseases, which would have prevented a real revolution in basic etiological ideas. Although stress is termed a "syndrome" and sometimes even an "epidemic" that is deemed to feature the uneasy modern times, it is not considered as an independent disease entity all by itself. Nevertheless, stress may have negative consequences in two ways. First, as the reserves of adaptation energy of organism are not infinite, wear and tear in the body will accumulate to constitute the signs of aging. Second, and most important, Selye suggests that general adaptation syndrome represented by the nervous and hormonal responses may sometimes become the cause of disease, especially if the state of stress is prolonged or intense. In general, the adaptive response can break down or go wrong because of innate defects, understress, overstress, or psychological mismanagement (ibid.). When such is the case, there come so-called diseases of adaptation, or more accurately, diseases of maladaptation. They are also termed stress-related diseases or stress diseases.

The value of the stress idea is thus not just in the theory of adaptation, but also in the conception of maladaptation, which gives an extremely important lead to the study of pathogenesis of all kinds of diseases. In real terms, it has spurred tremendous progress in physiological, psychological, medical, and health sciences. For example, stress is now evidenced to be a major contributor, either directly or indirectly, to six of the leading causes of death in the United States - coronary heart disease, cancer, lung ailments, accidental injuries, cirrhosis of the liver, and suicide. Yet, Selye (1982) further points out that no malady is just a disease of adaptation; conversely, there are no disease producers that can be so perfectly handled by the organism that maladaptation plays no part in their effects upon the body. Because of the universality of the adaptation syndrome in disease process, some researchers have come to the conclusion that even the label of stress itself is no longer needed. This notwithstanding, the relationship between stress and different kinds of diseases is not invariant. People seem to have especially heeded the pathogenesis of some singularly stress-sensitive disease entities by applying particularly to them the stress-disease terminology. The most common stress diseases include peptic ulcers in the stomach and upper intestine, high blood pressure, heart accidents, and nervous disturbances (ibid.). Stress also plays a role in aggravating such diverse conditions as multiple sclerosis, diabetes, genital herpes and even trench mouth. Recently, affective disorders, especially depression, have received more and more attention.

Although the emphasis on stress research in the mental health area is more recent, theoretical models in psychopathology have often assumed a construct of diathesis-stress (Rende & Plomin, 1992). Here diathesis refers to a predisposition to certain disorders. These models were first developed in theories of schizophrenia proposed during the 1960s, while most recently theories of depression have also explicitly adopted such forms (Monroe & Simons, 1991). The hypothesis in these models is that for a given disorder, there are specific factors (stress) that combine with the diathesis to trigger the onset of the disorder (Rende & Plomin, 1992). "The basic premise is that stress activates a diathesis, transforming the potential of predisposition into the presence of psychopathology" (Monroe & Simons, 1991).

It should be noted that the idea of diathesis or predisposition is congenital or constitutional in origin. Recent efforts try to incorporate diathesis-stress premises in theories of depression by invoking new domains of predisposition other than constitutional (e.g., cognitive or social vulnerability). By such an approach to conceptualization, important psychosocial factors are said integrated into the models and the diathesis' potential effects on stress are heeded (ibid.). However, in realistic terms, it does not seem that the originally biopsychological model is capable of allowing for the all too complicated psychosocial mechanics.

The stress buffering hypothesis

Although original stress research in physiology was not in a position to emphasize on a social dimension, the role of social environment and social relationship was heeded by many. And it turned out to be so important that physiologist Selye (1982) ended his article with a hearty advice: "Earn thy neighbor's love" (p.17). It is evident that the research interest in social support has advanced our understanding far beyond the traditional diathesis-stress paradigm. Conversely, it is the idea of stress in etiological thinking that has furthered epidemiological interest in social support.

The stress-disease hypothesis and the study of social support have now combined to dominate much of the social epidemiological dialogue as a momentous research program. The approach has suggested that social support may not contribute directly to health outcomes, but may "buffer" or "moderate" the deleterious effects of one's environment in times of stress (Bloom et al., 1991; Cobb, 1976; Cassel, 1976). In a flood of research interest in social support, theoretical and empirical work has focused mostly on such buffering hypothesis (Cohen and Wills, 1985; Thoits, 1982). Simply put, the idea of buffering assumes a model in which elevation in level of life stress place all people at risk for illness, but the impact of exposure to high levels of stress would be offset or "buffered" in the presence of adequate social supports (Bloom et al., 1991).

Empirical research, however, does not appear to consistently bolster the hypothesis. It is noticeable that research has been concerned with general life event stresses and mental health outcomes, but the association between the two does not come up as clear as expected. In view of such a situation, there are still strong arguments advocating a direct connection between social support and mental health. Generally speaking, this is a matter of whether the positive association between social ties and well-being is attributable more to an overall beneficial effect of support irrespective of whether persons are under stress or to a process of support protecting persons from potentially adverse effects of stressful events. Cohen and Wills (1985) term the former a main- or direct-effect model in contrast with the latter, the buffering model. Basically, the two models deal with different processes through which social support may have a beneficial effect on health.

In their review of the pioneering research on the subject, Cohen and Wills (ibid.) conclude that there is evidence consistent with both models. Evidence for a buffering model is found when subjective aspects of social support (perceived availability) are assessed which are responsive to the needs elicited by stressful events. Evidence for the main effect model is found when the support measure assesses a person's degree of integration in a large social network (ibid.). This conclusion is impressive indeed for it points out the differences in conceptualization and measurement of social support by examining the characteristics of method and analysis. Nonetheless, one of the fundamental issues remaining to be addressed is whether or not social support as *a* construct is scalable. After all, one has the reason to doubt that the role of social support could only be examined by losing its integrity, or all the positive evidence must be collected at the cost of conceptual consistency.

2   Issues in measurement and analysis

This chapter contains a discussion of the issues in measurement and analysis, which directs the reader's attention to the elements and dimensions of social support and reveals the "state of the art" of scale development. The crux is exposed to the reader by citing a resounding assertion in this field, "Social support, per se, is simply not a viable theoretical construct and it cannot be measured." My standpoint, then, is made clear: Such a stance is not substantiated with scrutiny into all the possibilities in measurement. In real terms, the combination of the subscales or different factors often makes good sense in research and clinical practice. Thus, the question is not whether a general scale is useful, but how such a scale can be constructed in a legitimate manner, or with approaches that are at least theoretically and empirically plausible. This is not unique to the conceptualization and measurement of social support; rather, it is a fundamental issue in all psychosocial scaling.

To give the reader a complete sense of the major issues, a more penetrating critique on theory and research about psychosocial determinants of depression is made. It is pointed out that behavioral and social investigators' modification of the meaning of stress has created much confusion. Especially, when stress is reduced to some life events, its capacity of representing the "psychosocial mechanism" of affective functioning and depression could be restricted to the minimum. Moreover, the issue of how to avoid overlapping the constructs of life stress and social support remains unresolved, since the demarcation line between supportive aspects and stressful elements is usually unclear. In terms of analysis, it is noted that recent progress in structural equations modeling has started to incorporate the measurement concern. Nevertheless, the technology puzzles practitioners and investigators not just with the complication of analysis but with a likely compromise in measurement. It seems only to confirm that all the original theoretical constructs would turn out to be unscalable unless they are broken down into some factors or "latent variables," which are often hard to use and depart from the original ideas in theoretical modeling. This certainly has imposed a serious restraint upon measurement tools available to both researchers and practitioners, as well as a barrier to analytic clarity and simplicity espoused by scientific tenets. Theoretical and practical workers, therefore, must look for a way out by maintaining the integrity of theory, the simplicity of analysis, and the validity of measurement. All these largely count on the manner in which they do their scaling. And the success of the advanced causal modeling strategy hangs on a breakthrough of the limits set with the "royal" unidimensional scaling and factor-based subscales approaches.

Elements and dimensions of social support

The conception of social support appears to be a major source of complexity, confusion, and controversy in current psychosocial research. Aside from enormous variations in definition, there are a number of ways to list its elements and dimensions. Cassel's (1974) original notion of social support, for example, only generally stressed the role of social ties and social feedback. Caplan (1974), in contrast, used the term "support system" to include not only family members and friends but also the "continuing social aggregates" like mutual-aid groups and neighborhood-based informal services. He also suggested three kinds of helping activities, corresponding respectively to emotional problems, demanding tasks, and specific stressors due to lack of materials, money, skills, and guidance. Another author, Cobb (1976), defined support singularly as information, though he proposed, too, three kinds of information that reflected emotional, esteem, and belonging supports.

If the picture portrayed by these early writers looked yet simple, the ensuing research has made the field of social support truly complicated by blossoming in a profusion of varieties (Vaux, 1988). Some analysts simply cited a number of possible measures; others provided rather refined classification schemes. For example, Kahn (1979) defined social support as "interpersonal transactions that include one or more of the following: the expression of positive affect of one person toward another; the affirmation or endorsement of another person's behaviors, perceptions, or expressed views; the giving of symbolic or material aid to another." Schaefer, Conyne, and Lazarus (1981) categorized social support into tangible support including direct aid or services, informational support that could help a person solve a problem and provide feedback, and emotional support that stresses intimacy and attachment, reassurance, and confidence in and reliance on another. All in all, writers from diverse disciplines have offered different views with their own terminologies. Those classification schemes have especially helped to delineate various ingredients of social support, though on the whole they appear to have failed to achieve a consonant understanding of the construct.

It is clear, however, that social support is a multidimensional phenomenon with seemingly too many elements that do not lend themselves to straightforward assessment. In empirical research, the reduction of the dimensions represented by all the variables lies at the center of the task of measuring social support. This is also true to the assessment of life stress, depression, personal coping, as well as many other theoretical constructs. Generally speaking, the simplification of the presentation of data is a fundamental issue of quantification in practice across all domains of behavioral and social sciences. In the study of social support as well as some other topics, there have been two major approaches to this concern followed by researchers knowledgeably or unconsciously. The first one is usually a primitive method using some variables as individual indicators of the degree of, say, social support, including demographic characteristics such as marital status or living arrangements. Sometimes multiple items may be scaled but they are not intended to be substantially inclusive. When these are used as measures of social support, however, investigators can be criticized for losing sight of other aspects that might also be important (Wallston et al., 1983). If a researcher were prepared with a sound theoretical rationale, she or he might justify the choice of items with thoughtfulness, which would make it an example of scientific reduction. However, as the field typically lacks a theoretical underpinning, this approach has often appeared to be problematic. Single-item indicators and indexes constructed from just a few items are therefore inevitably outmatched by more composite measures, namely, various multi-item scales. The approach to the latter is a comprehensive one aiming at aggregating all the information into a single measure. Typically, it is a broad scale which includes various aspects by weighting corresponding individual items. Nevertheless, scales can be not only too lengthy but unwieldy for many research and practical applications (Lubben, 1988). When we use a fairly comprehensive scale, the result of factor analysis can strike us with a pretty big number of dimensions. Yet they are an outcome that have already been simplified, or factor analysis would substantially lose its utility. Multidimensional scaling techniques including factor analysis, however, do not completely resolve the issue of multidimensionality, or multifactoriality. When all things are packed into a single measure, investigators can be questioned as to how and based on what they are legitimized to do that, since some aspects of social support seem so different in nature. Similarly, this approach is also theoretically difficult. Nonetheless, the first approach has its utility in focusing on a specific aspect of social support (as well as many other important phenomena and intervention methods), whereas the second approach is indispensable to their comprehensive research.

The state of the art of scale development

Vaux pointed out in 1988 that ten years before, social support was an idea that was both replete with meaning and nebulous. Yet, he continued to write,

> Over time, different approaches to the topic emerged that were, at first, thought of as different empirical operationalizations of a single construct. Now, most researchers recognize that social support is too complex an idea to be restrained as a single theoretical concept. (Vaux, 1988:296)

By viewing social support as a metaconstruct comprising several conceptual components, Vaux made the point that theorists and researchers need to be specific about their focus rather than using the term in a general way. He indicated three major approaches to social support studies nowadays. "These are support network resources, supportive behavior, and appraisals of support" (ibid.). In addition, in light of the functional forms of social support, "A consensus is emerging regarding the importance of six modes of support: emotional, advice/guidance, feedback, practical, financial/material, and socializing" (ibid.). Vaux noted that many measures focus on support network resources or support appraisals while fewer on specific supportive acts. In terms of measurement advances, Vaux summarized that "measures increasingly have reflected the conceptual distinctions noted above and have been designed with a more explicit focus" (ibid., p.297).

Vaux's writing provided some general grounds for the profusion of measurement choices in this field, with the conceptual differentiation of the phenomenon having been promoted by empirical studies. There are specific justifications for particular measures of social support as well. For example, some have argued that it is the sheer existence of relationships that is consequential for health, rather than their structural pattern or functional content (Syme, 1982). "The underlying idea here might be considered a social isolation hypothesis, although what exactly is consequential about social isolation is not spelled out" (House & Kahn, 1985:89). Others have claimed a logic that it is the quality of these relationships, particularly the perceived support they offer, that largely accounts for their effects (ibid.; Blazer, 1982; Grove, Hughes, & Style, 1983).

Individual assessment strategies used in various research projects are not without problems, though. Investigators focused on social network measures eloquently argue for the necessity of assessing network structures and interaction patterns unbiased by subjective conditions (Veiel & Baumann, 1992; Lieberman, 1986; Pearlin, 1989; Wellman, 1985). However, as pointed out by Veiel and Baumann (1992), such measurement approaches tend to be expensive, and may not always be feasible. And the solutions are not without problems of their own: "Breaking down complex transactions and relationships into concrete elements may make their assessment more immune to subjective biases but may miss essential supportive qualities" (ibid., p. 316). On the other hand, there are strong arguments for the advantage of reserving the term social support to refer to "perceived support" (Turner, 1992; Blaik, 1980; Cobb, 1976). However, "Scores obtained in this manner, as are most social support scores used in current research, are basically hybrids with unknown proportions of subjective-individual and social-environmental components" (Veiel & Baumann, 1992:317). In addition to the problem of confounding with other aspects of social support, such measures also have been shown to be confounded with important psychosocial variables other than social support itself (Dohrenwend et al., 1984). It seems that the genuine effect of social support measured in this way would be harder to detect especially in the mental health field.

Providing a theoretical framework for assessing the quality of measures of social support, House and Kahn (1985) contend that it is necessary to consider all three aspects of social relations - quantity (of integration or isolation), structure (of networks), and function (of support) - because they are logically and empirically interrelated. They write,

It is desirable on both substantive and methodological grounds that at least two, and preferably all three, of these aspects of social relationships be explicitly conceptualized and measured within a single study. Only then can the relationships both among these aspects of social relations and between them and health be understood. (ibid., p.85)

In their review of the diverse proposed measures, however, House and Kahn did not come up with any substantial scale that yields a single score yet embraces all the major aspects of social support. Nor did they seem to have favored such an approach, though they considered that it is critical to understand better how these aspects relate to each other. In fact, a more inclusive yet more differentiated approach is now preferred by the research community, though some primitive, one-sided indicators as well as some simply summated scales continue to be created and adopted. The result is a mainstream approach using multiple measures or a set of subscales in a single study (Sandler & Barrera, 1984; Lin, Dean, & Ensel, 1986). In the extreme, Vaux (1992:194) asserts that "Social support, per se, is simply not a viable theoretical construct and 'it cannot be measured." By viewing social support as a process whereby people manage social resources to meet social needs and to enhance and complement their personal resources for meeting demands and achieving goals, Vaux (ibid.) identified a number of social support constructs that are distinct yet measurable, including support resources, incidents, behavior, appraisals, and orientation. Although Vaux attended to the question whether these facets are combined in a measurement, he considered incorporating elements from a variety of facets as confounding constructs that quite likely operate distinctly in the support process.

Such a stance, however, is not substantiated by scrutinizing into all the possibilities in measurement. In real terms, the combination of the subscales or different factors often makes good sense in research and clinical practice. The question is thus not whether a general scale is useful, but how such a scale can be constructed in a legitimate manner, or with approaches that are at least theoretically and empirically plausible. This is not unique to the conceptualization and measurement of social support; rather, it is a fundamental issue in psychosocial scaling. By reviewing the general status of scientific inquiry in this regard, this book holds out a theme of unidimensionalization and considers it central to multi-item scale development. To clarify its meaning and see how it can be reasonably accomplished, however, a further methodological and theoretical reflection on scaling multidimensional constructs is instrumental. This will be related in chapter five.

Psychosocial determinants of depression: A critique of current practice in measurement and analysis

In writings focusing on psychosocial aspects of affective disorders (e.g., Becker and Kleinman, 1991; Freden, 1982), the scope of the topic can be very extensive. In the general models of psychopathology, however, there is not really much room for the so-called "psychosocial determinants." The central theme of a diathesis-stress provides congenital predisposition with an unequivocal position on the one hand and emphasizes on the role of life events on the other. The inclusion of other psychosocial factors, nevertheless, is a bit uncertain as to whether they should be considered as part of the diathesis or on the side of the stress. Because of the powerful influence of the research interest in stress, the part of the psychosocial variables seems to be made clear more in relation to stress than to diathesis. Nevertheless, stress in the eye of physiologists appears deviant from the conception of behavioral and social investigators; and their modification of the meaning has created much confusion. Especially, when stress is simply reduced to some life events, its capacity of representing the "psychosocial mechanism" of affective functioning and depression could be restricted to the minimum.

Fortunately, people now do not confine their thoughts to a single pattern of thinking like the diathesis-stress theory, although it is still used as a vehicle to convey their ideas. In terms of the effects of the social environment on affective disorders, Paykel and Cooper (1992:149) distinguish two main aspects: "life events, which represent recent major changes in the environment, and social support, one aspect of the supportive or stressful qualities of the environment not linked to recent change." It is worth noticing that in these words, both the supportive and the stressful qualities of the environment are mentioned. However, the issue of how to avoid overlapping the constructs of life stress and social support remains unresolved, since the demarcation line between supportive aspects and stressful elements is usually unclear. For instance, measures based on characteristics of social networks tend to implicate some stressful elements, such as marital disputes that are hardly isolated from the measure of family support. In general, there is a problem of confounding among the

32

theoretical constructs, which often blur their relationships with one another in empirical analysis. For example, depression is assessed at least partly in terms of its influences on all aspects of a person's functioning; the inclusion of some social aspects, however, would simply exaggerate the relationship between depression and social support or social stress. Therefore, certain rules need to be articulated and ways figured out to deal with such problems and dilemmas.

With the introduction of social support plus the original diathesis-stress model, the role of psychosocial factors in effecting depression still appears under-represented. In addition to the confounding problem, item sampling adequacy is rarely achieved in scaling those important theoretical constructs. For example, although social support had best be understood as a transactional process, support acts and behaviors have not been so well represented as support resources and appraisals in measurement literature. And people even try to justify the breakdown of some theoretically integral constructs as the major means to solve their measurement problems. On the whole, as "social support" is usually confined to the "informal" sector and "stress" reduced to some major life events, the part of many specific psychosocial factors, as listed by Becker and Kleinman (1991) and Freden (1982), would easily be ignored. Indeed, few, if any, have systematically connected the general, simplified models of "social support," "stress" and "diathesis" with those various, sophisticated "biopsychosocial aspects," such as health and socioeconomic status. It seems that investigators try not to be too inclusive even in introducing those general theoretical constructs, probably because they are too often embarrassed when more than one factor turn out to be involved in measurement.

The research community also seems to be preoccupied with a few popular notions. Especially, to some investigators, it looks like the only thing to do is to prove some simple negative impacts of stress and positive effects of social support. The pathways of those influences, however, are typically unclear or oversimplified. The role of some other variables has received relatively little study (Paykel and Cooper, 1992). In this regard, Kantor (1992:58-59) writes,

> Here-and-now-oriented clinicians sometimes do a superficial reactivity profile limited to catch-all concepts like "stress," "provocation," or "reality." They may overplay external factors, like the stress, and downplay internal factors, like anger. ... much stressology (the study of stress) presumes the primacy of the chicken (external matters) over the egg (internal matters), prematurely and arbitrarily settling an age-old problem.

Recent advancement somehow indicates the expansion of the stress-disease model to allow for the role of some important psychological variables such as personality and coping. Yet the integration of their separate models with the stress-buffering paradigm of social support remains to be addressed. In real terms, the role of social support is not isolated. A full understanding of social support necessitates the clarification of its interaction with other significant variables. And approaches like appropriate statistical control must be taken to distinguish the genuine contribution of social support to disease prevention and mental health promotion.

In this regard, let us examine a research example that is still well indicative of the state of the art of the research field. The most directly related work is Lin, Dean, & Ensel's *Social Support, Life Events, and Depression* (Academic Press, Orlando, FL, 1986). This work reported a specific research project conducted over 15 years ago in a tricounty area in upstate New York. Because the book also made valuable effort exploring conceptual and methodological issues, it has been cited by researchers in a wide range of disciplines. However, the book suffered from the following major deficiencies: (1) Lack of a comprehensive theoretical framework. The work was essentially interested in the role of social support; however, it defined social support from a dissection of the term itself and no broader theoretical context was explored. Wanting such a context, like many other works now available on social support, stress and depression, respectively, the relationship among the core constructs could hardly be teased out without confounding. (2) Limitation in measurement. For depression, it relied solely on the CES-D, and for stress, it simply subscribed to the idea of life events. This limitation is also a major target of my work for improvement. (3) Lack of theoretical and methodological grounds for treating social support as an integral construct. Although the book was heavily biased toward dealing with social support, the discussion focused on lower level constructs instead, including "confidant support," "instrumental-expressive support," "community support," and "network support." This indicated a FASEM approach to the use of the LISREL technique. It was mentioned, however, that the test "showed that multiple latent variables for social support...does not fit the data, as many indicators have substantial relationships with more than one of the latent social-support variables" (p.190). This, fortunately, lead to the avoidance of breaking down the construct in subsequent analyses. However, the reason for totally ignoring the results of dimensional analysis did not seem enough, and it was doubtable that specifying a single latent variable in such analysis was the best way to unidimensionalization. (4) Analytic complexity. The part of model testing was not suitable for exemplifying data analysis in most research courses. Various specific models as well as their testing appeared in a sporadic way, and variables beyond social support, life events and depression were not well-integrated with the basic models. Although the work contained more analytic details, my book is intended to bring breakthrough to the more fundamental issues.

Generally speaking, as researchers start to try some advanced techniques of statistical control like causal modeling, they may find the results more frustrating than encouraging. Traditional path analysis may fail to provide notable path coefficients suggestive of any remarkable relationship among the theoretical constructs being analyzed, not because of the absence of such relationships but because of the lack of valid measures comparable to the analytic advantages. Indeed, the conceptualization and measurement of social support, stress, depression and related constructs are fundamental issues in previous studies. Recent progress in structural equations modeling analysis has started to in-corporate the measurement concern, as is exemplified by the Factor Analytic Simultaneous Equation Model (FASEM) approach (Bentler, 1986) supported by some powerful statistical packages like the LISREL (Jöreskog & Sörbom, 1989).

Nevertheless, the technology as it does puzzles practitioners and investigators not just with the complication of analysis but with a likely compromise in measurement. It seems only to confirm that all the original theoretical constructs would turn out to be unscalable unless they are broken down into some factors or "latent variables," which are often hard to conceive of and depart from the original ideas in theoretical modeling. This certainly has imposed a serious restraint upon measurement tools available to researchers, and, at least in some situations, a barrier to analytic clarity and simplicity espoused by scientific tenets. On the other hand, the needs of practitioners for community assessment instruments would simply be ignored. Theoretical and practical workers, indeed, must look for a way out by maintaining the integrity of theory, the simplicity of analysis, and the effectiveness of measurement which counts on the manner in which they do their scaling. The success of the advanced causal modeling strategy, for example, hangs on a breakthrough of the limits set with the "royal" unidimensional scaling as well as the factor-based subscales approaches.

Research objectives

This volume will research into these fundamental issues by probing the psychosocial mechanism of affective functioning, with an emphasis on the role of stress and social support among elderly Chinese and Chinese Americans. The foregoing review of the general field shows that social support and stress are two leading approaches to contemporary psychosocial study of depressive disorders. The genuine effect of social support as well as its pathways, however, are not very clear under the predominant "stress buffering" as well as the "main (direct) effect" hypotheses (Cohen & Wills, 1985). Various knowledge gaps are left over among different approaches and models, with a complete theoretical scheme being typically missing while essential to the illumination of the intricate conceptual linkages. Most importantly, the variety of findings from social support and stress studies points to a fundamental issue of discrepancy in the conceptualization and measurement of the psychosocial constructs. This study, therefore, is aimed at advancing the art of both substantive analysis and scale development. The former involves integrating various elementary models and expanding to certain other variables, including aging and cultural variation; the latter features illuminating some befitting approaches to and strategies of operationalizing and scaling multidimensional concepts. To be more specific, the research foci are translated into the following individual yet interrelated objectives:

1) To establish an appropriate understanding of social support, stress, and depression by delineating a comprehensive conceptual scheme of social well-being, mental health, and quality of life, as well as, articulating a purpose-relevant approach to their conceptualization and operationalization.

2) To construct a causal model fitting in with the real-life psychosocial mechanism of affective functioning by building on the "stress buffering" as well as the "main effect" hypotheses on the role of social support, and taking into account some other main constructs and basic variables drawn from relevant research literature. Because of the characteristics of the research population, special regard will be paid to the impact of aging as well as the role of potential cultural differentiation.

3) To explore some theoretical and practical approaches to the standardized handling of multidimensional (multifactorial) constructs such as social

support, stress, and depression by elaborating on a central theme of unidimensionalization in psychosocial measurement.

4) To validate (or falsify) some basic scaling models by developing and applying specific sets of unidimensionalized scales.

5) To examine the role of stress in effecting depression and the moderating and mediating role of social support by testing some research hypotheses, with an emphasis on clarifying the functional pathways and controlling for other key variables.

3 Social well-being, mental health, and quality of life: A research framework

In the preceding chapters, critical issues in measurement were discussed with a detailed review of the social support field. Serious limitations in both summative scale instruments and factor-based subscales were indicated, so was the inadequacy of reducing life stress to merely some life events. In terms of analytical procedures, the necessity of applying statistical control was underscored while potential application problems with some advanced statistical techniques were signified. Previous research results about the psychosocial mechanism of affective disorders as well as some major theoretical and methodological problems will further be analyzed in this chapter.

Research workers often find that the immaturity of measurement technology as represented by various arbitrary scaling strategies has created tremendous incompatibility of research results. Beyond conventional understanding of the issue of confounding, a dilemma underlying all conceptual boundaries should also be recognized by relating to the practice of questionnaire design, in which reversing the coding of some items is methodologically favored. This suggests that a general demarcation line between stress and support (or well-being) is impossible, impractical, or unnecessary.

In this regard, an appropriate understanding of social support, stress and depression should be established by tracing the roots of confusion and delineating a comprehensive conceptual scheme of social well-being, mental health, and quality of life. Some logical requirements need be articulated for construct validity essential for a meaningful analysis in social and behavioral sciences, where the overlapping of constructs is unwelcome but not uncommon. In this chapter, it is suggested that a conceptual boundary needs to take root in the difference between different content areas, if two constructs cannot share the same content area simply because the quantitative and qualitative bounds will be ruined by reversible codings. This viable approach to clarification is based on the specific purposes of a study, and therefore certain flexibility in operationalization is indispensable and some variability in conceptualization should be envisioned. This perspective supplements the notion of validity in psychometrics by removing the rigidity of the construct to be measured. If the researcher allows some degree of overlapping of the constructs in a relational analysis, s/he must acknowledge this and interpret her/his results on that particular basis. On the other hand, if her/his constructs are mutually exclusive, then all kinds of scaling procedures could be tried and the multiple measurement results on the whole indicate the "true" relationship among the constructs. An idea of measurement power or scaling effectiveness is introduced to indicate the relative degree of success in attaining the maximum possible measure of the relationship under study. This directs research effort to the full exposure of specific relationships rather than aiming at some isolated, "absolute," but elusive individual constructs. With such understanding, definition of the key concepts pertinent to the specific research situation is offered, and operationalization made.

To prepare for a more complete theoretical modeling, the chapter further explores two special angles of viewing the issues under study, that is, "culture and mental health" and "aging and affective functioning." The material presented in these two sections would be especially useful to those who are interested in cultural issues and/or gerontological theories.

Dimensions of well-being, health and functioning and problems of confounding

A clear conceptual framework is indispensable for a discerning study. There is too much confusion, however, that prevents straightforward conceptualization in the psychosocial research field. Instead of delineating the concepts individually and making do some arbitrary definitions, I will approach conceptual clarity first by providing a bird's-eye view of such fundamental notions as well-being, health, and functioning, and then by considering some basic requirements for conceptualization in a sensible and competent causal modeling.

Conventionally, health has been considered either as absence of disease (a medical model) or as absence of illness (a sociological model) (Culyer, 1981). The definition of the World Health Organization (WHO) (1958), however, has promoted the notion to an ecumenical ideal by proposing a state of complete physical, mental and social well-being. This definition provides not only the conceptual linkage between health and well-being but also a comprehensive view of their major content domains, which have fashioned some standard dimensions for a general measurement scheme (McDowell & Newell, 1987; Kane & Kane, 1981).

Further insights have been gained in developing measurement tools in each province. Mainly in the physical aspect, a major achievement has been made in conceptualization by distinguishing disability from morbidity (Macintyre, 1986). This makes it possible to focus on functional status besides illness episodes or "health problems." In the mental area, although the concept of mental illness is no longer criticized by sociologists as was in the "anti-psychiatry" movement several decades ago, an emerging positive view of mental health has made "functioning" a more universal term for assessing mental status (Herzog et al., 1982). In this regard, Kane and Kane (1981) subsume most of the scales into two broad categories, namely, cognitive and affective functioning, in addition to some general measures of mental health. Depression is the major negative representation of affective functioning, the meaning of which is somehow narrowed down in practice (cf. Chapter One). It is noticeable that psychosocial studies often focus on the emotional or affective aspect while, in an extended sense, mental functioning is sometimes called psychological *well-being* (McDowell & Newell, 1987). However, it is in the social realm that the measurement has traditionally been made more often in terms of well-being or functioning than in terms of health (ibid.). No matter it is called social well-being, social functioning, or social health, measurement in this aspect typically involves two major constructs, namely, social adjustment and social support (Larson, 1993; McDowell & Newell, 1987; Kane & Kane, 1981).

Notwithstanding all the achievements in conceptualization and measurement, there have been considerable confusions inhibiting a thorough investigation. The distinctions among the three kinds of measures are often blurred (Kane & Kane, 1981); the conceptual lines distinguishing mental and social functioning are especially unclear. In real terms, the confounding between social well-being and mental health has seriously marred research findings. Most conspicuous is the equivocal position of so-called subjective, psychological, or mental well-being, which has to do with a number of constructs including happiness and life satisfaction. In the first place, this is often equated with mental health (e.g., McDowell & Newell, 1987), or positive mental health when distinctions are made between mental health and mental well-being (e.g., Herzog et al., 1982; Larson, 1993). In the second, it seems fully justified, too, to place subjective well-being in the category of *social* functioning (e.g., Kane & Kane, 1981). From a comprehensive point of view, however, anything dealing with overall quality of life could be held as a global measure outclassing any single domain. In addition to some general indicators of subjective well-being, most scales of life stress also serve as the examples. Under certain circumstances, though, it is not totally unreasonable to regard subjective measures of well-being such as life satisfaction as an indication of mental functioning; and vice versa (e.g., Acosta-Cooper, 1989). The point is, any discussion and arrangement can hardly avoid being arbitrary without purpose. In the following, I will explicate how research objectives should serve as the logical yardstick.

The logic of relational analysis and the requirement for construct validity

The case in the above may not be a problem by itself in merely theoretical reasoning. Even in the operationalized measurement of a specific domain, such as depression, it is often not unreasonable to simultaneously tap other aspects (as precedents, concomitants, or consequences) to enhance the discriminating power of a scale, such as the CES-D. However, this approach is not always worthwhile or even logically sound. When we talk about social support and depression, for example, we consider the two constructs as essentially different from each other; therefore, we are interested in seeing any significant relationship between them. If, at the same time, we allow either measure to include a portion of the content of the other, the relationship between the two would immediately be obfuscated. If the operationalized measures substantially overlap each other, the results can be highly exaggerated, or offset, and yet all could literally be meaningless.

A logical requirement for any meaningful causal modeling or even simple relational analysis, therefore, is not just facial intelligibility, or content validity in terms of operationalization. And the conventional idea of construct validity may appears too vague in effect. What should be stressed are conceptual accuracy, in terms of the mutual exclusiveness of the measures, and theoretical clarity, in terms of the authentic relationships among the constructs. It should be pointed out that this requirement is not absolute. If, in theory, we allow some constructs to overlap one another to some extent, then their measurement should allow for some "confounding" accordingly. However, research conclusions drawn from the subsequent findings must clearly reflect such a theoretical understanding as well as the specific logic of reasoning. The logical requirement, therefore, is objective-specific. That is, it depends on the purpose and research design of a specific study. For instance, it may not be a big problem for one to use depressive symptomatology as an indication of "subjective well-being" (e.g., Acosta-Cooper, 1989), if s/he is only interested in its correlations with constructs or measures other than "depression." Especially, in studying the potential relationship between social support and depression, it is no harm to include in a depression scale items tapping its *somatic* symptoms verified by biomedical studies. However, it will be contaminative to include in the scale items drawing upon the indirect *social* representations of depression (e.g., familial and other interpersonal problems). This would confound the scale with the measure of social support or stress, which is usually not allowed by both theory and specific research purpose. Once the relationship in between can be considered as established, nevertheless, the social items may be included as well in assessment tools for the purpose of mental health practice (e.g., clinical diagnostic schemes). However, this should not be the case before any such relationship is validated, especially in a research whose focus is exactly on doing this. Thus, even if some "contamination" is inevitable, one should at least be aware of the violation of the logic rule and take care of the issue accordingly.

Definition of depression, social support, stress, and related concepts

With the above understanding, the major terms employed in this study could be clarified in the interest of both conceptual clarity and analytical meaningfulness.

Depression

Depression can be a brief negative mood, an interrelated set of symptoms and experiences, or a medically-defined syndrome (Gotlib & Hammen, 1992). As a syndrome or disorder, "depression is defined as depressed mood along with a set

42

of additional symptoms, persisting over time, and causing disruption and impairment of functioning" (ibid., p.2). This definition of clinically significant depression, however, has limited utility in a community mental health survey study that aims beyond the very few patients identified with certain specific diagnostic criteria (e.g., American Psychiatric Association, 1987). It is especially awkward for application to the research population in this study for reasons explicated earlier. In general, researching *symptoms* of depression rather than *syndromes* of depression is considered as advantageous because

> ... (a) current psychiatric diagnostic systems produce data of questionable reliability and validity; and (b) syndromes, as they are currently identified, are such intricate yet loosely defined concepts that the professional who finds significant environmental and biological correlates of the syndromes does not know what causal mechanisms are involved or even where to look for them. (Costello, 1993:1)

Besides, the syndrome approach makes the problem of confounding worse by defining a disorder based on its association not only with present distress (a painful symptom), but also with disability (impairment in one or more areas of functioning) (American Psychiatric Association, 1987). Nevertheless, Costello (1993) emphasizes that the investigation of symptoms of depression should not become an end in itself. "The goal of such research should be to establish the syndromes of depression on a firm research footing" (ibid., p.15).

For the purpose to include and focus on minor depressive symptoms in the present study, a broader scope is proposed here for a definition starting from the normal (optimal) state of affective functioning while containing the most seriously depressed cases as its extreme.[1] This would allow for the strategy of examining changes and variations as well as associated factors without being embroiled in an arbitrary decision of a yes-or-no cutoff point in a community survey research situation.

There is some question with this catch-all definition, however. Continuity has been an issue in mental health studies. The question is, are symptoms and syndromes on the same dimension? "Or, are there qualitative differences between mild depression and more severe clinical syndromes?" (Gotlib & Hammen, 1992:6). The available answer is, "*continuity* between mild and severe levels of depressive symptomatology differing only in degree may occur, but high and low scorers on depression measures may differ on various other characteristics as

43

well" (ibid.). In other words, "while depression can certainly be scaled on a single dimension of severity, qualitative differences exist that distinguish more severe, persisting, diagnosable depression" (ibid., p.7). Note here a more general issue of *generalizability* of depressive symptomatology is introduced in terms of the possibility of a global scale. The current state of the art is, beyond numerous clinical classification schemes and diagnostic categories, people have come up with some generalized, global depression measures. And most depression scales are highly sensitive, though not very specific. In particular, it has been recognized that elevated self-report scores such as the CES-D may indicate nonspecific negative affect that underlies emotional distress (ibid.). This, indeed, has made possible a majority of community mental health studies dealing with the general psychosocial mechanism of depressive disorders; it also renders an instrument for the present study with some solid grounds. On the other hand, as Gotlib and Hammen (1992) point out, scores on the scales indicate severity of current symptomatology, but they do not necessarily translate into diagnoses of depression in the DSM-III-R usage. They suggest,

> According to this view, clinical depression includes a core of nonspecific negative affectivity, but also includes other characteristics of the person that may be specific risk factors for an episode of depression. (Gotlib & Hammen, 1992:6)

The inclusion of the various risk factors, however, is often unjustified in research assessment in contrast to clinical diagnosis. As has been shown above, this often invites confounding in measurement, which, in turn, results in less meaningful or even meaningless analysis. Specifically, in studying psychosocial factors that may effect depression, measurement items that directly reflect or draw on the substance of social support, stress, coping style, and so forth should not be included. Yet most "standard" instruments, like the CES-D, are not amenable to such specific research purposes. Therefore, it is essential to demonstrate the application of the articulated perspective by modifying measurement instruments for the specific purposes of a study.

Social support

Generally speaking, social support is "support accessible to an individual through social ties to other individuals, groups and the larger community" (Lin

44

et al., 1979). Although helping professionals are also interested in support accessible to a family or other kinds of groups of individuals, this book will not change the definition since elderly individuals constitute the focal-point analytic unit here. The "social" sources of support, however, are not clear by this definition, and thus needs to be further clarified.

A theoretical construct relevant to the issue is a "social support system." Caplan (1974) defined it in terms of

> ... continuing social aggregates that provide individuals with opportunities for feedbacks about themselves and for validation of their expectations about others, which may offset deficiencies in these communications within the larger community context. (p.154)

What deserves attention is that social support systems can be classified into two different categories, that is, the formal and the informal. A formal system is made up by agencies consisting of a range of incorporated or public bodies, mainly governmental welfare departments and voluntary organizations. Private market-based services (commercial system) are also included in the formal system together with the statutory and voluntary segments. An informal support system is the array of nonprofessionals who provide assistance and support to individuals (Dobelstein & Johnson, 1985), which is also referred to as a "natural support system." Here "natural" means less organized, structured, and governmentally mandated or sponsored, and with less expertise basis. It includes family members, both physically close and extended family, who are available to respond to a need for care. It also includes friends, neighbors, and a widely diverse group of people who have established a relationship over time that provides reciprocal support but whose primary relationship to the person in need is not as helpers with personal problems. It should be noted that there is no absolute distinction between formal and informal systems, and sometimes such a term as "quasi-formal" may be more suitable to describe some transitive form of the support system. The point is, the term social support often refers exclusively to the informal sector. In recent years, informal care, informal welfare, and so forth have been moving up the Western welfare agenda (Pinker, 1979), which in turn has pinpointed the enthusiasm of studying social support in such "informal" sense. However, it is important to keep in mind that social support thus defined is not everything of a person's social functioning, no matter how policy concern and scientific interest have intensified its position.

As one scrutinizes into the notion of social support, more conceptual issues arise that demand clear answers. In addition to the question of who are responsible for support, where should support be provided has been an important matter, and both together have propped a long-standing debate over the subject of community care in the West (Chen, 1996). How to promote social support by professional intervention is another issue, which hangs on the networking strategies in community organization as well as practice skills in gerontological work with the elderly. These, however, are not the issue or the focus for the present study. Here the conception of social support is based on the "informal" connotation and is in line with the idea of community care. And my aim is to research into the function of social support other than to figure out social support intervention strategies before its role is verified. More important to the present study is, therefore, how to make the conception and measurement meet the logical requirement as discussed earlier.

The content areas of social support and its dimensions for measurement will be dealt with at length later. What should be emphasized here is that a growing portion of literature has observed detrimental aspects of social relationships following the rush of research interest in social support. This reflects a desire of people to recall the emphasis in early social research to view the environment as a source of problems (e.g., Levine & Scotch, 1970), in order to balance a one-sided notion of social milieu solely as supportive resources (except for some obviously stressful life events) (Heller, 1979). It not only reconfirmed the observation that social networks are not equal to social support, but also further clarified that existence of networks can be even worse than simply "nonsupport." The implication to measurement is that support is potentially clouded by stressful social processes when it is operationalized in terms of some network characteristics. For example, having a large social network can make experiencing the death of a relative or friend more likely (Moos & Billings, 1982). Indeed, when negative social exchanges and events are implicated in the conception and measurement of social support, it is readily to be confounded with the other construct social stress.

Summarizing efforts to improve validity in this regard, Rook (1992) articulated three different strategies in previous research to understand how such exchanges affect psychological well-being. That is, a) to contrast the effects of positive and negative exchanges on various aspects of emotional health and functioning, b) to conceptualize such negative exchanges as stressors and compare the impact of interpersonal versus noninterpersonal stressors, and c) to contrast the stress-alleviating effects of social support with the stress-exacerbating effects of social conflict. Basically, these are an attempt to distinguish between social stress and social support, social stress and other stress, as well as social stress and social support as mediators of other life stress. Social support and *social* stress in such a sense, however, can be regarded as being on a single dimension while representing two opposite directions. In other words, they indicate the positive and negative impacts, respectively, of the "informal" social environment upon human health and well-being. Therefore, in the measurement of social support, it is not necessary to exclude all the items that implicate social stress, but their codings must be reversed in order not to offset the positive ratings of support items. The key point is to distinguish as clearly as possible between positive and negative elements of social networks, and reconcile their functions in a unified scale by assigning different coding orders indicative of the valence of various relationships. In such case, the scale actually becomes a social support-social stress scale, and the zero point of the scale may not necessarily be "neutral" indicative of both non-support and non-stress in the "social" and "informal" sense. In other words, social support and social stress áre treated as two relative constructs.

As a matter of fact, in designing any measurement scale using paper-and-pencil instruments, research methodologists would suggest to purposively reverse some of the questions and answers for certain reasons. This raises a question as to how to avoid the confounding between *life* stress and *social* support in this case. Since some of the "supportive" items could and should be arranged in the different format or opposite direction, that is, as "stressful" items in the scale, the demarcation line distinguishing the two constructs cannot be determined simply by that stress-support difference. Similarly, the life stress scale may also contain some reversed questions, that is, some items that appear to be indicative of "well-being," or "supportive." It seems, therefore, that the conceptual boundary can only be determined by their different content areas and foci. That is, anything that has to do with the supportive or stressful properties of the *informal social* relationships can be designated as the content of the social support-social stress scale, and thereby should not be included again in the life stress measure, or more accurately the life stress/ well-being scale. All in all, it is essential to distinguish the "informal" social portion from the life stress/well-being measure tapping the overall quality of all the remaining aspects of life, for the purpose of examining the "stress-buffering" hypothesis. This understanding will not only help to meet the logical requirement for accurate conceptualization and measurement but provide useful insights for a pertinent causal modeling.

Life stress and quality of life

The original meaning of stress is provided by Selye (1982) as the common result of any demand upon the body, be the effect mental or somatic, which has been discussed in detail earlier. More succinctly, it is "the rate of wear and tear in the body" (Wallis, 1983). Many investigators, however, persist in using the term to refer to any external stimulus that causes wear and tear, or to the resulting internal damage. This has led to considerable confusion. As one researcher has put it, "Stress, in addition to being itself, and the result of itself, is also the cause of itself" (cited from Wallis, 1983:49).

Although Selye's general conceptualization is criticized as short of insight into psychological phenomena accompanying stress and lacking attention to individual differences that might be products of these psychological processes (Hobfoll, 1988), it provides a baseline for further pondering on its consequences, causes, concomitants, as well as mediators. In general, the book accepts Selye's view, and therefore the external stimulus that causes stress can be declared as a "stressor." Nonetheless, social investigators in the health field rarely inquire into the physiological or psychosomatic process. Rather, when they talk about psychosocial mechanism of a stress-related disease they are really interested in the direct connections between the disorder and various psychosocial stressors other than stress itself as defined in physiological terms. Thus, most of the time, the stress they are measuring is actually some common disorder-precipitating property of all kinds of stressors instead of a "general adaptation syndrome" (Selye, 1982). As a matter of fact, it is this shift in meaning that has allowed for many studies of so-called "psychosocial determinants" of disorders under the name of stress. For all reasons like such, the meaning of life stress is specified in this book as *the attribute of various life stressors that generates the "general adaptation syndrome" as described by Selye (1982) as well as the "stress-related diseases" as substantiated by pathological studies.* Here life stressors are viewed as typically developing from a combination of personal and environmental factors, including relatively discrete, short-term life events, as well as longer-term, sequential stressors and chronic life strains (Moos & Billings, 1982).

The above definition of stress represents a break-through of two stereotypes of stress. First, it is not a bodily syndrome, but rather, it can be regarded as stimulus-oriented (Lazarus, 1966). An advantage of this approach is that stress defined in this way, unlike the response-oriented approach, will hardly be confounded with disorder consequences such as anxiety or depression. Indeed, by Selye's delineation, or in the psychosomatic sense, it is often hard to distinguish between the two things. On the other hand, however, this definition is prone to confounding with social support, especially when positive life events are included in its measurement. Criticism may also be incurred from the interactional point of view (ibid.). However, the mediating characteristics that form the basis for individual differences stressed by the transactional approach are indeed the focus of the present study, though they are pursued as important psychosocial mechanisms of affective functioning without solely banking on a somewhat overloaded stress construct (as defined as a particular relationship between the person and the environment) (Lazarus & Folkman, 1984; Mc-Grath,1970).

The problem of confounding stress with social support is the other aspect of the same issue as was discussed in conceptualizing social support. Here it is advisable to relate the stress concept with some fundamental theoretical constructs discussed earlier to further unfold the point. It is a wonder that although there have been strong arguments against the inclusion of positive life events in the scales of stress, few, if any, have advocated their involvement in the measures of well-being and health. Rather, it is "stressful events" that have been taken as one of the objective conditions indicative of the state of well-being (e.g., Wilkening & Ahrens, 1979). This looks quite bizarre, though it demonstrates the possibility of refining the measurement of well-being by taking into account the role of life events. Although it seems to be more reasonable to express the role of life events in positive terms in this case, it is logically not a problem if stress is viewed as the negative portion of an extended measure of well-being.

All this indicates that well-being and stress (or beneficial and stressful) are relative constructs. Their positions may be switched by reversing their coding signs. In this view, not only positive and negative life events can be included in a same scale but any stress or well-being scale can be considered as a stress/well-being scale, provided that the signs and weights of different items are adequately arranged and reconciled. To gain in conceptual clarity for the purpose of appropriate operationalization, Campbell's (1974:11) delineation of the quality of life as "the rewards and disappointments which make up the experience of living" is of main interest. Investigators have typically used the terminology of well-being as well as health to approach this most comprehensive and ambitious construct in psychosocial studies, as is indicated by Campbell (ibid.) who points out that

> The challenge which we now face is to look beyond the material conditions of life which we have traditionally accepted as criteria of *well-being* [italicized by the quoter], into that far less easily measured world of feelings and emotions where the quality of life is ultimately determined.

The interesting thing is that not only researchers like Campbell have taken for granted the inclusion of the "disappointments" or stressful life events in the notion of well-being, but others have persisted in embracing all the events, whether negative or positive, in the idea of stress. By integrating the two subjects, I would argue that stress and well-being are two approaches to the same topic of quality of life. While each has tried to incorporate the major perspective of the other, they had best be distinguished as representing two different directions. In other words, when the two concepts are considered relative to each other on the same dimension, "well-being" may take on only positive values indicating higher standards of living, but allow for the effects of positive life events and the states of "eustress" (Selye, 1982). On the other hand, "stress" in the sense of distress may cover only negative events and aspects, marking the lower or under qualities of life expressive of the states of distress. Under this conceptual framework, measures of life events, material conditions, and subjective well-being (e.g., life satisfaction) will be regarded as complementary to one another in forming a unified stress/well-being or quality of life measure. This is to view stress and well-being as relative concepts, which would not only facilitate research but also provide a unified basis for analyzing service needs in helping practice.

An significant feature of the definition of stress in this book is that it is very comprehensive, including all the specific disorder-precipitating factors while measuring them at the very general, unified level. However, it must mutually exclusive in content with the disorder (depression), social support, and some other major constructs for the purposes of this specific study (e.g., excluding the part of informal social support-social stress, as discussed above, in the interest of analytic meaningfulness in studying "the relationship between social support and stress"). On the other hand, if we unduly confine ourselves despite of the advantage of theoretical generalization, the opportunity to triumph over or include studies based on individual facts like socioeconomic status and health and physical conditions would simply be missed by reducing the stress concept to some mere life events.

Personal coping

While social scientists are preoccupied with the role of social support in relation to depression, psychologists consider that coping resources play a central role in contemporary theories of stress (Moos & Billings, 1982). Comprising social network resources as some aspects of environmental coping resources, the broad construct of personal coping focuses on both personal resources and appraisal and coping processes (ibid.). With regard to appraisal and coping strategies, Moos and Billings (1982) organized the major dimensions into three domains according to their primary focus, that is, appraisal-focused coping, problem-focused coping, and emotion-focused coping. As for personal coping resources, they are "relatively stable dispositional characteristics that affect the coping process and are themselves affected by the cumulative outcome of that process" (ibid., p.215). There are numerous variables involved in this domain, such as ego development; self-efficacy, social competence, and related beliefs; cognitive styles; and general problem-solving abilities. Among all such concepts, self-efficacy, hardiness, locus of control, and behavior pattern are less self-explanatory. According to Bandura (1982), self-efficacy concerns how effectively one can execute courses of action necessary to deal with situations involving unpredictable and stressful elements, which can be used to predict a wide range of adaptive life behaviors, such as coping behavior. Hardiness is a constellation of related personality dispositions of control, commitment, and challenge (Kobasa, Maddi, & Kahn, 1982). Related to this, locus of control is a generalized belief concerning personal control over important outcomes (Rotter, 1966). Finally, there are two major behavior patterns: Type-A behavior is characterized by excessive competitive drive, impatience, hostility, and accelerated speech and motor movements, while the Type-B pattern is defined as the relative absence of these characteristics (Cohen & Edwards, 1989). In addition to all these constructs, there are still more terms that can be used to describe personality traits or personal coping resources (e.g., Moos & Billings, 1982).

The so-called personal resources seem to be a construct too complicated to be included in a causal modeling analysis. In this regard, Holahan and Moos (1985:739) indicate that "Especially relevant is the personality disposition underlying the related variables of self-efficacy, self-confidence, and perceived control." As a vague idea involving hardiness, locus of control, self-esteem, private self-consciousness, and behavior patterns (Cohen & Edwards, 1989), personality has often served to represent all of such resources. However, according to Moos and Billings (1982), personal resources are a complex set of personality, attitudinal, and cognitive factors that provide the psychological context for coping. The role of either a coping strategy or a personality has been explored quite thoroughly with such understanding, but the part of "attitudinal factors" seems to be typically overlooked.

Although specificity is desperately needed to sort out research findings based on these various notions, some general modeling has been made to account for the dynamics of psychological process involved in stress response. Strictly speaking, coping refers to behaviors that are employed for the purpose of reducing strain in the face of stressors (Hobfoll, 1988), whereas appraisal is the cognitive basis for any kind of behavioral coping (Lazarus & Folkman, 1984). Although the above analysis introduces an overwhelmingly complex picture, what researchers are usually interested in under the rubric of coping are so-called coping strategies or styles, whereas personality is sometimes taken as another separate category. And the focus is a simplified dichotomous variation, that is, the difference between a generally positive, problem-focused coping (called the approach strategy) and a generally negative, emotion-focused coping (called the avoidance strategy) (Holahan & Moos, 1985). Moos and Billings (1982) have preliminarily described nine specific situations (content areas) for such process oriented measures of coping, which "encompasses the major types of responses identified by existing measurement devices and can be used as a guide in constructing new procedures" (ibid., p.225).

The point is, however, when we assess coping behaviors in terms of some social activities we should heed the potential confounding problem, since social support may also involve such activities of the focal individual. On the other hand, personality traits like self-esteem should be treated with care, since they can be important indications of depressive symptoms and disorders.

Culture and mental health

This section is concerned with how the general perspectives on psychosocial mechanism of affective functioning can be applied to a specific cultural context, which is literally different from the ones having forged this kind of expertise. The available literature and my personal experiences render a working basis for unraveling these issues. First, I shall consider a general question: What are the characteristics of Chinese culture? Then, I will concentrate on relevant conceptual and measurement concerns, such as, how such cultural features influence mental health in general and affective functioning (depression) in particular?

By asking what is prototypically Chinese, Tseng and Wu (1985) abstract some of the common features of Chinese culture shared by all ethnic Chinese, whether in the homeland or other settings. They are family and collective responsibility, emphasis on the parent-child bond, the art of social interaction and the importance of the personal network, control of emotion and cultivation of morality, and the value of education and achievement. Dominating all these features, familism has traditionally occupied a central position and played an extremely important role in providing support for the elderly (Chen, 1996). However, in mainland China there have been a number of major historical events since 1949 (ibid.), which has been regarded as a cultural transition (Chu, 1985). "The traditional patterns of social relations that espoused filial piety and respect for elders and that deterred innovation no longer dominate life in contemporary China" (ibid., p.26). Nonetheless, research suggests that after decades of ups and downs many cultural values are now regaining their position in mainland Chinese society (Chen, 1996).

In terms of the cultural influences on mental health, it is suggested that the Chinese are not inclined to talk to outsiders about their private lives, feelings, as well as emotional matters with family members (ibid.). Although the Chinese do convey personal emotions, they rely a great deal on nonverbal communication or symbolic figurative expression. Due to this cultural characteristic, psychotherapy relying on verbal communication as the sole or major tool has been found difficult for Chinese people to accept (ibid.). On the other hand, the somatization of symptomatology seems to suggest that people tend to talk about their ailments in terms of physical stress rather than psychopathology. This has undergirded a medical belief putting emphasis on organic causation of mental illness. Note there is a view that no unified psychiatric theory has been developed by the Chinese on the causation, symptom manifestation, or course and outcome of mental illness; nor is there a definite, culture-specific system of classification of mental disorders (Tseng & Wu, 1985). It should be pointed out, however, that the theoretical basis of mental disorders can be discerned in the Chinese medical thought that emphasizes on the body-mind unity. This psychosomatic integration characterizes the relationship between psychological and physiological functions. The imbalance of emotions disturbs the functioning of the internal organs; excess and lack of harmony of emotions are regarded as pathogenic. High value is thus placed upon moderation and inhibition of emotions or affective expression (ibid.). Traditional Chinese medicine has wielded a pervasive influence on the symptom formation of mental illness and mental health-related behavior of patients and their families. Indeed, it should be recognized that the Chinese do have a system of psychiatric knowledge closely related to Chinese culture.

One of the characteristic features of Chinese patients' psychopathology is the low prevalence of depressive disorders with their predominant symptomatology of somatization. In addition to the cultural differences in definition and diagnosis (Altshuler et al., 1988; Nakane et al., 1988, 1991), Lin (1985) provided several reasons to account for the low prevalence in epidemiological reports: a) Confined to the traditional concept of madness in Chinese society that emphasizes outward antisocial or bizarre behavior as pathognomonic features, the people with dysphoric conditions neither seek psychiatric help nor are they reported in the surveys; b) The Chinese reluctance to express or discuss one's feelings, especially to anyone outside of one's family, may also play a part in inhibiting the manifestation of a depressive condition; c) Somatization, which is more culturally acceptable, plays an important role in influencing the diagnosis of depression; and d) The Chinese people possibly suffer really less depression because pathogenic conditions for depression, such as divorce and drug abuse, are less prevalent, whereas mutual help through an extended family or neighborhood alliance is more readily available for those under stress in Chinese society.

On the other hand, however, it is proposed that there are basic similarities in the psychopathology of mental disorders between the Chinese and the people of Western and other cultures. Two major similarities have been observed and reported by various investigators (ibid.; Altshuler et al., 1988). First, the entire range of symptomatology observed in Western or other cultures have also been observed in the Chinese. Second, all types and subtypes of mental disorders as discussed in Western literature and textbooks have been identified among the Chinese when standard Western diagnostic criteria are applied. Undoubtedly, the confirmation of these similarities is of fundamental importance to psychological anthropology and cultural psychiatry, which in turn guarantee the applicability of the general body of psychopathological knowledge to the study in Chinese cultural settings with all the insights demonstrated above.

It is noticeable that Lin's (1985) last point (see above) reveals some characteristics of social support in Chinese societies, with familism being the earmark. The emphasis on family and collective responsibility and the accent on parent-child bond, as well as the art of social interaction and the importance of the personal network, have cultivated the value of education and achievement as well as the worth of morality and control of emotion. It is likely that mutual help through an extended family or neighborhood alliance is more readily available for those under stress in Chinese society. And family support carries a unique weight. Nevertheless, psychological problems may also be generated in a seemingly closely knit family. Hsu (1985) lists the following as common problems in the Chinese family: inadequate parent-child communication, the generation gap, split loyalties, and sibling rivalries. He holds that these problems may be considered inherent in Chinese family relations, especially as they concern relationships between parents and children.

Generally speaking, Chinese culture emphasizes harmonious interpersonal relationships, interdependence, and mutual moral obligation or loyalty for achieving a state of psychosocial homeostasis or peaceful coexistence with family or other fellow beings (Lin, 1985; Hsu, 1971). Indeed, a harmonious family life was the ultimate ideal of the traditional Chinese familism (Chen, 1996). Researchers have stressed the value of *Xiao* (filial piety) and considered it as oppressive in Chinese culture. In studying the traditional approach to elderly support, however, it is argued that this one-sided viewpoint of the Chinese familism based solely on filial piety, especially when it is interpreted as an oppressive *Xiao*, is misleading (ibid.). Another forgotten value, *Ci* (parental caring responsibility), should be put in place to represent the reciprocal nature of intergenerational support and the true mechanism of so-called family and community care for the elderly (ibid.). On the whole, under the ancestral doctrine of *the* familism, people tend to look for not only the cause of their stresses but also the help they need in their relationships with people, rather than in themselves (Lin, 1985). The Western concept of personality rooted in individualism, in contrast, has been criticized as overlooking man's relationship with his fellow men, which is argued by Hsu (1971) as the central ingredient in the human mode of existence. Yet, interesting enough, Western medicine, psychiatry, psychology, and epidemiology seem now all turning to a similar psychosocial dimension as has been consistently stressed in the Chinese culture. This trend is evidenced by the rapid growth of stress and social support literature in the West as has been reviewed in the preceding chapter.

55

Aside from the characteristics in the manifestation of depression, social support, and stress as well as the underlying knowledge and value bases, the Chinese are also characterized by their coping styles and help-seeking behaviors. Although they are marked with insights into social life for punctuating the part of social support and social stress (not necessarily articulated as such), the Chinese surprisingly seem to prefer a so-called avoidance strategy, that is, an emotion-focused coping. *Ren*, or tolerance, is highly appreciated as a great virtue in traditional cultural teaching. As this approach is generally considered negative as opposed to the generally positive, problem-focused coping (the approach strategy),[2] the recognition of this cultural attribute has a profound implication for mental health studies in Chinese societies. Other things being equal, the Chinese may suffer even more widespread depression (at least in terms of its minor forms) than other nationalities because of the less outgoing national character shared by average people. However, it is hard to detect its existence because they are so reluctant in psychological help seeking.

The influence of culture is ubiquitous. Under the Chinese cultural prescriptions, even some basic variables have got quite distinctive implications. In contrast to the ageism that has ever featured a trend in Western nations, the so-called "gerontocracy" seems to have typically prevailed the Chinese family and society. Although this view can be criticized as one-sided, a cultural difference in the meaning of age is obvious. On the other hand, in contrast to the function of age, the modern Western notion of "sexism" may particularly be suited to depict the differentiation of role by gender in traditional Chinese society. Generally, the cultural influence may be manifested by some observable facts. For example, in terms of living arrangements, the Chinese elderly have distinctively tended to choose staying with male offsprings, especially with sons (Chen, 1996). Cultural influence may also be evidenced in the subjective meaning of specific measurement items, such as those tapping even merely physical functioning (Ikels, 1989). It should be pointed out that the influence of culture is not only pervasive but can be very subtle, which makes the assessment of the service needs of Chinese people full of pitfalls (Chen, 1996). All in all, in conceptualizing, measuring and analyzing the key constructs, a cultural perspective is essential to make the study specific and relevant. When we eventually seek to make a case of the Chinese and Chinese-American elderly, the strong influence of a unique cultural heritage must not be ignored.

Aging and affective functioning

With regard to this special angle of study, Murphy and Macdonald (1992) set out by advising that "Explorers of affective disorders in the elderly will find familiar country - the same signs, symptoms, treatment and responses as in younger patients, yet they will find differences, ..." (p.601).

As Murphy and Macdonald suggest, the most surprising finding in epidemiology of affective disorders in old age has been that the prevalence rates amongst elderly people for most nonorganic mental disorders are similar to or even slightly lower than other age groups (Myers et al., 1984; Gurland, 1976). Therefore, it is important not to exaggerate the magnitude of depression in the older population. This is especially true when the usual diagnostic criteria are used which confine the concept of depression to a disorder lasting for at least some weeks, characterized by symptoms of mood disorder, and physiological and cognitive disturbances. Potential qualitative difference captured the attention of scholars who pursued the issue of whether depression in old age represents a separate category of illness from that affecting younger people. However, no efforts trying to establish such a separate category have been supported by empirical research, and the current view is that no distinction exists between depression of the elderly and the younger populations (Murphy and Macdonald, 1992).

This notwithstanding, late-onset affective disorders are harder to classify, and episodes of illness may become more frequent and prolonged with age (ibid.). The symptoms of depression in old age have some characteristics, too. Most importantly, there is a basic question on how to define the distinction between depression as "depressive illness" and depression as a normal, understandable response to unhappy circumstances (Murphy & Macdonald, 1992). This question has particularly bedeviled epidemiological surveys of the elderly, in which those who have investigated the extent of simple depressed mood and other minor symptoms unaccompanied by biological changes find a very high prevalence in elderly people compared with younger counterparts (ibid.). This has given rise to problems in comparing results between studies. Therefore, we should distinguish clinical diagnoses from the results using low threshold criteria with self-rating scales or standard questionnaires (Zung, 1965; Srole & Fischer, 1980).

All these have significant implications to research design concerning affective disorders among the elderly in terms of goal setting and the measurement of functioning. It seems that researchers should no longer confine themselves to cases that are clinically severe enough when studying the older population. When we make the statement "Affective disorders are the commonest psychiatric conditions encountered in elderly people" (Murphy, 1986), we must include their minor forms that are most frequently seen. Here the idea of continuity in affective symptomatology is especially important to research measurement.

When one sets about to build a continuous scale of affective functioning, however, an issue will be confronted as usual: Which point or interval should we consider as "normal"? And if age makes any difference, a more general issue will set in: What is "normal aging"?

The first issue is not really a question for the inquiry here because I am more concerned with a wide range of assessment than a cut-off clinical diagnosis to which the criteria for admission to treatment are more important than the pursuit of etiology. The approach to the latter is more based on a continuous or spectrum-type measurement while the cutoff point for yes-or-no diagnosis can be left for clinicians and health care professionals to decide. For the ultimate purpose of mental health and well-being, I can define the "normal status," if need to specify, as the absence of any major symptoms of affective disorders whether or not they constitute a clinical case. The utility of the measurement in the present research, however, is not in the absolute values or scores but in the comparative differences associated with various facts.

The issue of normal aging lies at the center of gerontological investigation, which carries special weight today in face of the "greying" of the population. Gerontology is the multidisciplinary study of the biological, psychological, and social aspects of aging. It not only delivers phenomenal practice but also is equipped with its own theories. Biochemical and physiological theories provide the understanding of normal changes in major organ systems and how they influence the elderly person's functional ability. One major conclusion is that there are many normal changes in these organ systems that do not imply disease, but in fact may variously slow down older persons (Murphy and Macdonald, 1992). However, it is also evident that many older people have chronic health problems that compound the normal changes that cause people to slow down. Psychological theories focus on mental changes with aging. Similar to the physical process, there are both normal and abnormal alterations. Whereas some changes in cognitive and affective functioning are due to the effects of diseases, others may be primarily a function of normal aging. Specifically, Shulman (1989) postulates that depression is a final common pathway for central nervous system dysregulation, which seems to challenge the concept of depression in old age as a primary mood disorder at all. In practice, depression in old age has frequently been perceived as a predictable, understandable response to the losses and declines in the last season of life. And "the wintry themes of aging and sorrow have been closely linked in our minds" (Murphy and Macdonald, 1992: 601). However, research suggests that normal aging does not result in significant declines (ibid.). Surveys in a number of different communities have shown that the great majority of older people do not feel depressed. "Indeed, most old people feel that life has turned out better for them than they expected" (ibid.). Therefore, some gerontologists believe the effects of the aging process itself have been exaggerated, although they do not deny average age-related losses.

Scrutinizing into the notion of normal aging in general, Rowe and Kahn (1987) emphasize on the modifying effects of diet, exercise, personal habits, and psychosocial factors. A distinction is made between usual aging, in which extrinsic factors fortify the effects of aging alone, and successful aging, in which extrinsic factors play a neutral or positive role (ibid.). Rowe and Kahn's (1987) idea of a transition from usual to successful aging has significant bearings on a continuous measurement of affective functioning. If we confine ourselves to the diagnosis of clinically severe cases, we would only get involved in the issue of making a distinction between clinical categories and clinically negligible symptoms. By articulating the goal of successful aging, however, we are required not only to assess the usual status but also the optimal level of affective functioning. This expansion coincides with an emerging view of positive mental health that complements the traditional negative perspectives in the field (Herzog, Rodgers, and Woodworth, 1982). Furthermore, the distinction between usual and successful aging exhibits the role of extrinsic factors in health which has a wide range and includes important psychosocial variables. In the study of affective functioning and disorders, this is very insightful and indicates a variety of gerontological approaches to theoretical modeling and research hypotheses formulation.

Notes

1   This is also why the term affective functioning is used whenever it is needed to avoid confusion with the narrow clinical sense, other than to implicate other forms of affective disorders.

2. Nevertheless, *Ren*, if viewed as a personality trait or part of the national character other than simply a coping strategy, has positive meaning in impulse control etc.

4 Modeling psychosocial mechanism of affective functioning

In this chapter, a causal model will be created by integrating the research assumptions in the literature dealing with the major theoretical constructs discussed in preceding chapters. The potential impacts of aging, gender, and cultural differentiation will also be taken into account.

Social support, stress, coping, and depression

Social support, life stress, and personal coping are three building blocks frequently exploited for modeling psychosocial mechanism of psychological disorders in research literature. To create an analytical model for the purposes of the study, I shall begin with these major constructs by building on previous theoretical and empirical work and demonstrating the logic of causal modeling. This logic can be related in terms of a few hypotheses regarding the relationships among the key concepts, as well as, their integration into an organic body of all the speculative understanding.

Social support and depression

The relationship between social support (SS) and depression (D) is provided by the hypothesis that "the probability of developing depressive symptoms is higher in persons who are conspicuously deficient in social support" (Henderson, 1992:85). This hypothesis has attracted by far the most research effort in the social support area (ibid.). It can be diagramed as follows:

$$SS \longrightarrow D$$
$$(-)$$

Diagram 4.1 The relationship between social support and depression

This diagram represents the dominating concern of the research literature about the impact of social support upon mood disorder.

In contrast to some claims of broad effects (including physical health consequence) of social support, the proposition that supportive social relationships confer some degree of protection against depressive symptoms and depressive disorder "does have a plausible theoretical basis" (ibid.). For the purpose of summarizing empirical evidence, Henderson (ibid.) carried out a search of the English-language literature by selecting those publications that addressed social support and depression and that were conducted on community or other untreated samples. Thirty-five studies were identified; yet an intended meta-analysis turned out impractical due to unmanageable variability in the measures of the constructs as well as the characteristics of the samples. Alternatively, Henderson examined the individual studies reported and the significance of their findings. Noticing that only four studies found no evidence for the protective effect of social support, Henderson (1992:86) concluded that

> Across this melange of study characteristics, two findings emerge with remarkable consistency: (a) there is an inverse association between social support and affective symptoms, and (b) there is a buffering effect in the presence of severe stressors.

On the whole, as Henderson held, "a case can be made that the hypothesis about depression should be accepted - that is, that deficient social support increases the risk of developing depressive symptoms" (ibid., p.87). Where this hypothesis is considered unconditional, the lack of social support would contribute to depression whether or not severe life events also takes place (the "main effect" hypothesis). Finally, it was also pointed out that "The difference that one would expect to most influence the results is in how depressive symptoms and social support were measured" (ibid.).

Although the association was usually not a strong one, the above hypothesis can be further specified according to whether a direct or a buffering effect is proposed. Before the stress-buffering hypothesis can be introduced, however, depression should be articulated as a stress-related disorder. In other words, the relationship between stress and depression should be clarified first. The belief has long been held that depression can be provoked by life stress, as indicated by traditional diathesis-stress theories of psychopathology in general and the distinction between "reactive" and "endogenous" depression in psychiatry in particular (Monroe & Simons, 1991; Brown & Harris, 1989). Although too often the etiological theories implicate various other variables, the part of stress (S) in effecting depression (D) has been made fairly clear. Therefore, when it is isolated from others in preliminary analysis, the simple hypothesis can be expressed as follows:

$$S \longrightarrow D$$
$$(+)$$

Diagram 4.2 The relationship between stress and depression

There is ample evidence on the role of stressful life events and circumstances as factors in depression, and this approach has undergone considerable methodological and theoretical evolution (Hammen, 1992). On the other hand, important limitations of the stress approach are nevertheless evident and, after all, no definitive conclusion is available regarding the stress-depression connection (for example, the effect size is generally below 0.30, accounting at best for 9% of the variance in illness) (Holahan & Moos, 1985; Cohen & Edwards, 1989). Here, treating stress disease as a relative concept is considered a key to linking stress research with the investigation of illness in general and with the study of depression in particular.

Generally speaking, there is no fixed threshold or critical point by which a judgment can be made straightforward as to when stress will trigger a disease. Because of the conditions under which stress leads to disease, Selye (1982:14) used the words of "indirect production of disease by inappropriate or excessive adaptive reactions." In other words, the effect of stress should be pursued in relation to other factors in terms of susceptibility to disease (Frankenhaeuser, 1986). It can be mediated by various biological, psychological, and social mechanisms. Before research interest in social support produced the stress-buffering hypothesis, theoretical models of psychopathology had usually assumed the construct of diathesis-stress as was mentioned earlier. It was basically a physiological or psychosomatic notion that used to give little regard to the "psychosocial" factors mediating between stress and disease.

Diathesis-stress models

"The hypothesis in these models is that for a given disorder, there is both a predisposition to the disorder (i.e., *diathesis*) and specific factors (*stress*) that combine with the diathesis to trigger the onset of the disorder" (Rende & Plomin, 1992:177). "The basic premise is that stress activates a diathesis, transforming the potential of predisposition into the presence of psychopathology" (Monroe & Simons, 1991:406). In the case of depression (D), this diathesis(Di)-stress(S) interaction hypothesis can be diagramed as follows:

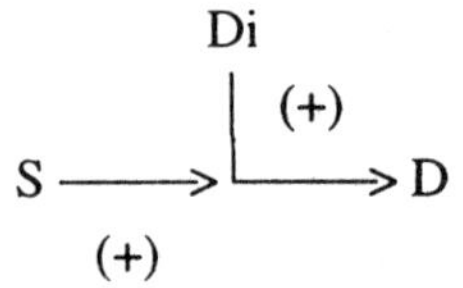

$$
\begin{array}{c}
\text{Di} \\
\quad\Big|\ (+) \\
\text{S} \longrightarrow \ \llcorner \longrightarrow \text{D} \\
(+)
\end{array}
$$

Diagram 4.3 A general diathesis-stress model

Despite the long-standing appeal of diathesis-stress concepts, however, the manner in which diatheses and stressors interact to produce disorder remains poorly specified (Monroe & Simons, 1991). As Monroe and Simons (ibid., p.412) indicate,

There are two levels of ambiguity that cloud the issue of interaction in diathesis-stress theories. The first level concerns common assumptions about the nature of the diathesis-stress interaction. The second level ... involves assumptions about the nature of the diatheses and stressors, respectively, that underlie the interaction.

Based on the clarification of these assumptions and hypotheses, Monroe and Simons point out that the challenge is to maintain a focus on the meaning of interactions between diatheses and environment, and ultimately among other contributing factors, without falling into the looseness that such thinking can engender. Two approaches to the application of the diathesis-stress model are articulated. They call the first interactive analysis, which implies a more restrained focus and an in-depth probing of associations between the components of the model, often multidirectional and transpiring over time. Complementarily, the second is to think in extensive terms and comprehensive theories, with a broad view of possible correlates, often sweeping and possessing functionally interchangeable components, that can combine in nonspecific ways. As they recapitulate,

> The first approach suggests an intensive study of specific factors and their integration over time within focused, prospective studies. It describes developmental dynamics: specific processes. The second approach suggests extensive study of suspected etiologic influences and their respective contributions. It describes linear, additive, and atemporal associations: nonspecific arrangements. (Monroe & Simons, 1991:422)

Monroe and Simons (1991) indicate that both approaches have their place, but that the intensive rather than comprehensive focus on concepts, measures, and interactions most closely exemplifies the spirit - and may help to realize the promise - of diathesis-stress concepts in psychopathology research. However, in my opinion, the potentialities of the comprehensive approach are somewhat understated. The present study falls in this class because, wanting longitudinal data for interactive analysis, it is interested in exploring some opportunities for generalized measurement and comprehensive analysis. In pursuing such an approach, I shall introduce some other variables, step by step, with a broad psychosomatic conception of a diathesis. To stay with my research emphasis, I will proceed with the two major hypotheses mentioned earlier on the role of social support. After taking into consideration the function of personal coping, I shall then try to integrate all of them with the general diathesis-stress model.

Social support as stress buffer

In modeling the effects of social support in relation to stress and depression, Lin

(1986) identified three classes of the variables' temporal sequence in terms of the effect of social support preceding life events, the contemporaneous effects of social support and life events, and the effect of social support subsequent to life events, respectively. For each temporal sequence, there are three plausible additive models and one plausible interactive model, illustrating the so-called interactive (conditioning), mediating (suppressant), counteractive (vulnerability) and independent effects of social support. To view the modeling effort as a whole, Lin's first and third classes of the sequence correspond to the idea of elaboration in multivariate analysis (the explanation and the interpretation models), whereas his second class of the sequence (in a sense also the independent effects hypotheses) incarnate the notion of multiple causation in social statistics (Li, 1988). These are two basic approaches to causal modeling dealing with individual causal pathways and links. The customary statistical control and multiple regression (as well as ANOVA etc.) methods are based on these approaches, which are very useful in preliminary analyses. The present study, however, is interested in expanding the basic causal models along the dimension of a truly multiple causation, or forming a causal network that is more complex yet more becoming to represent the reality. Statistically, this involves the techniques of path analysis or structural equations modeling combining the aforementioned two kinds of analytic methods.

Simply put, a causal network is a complex hypothesis, and the purpose of structural equations modeling or path analysis is to test the hypothesis using empirical data. The application of path analysis, however, is conditioned on some restrictive requirements for analytic models, especially when it is to be performed with simplicity. To comply with the major assumptions on linearity, additivity, and independence of residuals, Lin's basic models need to be culled, in conjunction with a consideration of their actual significance, for the purpose of further model building. It should be pointed out that these requirements can be loosened because of the availability of more powerful statistical packages recently developed. However, it is helpful to follow this line for the moment in the interest of simplicity of the resulting models.

The independent effects models, though somewhat oversimplified, constitute the usual assumptions underlying most simple bivariate analyses and will serve the same purpose of preliminary data analysis in the present study. The interactive models, on the other hand, pose extraordinary difficulty in the kind of analysis, and more notably, have been found to have no empirical significance (Lin, 1986). Therefore, my focus will be placed on the other additive models,

66

which can be generalized and presented, mainly by combining Diagrams 4.1 and 4.2, as the diagram below. The relationships among the variables need to be further explicated, however, especially regarding the relationship between social support and stress.

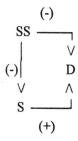

Diagram 4.4 Social support as stress buffer
(Combined with its direct effect)

The meaning of "buffering" needs to be clarified first in the interest of specificity in causal modeling. Alloway and Bebbington (1987) point out that the term has been used to describe at least three types of relationship; this confusion arises partly because it is possible to look upon a variable as either adding to or multiplying the strength of a relationship between two other variables. In reviewing the basic models in the above, I have made clear that the focus of the present study is on the additive other than the truly "interactive" (multiplicative) archetypes. Nevertheless, as Alloway and Bebbington further point out,

> Some workers ... have used the term "additive" to cover situations where factors have only independent effects upon the dependent variable. By this they mean that factors add independently to the *risk*, rather than to the *effect* of another factor upon risk. (ibid., p.93)

In the present study the two different meanings of "additive" are taken to serve two different foci in regard to the "main" or direct effect and the "stress buffering" hypothesis. The former is the effect of social support directly exerted on depression, which offsets the depressive consequence of stress by virtue of an additive (or subtractive) relation between stress and social support in effecting depression. This effect is completely independent of stress. The latter

67

is not the direct effect of social support on depression but its influence (mediating effect) over stress (also in an additive manner). Yet this influence may be exerted either on stress itself or on its depressive consequence. Therefore, the chained pathway in Diagram 4.4, which can be redrawn as follows,

$$\text{SS} \xrightarrow{(-)} \text{S} \xrightarrow{(+)} \text{D}$$

symbolizes both components of the "stress buffering" effect of social support.

It should be noted that there is a significant confusion in routine diagrammatic denotation of the meaning of "buffering" in relation to a disorder. This "buffering" hypothesis is often chained as

$$\text{S} \longrightarrow \text{SS} \longrightarrow \text{D}$$

which makes good intuitive sense (as a flow chart indicating the interactive process as something like mechanical force). In the language of causal modeling, however, it is not logical to put the symbols this way, which gives no indication of the impact of social support (SS) on stress (S). By the causal modeling conventions (Davis, 1985), it would be much more relevant, though less intuitive, to redraw the diagram as follows, which is actually part of Diagram 4.4,

$$\text{SS} \xrightarrow{(-)} \text{S} \xrightarrow{(+)} \text{D}$$

in which the buffering role of social support ought to be understood in terms of its mediating effects on the incidence and severity of stressors and/or their disease consequences (or simply stressful symptoms).

The interaction between social support and stress is additive, and therefore it is not to be confused with the higher level interaction symbolized by the interactive (multiplicative) models mentioned above. While stress may also influence social support as indicated by some of Lin's models, this diagram simplifies the situation since simultaneously pursuing the two directions will usher in too much technical (nonrecursive) complication that goes beyond the objective of this book. On the other hand, a separate pursuit of the other direction is unnecessary, too, for there are already ample efforts in doing this (e.g., Lin, 1986). Similar considerations apply to the relationship between stress and depression. Finally, it should be noted that there are hypotheses proposing the effects of social support on stress and disease *not* as a protective "buffer." Rather, they can be inauspicious for mental health, such as the "vulnerability" models (ibid.). And, as Henderson (1992:87) writes, "Particularly noteworthy is the unexpected finding of Husaini, Newbrough, Neff, and Moore (1982) that support from relatives and friends, in the presence of adverse life events, was directly associated with higher levels of symptoms." In such cases, the signs of the valence of the relationship between social support and stress, and possibly between social support and depression as well, would be reversed (i.e., be switched to the positive ones). This book, however, is not intended to go beyond the issues concerning the most salient stress buffering as well as the direct ("main") effect hypotheses.

Personal coping as a moderator between stress and depression

Probably the most well-known and basic model in this respect is Lazarus and Folkman's (1984) paradigm, in which cognitive appraisal and behavioral coping are viewed as mediators of stress and stress-related adaptational outcomes. By linking potential stressful events with illness and/or illness behavior, Cohen and McKay (1984) incorporated the role of personal resources into Lazarus and Folkman's appraisal and coping model, proposing that there are two major points at which social or personal resources may influence the effects of psychosocial stress on health. These two points are corresponding to Lazarus and Folkman's concepts of primary and secondary appraisals. According to all such theoretical propositions as well as their supporting evidences from empirical studies, a causal link starting from stress (S) through depressive illness (D), mediated by the process of appraisal and the strategy of coping (C) on the basis of personal resources (P), can be hypothesized for further testing with the particular sets of empirical data. Since the study is not designed to go into the details of personal coping by distinguishing between appraisal and behavioral efforts as well as between the two forms of appraisal, the hypothesis can be generally shown with the following flow chart,

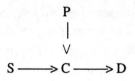

in which coping is generally defined as cognitive and behavioral efforts to master, reduce, or tolerate the internal and/or external demands that are created by the stressful transaction. And similarly, this simplified, intuitive, yet "mechanical" chart should be redrawn to form a causal link (path) using the normal modeling language and logic (suppose personality and coping are measured by some continuous scales):

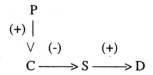

Diagram 4.5 Personality and coping as stress buffers

Integration of basic models and incorporation of
Physical, psychological, and social buffers

The foregoing discussions lay some necessary groundwork for further causal modeling. My objective at this stage is to construct a relatively comprehensive path model by integrating those basic models. The key point is to incorporate the separately hypothesized physical, psychological and social moderator or "buffer" variables. Since the social support buffer model (Diagram 4.4) is the expansion and incorporation of Diagrams 4.1 and 4.2, the operation to be performed is only to combine Diagrams (Models) 4.3, 4.4, and 4.5. To clearly demonstrate the process, this is done in two steps. The first step is to incorporate the physical and psychological moderators in Diagrams 4.3 and 4.5, which results in the following intermediate form of the model:

70

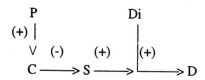

Then, the second step further incorporates the role of social support (Diagram 4.4) into the paradigm, with the resulting model outlining and integrating the major hypotheses established in theoretical and research literature.

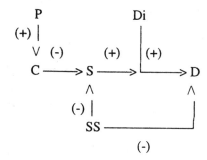

There is yet something missing. Remarkable modeling efforts can be seen in the literature to link social support with personal coping (Gore, 1981; Sarason & Sarason, 1982; Gottlieb, 1983; Cohen & Wills, 1985; Vaux, 1988; Schwarzer & Leppin, 1992). This pathway should be added and, as a result, Diagram 4.6 gives a more comprehensive and relatively complete causal network. The model, however, reflects my emphasis on, or bias toward, the role of social support in relation to depression; the function of other variables is comparatively more simplified (or omitted to avoid unnecessary complication of the model).

It should be noted that this result is not just a logical synthesis of the foregoing analysis, but also can be corroborated with some other comprehensive modeling efforts (e.g., Pearlin & Aneshensel, 1986; Monroe & Steiner, 1986). However, prior psychosocial modeling has typically failed to incorporate the part of physical moderator (diathesis) on the one hand, and distinguish between the pathways of personal coping and social support on the other. The venture of causal modeling here, therefore, furnishes succeeding empirical enquiry with a more appropriate theoretical framework.

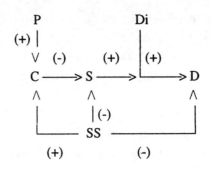

D:	Depression	SS:	Social Support
Di:	Diathesis	C:	Coping Strategy
S:	Stress	P:	Personal resources

Diagram 4.6 An integrated model

At this juncture, it should be pointed out that although epidemiological research has examined a variety of risk factors on depression, theoretical modeling in the psychosocial domain has typically failed to incorporate and take control over some other significant variables beyond those mentioned above. Researchers might be ignorant of the relevance of many other factors, such as sociodemographic characteristics as well as prior health and illness history, to the topic; but most of the time, it is some specific and particular purpose, emphasis, or bias of the investigator that constitutes the grounds of choice. Too much complication is also a major issue, and for this reason even as researchers desired to be all-sided they would turn to examine some separate models in terms of a number of factors, such as age, sex, marital status, social class, and history of prior illness. However, although simplicity is an important scientific principle, it cannot be achieved by loosing sight or giving up control of some essential variables while putting focus on some others. To make the results most meaningful and accurate, all the major factors must be dealt with together, though the analytic strategies can be diverse (some of which may even look like separated analysis methods, e.g., Lin, 1986). Indeed, the major contributions and limitations of various approaches examined earlier all reflect this focal issue. In the following, I shall try to expand the "integrated model" by taking into account some other important person and environment variables. Before I proceed, however, the relationship between social support and depression shown in the above model needs more elaboration.

Subjective aspects of social support and cognitive processes in depression

It is important to note the fact that "virtually all measures of support are self-report instruments, presented in interview or questionnaire format" (Vaux, 1988:34). Although social research methods texts frequently mention the inherent limitations of such instruments (e.g., Sommer & Sommer, 1991), few go into detail of their consequences bearing on research results. However, one who engages in mental health surveys cannot be simply advised not to use the tools at all when the respondents are mentally infirm. Here the point is, if such measures are to be used, we should be aware what the impact of affective disorders, if any, would be like in order to figure out how to appropriately deal with it. Without resolving this problem, it is not likely that the true associations of the symptomatology could be detected as well as the validity of many other measures based on self reports be established.

The cognitive psychology of depression provides the understanding of the dynamic interaction between dysfunctional cognitive styles and the psychosocial environment in producing depressive information processing. The cognitive models not only emphasize that depressed and depression-prone people think negatively but also that such individuals may systematically misinterpret and distort reality (Alloy, 1988). The mechanism is revealed in light of a variety of maladaptive self-management, inference, and memory processes in depression. The maladaptive inferences, in turn, are hypothesized to be the result of the operation of pervasive negative schemata or cognitive styles (ibid.). The cognitive models seem to fit in well with the conventional wisdom about the distortion of reality by depressed people.

While traditional cognitive theories highlight the idiosyncratic meanings or inferences depressed individuals derive from life experiences, the central notion of distortion in depression has been challenged in recent years. The emerging findings of "depressive realism" and nondepressive biases seem to suggest that depressed people's perceptions and inferences are often more accurate or realistic than those of nondepressed people (Mischel, 1979; Abramson & Alloy, 1981). This poses a deadly threat to the theoretical basics of psychopathology, especially the cognitive models, as well as a great puzzle to everyday intuitions. Absolutely, the findings have provoked tremendous controversies, and more importantly spurred cognitive psychologists to look for theoretical outlets and plausible explanations. Four perspectives are then offered: the naive, the ironic,

73

the comic, and the tragic (Alloy, Hartlage & Abramson, 1988).

Notwithstanding the controversial yet intriguing conclusions that the perception of depressives is more realistic while the optimistic biases and illusions of nondepressed individuals are more adaptive (ibid.), it is for certain that affective symptomatology does make a difference in the process of cognition. However, in screening or assessing the symptomatology itself, subjects are often expected to "describe" their feeling state, in spite of the fact that their so-called "privileged" position may turn out to be an unexpected source of variation. Paykel and Norton (1986) reviewed the similarities and differences between self-rating scales and observer scales. Summing up the limitations in the applicability of self-rating scales, they point out that severely ill and psychotic depressives appear to underrate themselves whereas neurotic patients overrate themselves. And the "trend in clinical research in depression seems to have followed the Paykel and Norton statement that self-rating scales have their main applicability in the minor forms of depression" (Bech, 1992:8).

As for the assessment of social support in the form of self-reports, the problem in a sense becomes more complicated. Vaux (1988) writes that one of the most striking features of the literature on social support is the astonishing diversity of measures used in research. Regarding this situation, a number of reviewers have pointed to a problem of inadequate conceptual and theoretical preparation in various research as well as the prematurity of the realm in general. When one sets about to tease out a clear construct of social support, however, there emerge a variety of ideas that do not lend themselves to straightforward overall measurement. Literature suggests the components of social support can be categorized as practical vs. emotional, instrumental vs. expressive, and behavioral vs. affective. Its measurement, however, entails more refined considerations.

The issue emerges when the relationship between affective functioning and social support comes to our attention. Mental health investigators are frequently confronted by problems of inference when examining the effect of social support on affective disorders. The measurement of social support is believed to be distorted by the existence (or non-existence) of a symptomatology. So is social stress. As Alloway and Bebbington (1987: 95) state,

> One of the consequences of depressed mood is a change in perception of the social world. If adversity and social support are measured at a time when the subject is depressed, a mood-related pessimism may increase

74

both the recall of misfortunes and the negative assessment of current circumstances.

However, we should not forget that social support has various components which could be much differentiated in nature. Therefore, it is advisable to consider which might be more impacted than the others. Intuitively, those aspects depending on the evaluation, appraisal, rating, or judgment implicating the affective disposition of the subject would be more prone to the influence of the symptomatology. The other aspects determined by more objective characteristics, such as the number of network members, should be less affected albeit they are based on self-reports as well while entail only simple cognition of the facts. In real terms, the difference between the two kinds of support measures in light of the process through which social support is related to health is evidenced (Cohen and Wills, 1985). The causal direction of the relationship, however, has not been illuminated in terms of this measurement issue.

Turner (1992) argues that there would be significant advantage to reserving the term social support to refer to perceived or experienced support, which has been most clearly described by Cobb (1976). Another writer, Blaik (1980), suggests that perceived support may be of particular value in late life, when the environment exerts a great influence on disease onset and perceived vulnerability accompanying the aging process may increase. This interest in the perception of social support by the subject seems to have prevailed and been maintained by the axioms of social psychology (Turner, 1992). However, except for some particular "pure" social studies, social support is not the ultimate goal of our inquiry. In relating it to well-being and health especially to mental functioning, the genuine effects of the more subjective measures (e.g., perceived social support) would be harder to detect as the causal pathways become nonrecursive due to the impact of mental functioning on the evaluation of support. As a matter of fact, our assumptions about the causal directions are largely not validated not simply because most of our studies are cross-sectional in nature. Biological studies contributed much to the establishment of the causal hypotheses on the role of social support (Cohen and Wills, 1985). However, animals and human body do not think and feel as does our mind. The issue of subjective measurement is unique and demands special theoretical attention and methodological treatment in psychosocial studies.

The implication is, in measuring social support as well as other constructs in relation to depression, we should use multiple indicators and avoid a total reliance on the self perception of the subject. In using questionnaire survey data, the inevitable influence of mood states should be considered in measurement. In addition, possible impacts of depression on social support and etc. should also be incorporated into deliberations of causal modeling.

Cultural differentiation:
A new perspective

Earlier in discussing cultural issues in conceptualization, measurement, and analysis, the major features of the Chinese culture as well as their influence on mental health in general and on depression in particular are described in contrast to the Western prototypes. The kind of cultural awareness has become more and more important in the advancement of research and practice (Sue & Morishima, 1982). This study, however, is not in a position nor intends to pursue a cross-cultural comparison. Although the cross-cultural design makes the best sense in revealing the significance of cultural difference, observing the within-group variation is also of relevance (ibid.), especially when this is typically overlooked. The advantage of this viewpoint is that it views a given culture as a dynamic process, rather than a fixed pattern with some rigid boundaries. Here it should be pointed out that in studying the bordering or interface issues of a multicultural system, a dynamic perspective has been in place to view the most prominent trend as a process of assimilation or acculturation (Gordon, 1964). The acculturation or assimilation model, however, does not seem best suited to study the cultural issues herein. This is not only because the majority of the research population were not immigrants or descendants of immigrants, which makes the acculturation or assimilation model largely irrelevant to this study, but also because there are several problems with the model itself. First, by assimilation and acculturation, this model may easily be taken to presume a "standard," "criterion," "normal," "model," or "ideal" pattern of culture for a country like the United States, which means, at best, *an* "American" prototype, or, at worst, *the* Anglo-Saxon or white Protestants origin. For example, investigators have typically used the ability to speak English as an indicator of the degree of acculturation in this country, yet seldom, if any, also considered Spanish as a criterion, though no one would deny the multilingual and multicultural features of the American community. As a matter of fact, the real emergence and the very idea of a pluralistic society have been posing more and more difficulty to such

76

a vague "melting pot" model. What seems promising has been an alternative approach to intergroup relations by focusing on each particular ethnic group, including the white Protestants as such a sociologically definable entity, as did Gordon in the capacity of General Editor of a series of such books (e.g., Kitano, 1969). As yet, this approach is still under the shield of assimilation theory. However, it allows the author, without presuming a very likely biased "standard" (in terms of the majority or a mainstream) to be approached, to start from the traditionally or historically recognizable modal characteristics of each culture, and pursue its evolution into a subculture in a pluralistic society, as did Kitano (1969) in studying Japanese Americans and Lyman (1974) on Chinese Americans. The two concepts of cultural and structural pluralism used by Kitano to conclude his work are especially instructive, although he considered them as the most significant factors in the Japanese "acculturative" process (ibid.).

Following Kitano's idea of the pluralistic development of a congruent original culture, this book holds out a theme of cultural differentiation, as a strategy in contrast to the conventional approach of assimilation or acculturation, for the study of contemporary cultural issues. In addition to the advantage of avoiding the potential bias mentioned above, this perspective is suitable for studying the evolution of either *a* culture of a nation or a subculture in a pluralistic society. This makes it possible to connect the cultural issues embedded in the elderly Chinese living in their homeland with those facing the Chinese Americans in the United States, and also allow the present study to approach them simultaneously. Even if there is a phenomenon that may be called "Americanization" among the Chinese-American elderly, it can be viewed on the other hand as a consequence of the cultural differentiation of the Chinese community resulted from interacting with all other cultures, not just the Anglo-Saxon civilization. With such a perspective, different ethnic groups assimilating one another can be observed as a trend of multidimensional convergence. But finally, this approach relates the kind of empirical enquiry to the idea of alienation in some thought-provoking philosophical reflection on man and culture.

Affective disorders in old age:
The gerontological approach

One class of person factors with which the occurrence and the meaning of depression have been extensively associated is demographic background. Characteristics in this aspect serve to place people at increased or decreased risk for affective disorders. Among the few major variables, age has special theoretical significance in studying the aging population, and therefore its role should be scrutinized in greater detail. It is noted, however, that age as an elusive variable in social research "is almost always collected but very often not used - or at least, not used to any real effect" (Finch, 1986:12). In this section, I shall try to connect the general body of knowledge reviewed above with the study of aging by exploring the utility of gerontological theories.

The role played by age as a general risk factor of affective disorders has been reviewed in the introductory chapter. By singling out the elderly group, the difference that the age factor makes would hopefully be controlled. However, it has been made very clear that the elderly population is itself tremendously heterogeneous, and among all the reasons age might still play a part. Therefore, there is the subtyping of older people into the young old, the middle old, and the old old, which helps to remind us of the potential role of the aging process in the shaping of affective disorders. The materialization of a gerontological approach, however, involves the issue of how to integrate gerontological theories with the general perspectives reviewed in the preceding sections.

The caveat is about the relevance of the theories to a specific research like such. Generally, gerontological theories attempt to answer the question as to what makes for successful aging (Hooyman & Kiyak, 1991). All of the theories address the basic issue of determining the optimal way for older people to live their life. Now the body of gerontological expertise is so inclusive that all the approaches and perspectives discussed in this part seem able to find appropriate places in its texts (e.g., Hooyman & Kiyak, 1991). Nevertheless, even well-established as theories in their parent disciplines, they mostly serve as "contexts" in gerontology. What are up to the theoretical standards of its own are those conventionally accepted and labeled as "theories of aging" or "gerontological theories." In the area of psychosocial gerontology, these include role theory, disengagement theory, activity theory, continuity theory, subculture approach, interactionist perspective, social exchange theory, political economy approach, and age stratification theory. None of these theories thus far adequately explains psychosocial aging (Hooyman & Kiyak, 1991). Although the various models are credited as a framework for research directions, their applicability to specific studies should be further scrutinized.

First, these models are designed at a very general level, all aiming to explain the aging process and why some people age more successfully than others

78

(ibid.). Under such a sweeping rubric, the boundaries of the variables involved can be rather vague, although the deemed deciding factors may be made somewhat more specific. In terms of successful or problematic aging, different languages are used, such as the roles, position, and status of older people in society, or their adjustment and adaptation to environment or to aging itself. The well-being of the elderly, however, tends to be assessed mainly in terms of their subjective well-being or satisfaction. Obviously, not all studies on aging will adopt this indicator as the criterion or dependent variable, and therefore the models do not appear pertinent to all of the research foci (the relationship between satisfaction and depression has been mentioned earlier). Nevertheless, some models variously address other aspects of the aging phenomenon as well. For example, the role theory indicates that unjust age norms may cause depression in the elderly, which helps us to search for its implications in a specific cultural setting. It supplements our understanding based on epidemiological investigation of depression by expanding the idea of risk factors to include not only age but also the social and cultural variable age norms. Even though some other theories do not specifically and directly attend the issue of affective disorders, their insights on the generally operating factors can be taken as valuable input to current research. For instance, the continuity theory may supply an account for the similarity in the epidemiology and symptomatology of depression in the elderly and the other age groups. Besides, it reminds us of the role of personality in modeling the disease process.

Second, although the theories are neither able to fully explain how and why associations occur among the concepts being studied nor sufficiently tested, each theory suggests some important factors that may be related to aging (Hooyman & Kiyak, 1991). In particular, these theories add special insights to the study of affective disorders when it comes to the elderly population, which enrich our understanding of the role of aging in influencing affective functioning and effecting depression.

Gender comparison: A feminist viewpoint

Morgan (1986) considers gender as a key variable is both ubiquitous and hidden. Morgan wrote,

It is ubiquitous in that it is one of the most common "face-sheet" variables ... and yet hidden in that, despite this commonness, it is often ignored or buried beneath some other more inclusive category such as "children", "rate-payers", "professionals", or "students". (ibid., p.31)

It is noted that the higher realms of sociological theory remain apparently gender-free; and the higher the level of generality the more likely it is that gender differentiation will yield to more abstract categories such as "role," "social actor," "organization," "class," and "system" (ibid.). However, feminist theory insists in that "gender belongs up there with the more familiar categories of sociological discourse" (ibid.). As Morgan (1986:32) indicates,

In addition to being part of everyday descriptive documentation and to its deployment as an explanatory variable, gender's status is also enhanced by political and ideological considerations. Feminist sociology has reminded us that the inclusion or non-inclusion of gender in a research project is as much a political decision as a theoretically-based choice.

By distinguishing the social/cultural term "gender" from the biological term "sex," feminists urge a recognition of the "socially unequal" nature of the feminine and masculine dichotomy. This advocation of awareness is especially pertinent to the conduction of research in Chinese community settings, since the Chinese cultural tradition has prescribed remarkable discrepancy in gender situation. Nonetheless, "... the value of feminist critiques to the discipline of sociology lies in the accumulating evidence that gender is not a good index to understand the social world" (Matthews, 1982:29; cited from Morgan, 1986:41). Morgan (1986) thus suggests that

In data analysis, where gender is used as an independent or test variable, always note non-significant findings as well as those deemed to be significant. (p.32)

Psychosocial determinants of depression among elderly Chinese and Chinese Americans

Although there are still many other variables that deserve one-by-one discussion, I will stop here for mainly three reasons. One is that my major purpose is to explore the role of social support in maintaining normal and successful affective functioning in terms of the moderation of depression. Although the functions of other variables are also (may be even more) important, they are taken into consideration mainly in the interest of appropriate analytical control. Second, the major pathways of the effect of social support have been clarified (and also simplified) in the integrated model (see Diagram 4.6), by including all the primary variables identified in previous research. The inclusion of more facts may be necessary, which is the issue I have been dealing with since the model was built; however, their functions are relatively minor, needless to involve further complication of the paths. Therefore, they will only be simply connected to depression state even if incorporated into the model. Third, the role of most person and environment factors effecting depression can be expressed through the very broad conception of stress, which is one of the primary mechanisms established not only in the biopsychology but also in the sociology of mental disorders (Eaton, 1986). I will further develop this point later by considering the measurement issues of relevant constructs like stress. Indeed, there are few variables left after stress as well as all the buffering mechanisms like diathesis, personal resources, and social support are considered. For example, the role of previous illness history can be considered on the side of stress. Here, only three basic variables, namely, gender, age, and study site (reflecting the influence of cultural differentiation), are given independent positions in the causal model (see Diagram 4.7).

The negative sign assigned to the effect of age on depression is based on the protective-aging assumption suggested by previous research, as has been reviewed earlier, as well as on the proposition of a "gerontocracy"-like Chinese cultural norm. It should be noted that this does not indicate my preference for this assumption, as intuitively I may suppose some negative impact of aging as well. However, I can subject either hypothesis to empirical test to detect the actual effect of aging. The two other variables are categorical, which need special statistical treatment, and therefore their relationships with depression cannot be given any signs. In addition, the impact of depressive states on social support as discussed above is considered by adding an arrow starting from depression (D) toward social support (SS). Because this study intends to focus more on social support, the negative impacts of depression on other variables are not considered.

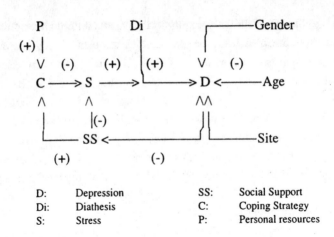

D:	Depression	SS:	Social Support
Di:	Diathesis	C:	Coping Strategy
S:	Stress	P:	Personal resources

Diagram 4.7 Psychosocial determinants of depression: A theoretical model

This model has certain limitations, which will be stated, along with the restrictions in some other aspects of the study, in summarizing the findings of the book. But here the reader may immediately judge the model as oversimplifying the reality. Compared with the familiar practice of applying quantitative techniques in social studies, however, this has been much more accurate than the usual statistical designs like a single, though elaborated, regression model, which, after all, cannot clarify the interrelations among the key constructs as the path model does. In fact, the path analysis involves several regression models rather than just one (Pedhazur, 1982), which gives a more precise delineation of the psychosocial mechanism of affective functioning (depression) among elderly Chinese and Chinese Americans.

The point is, in a single study, one must strike a balance between the requirement for accuracy and the requirement for simplicity. With this model as a framework providing appropriate analytical control, individual research hypotheses can be made more meaningful. Table 4.1 summarizes all the elementary hypotheses involved in the model, with each being marked by the symbols used in the model indicating each pair of variables linked by the corresponding pathway. The basic assumptions underlying the model and the hypotheses are: a) The theoretical constructs are scalable at the general level as they are defined (otherwise a FASEM approach would be preferred, see next chapter); b) There is no substantial overlapping between any two of the constructs, which precludes the confounding problem by setting the principle for subsequent scale development.

Table 4.1 Summary of individual hypotheses involved in the theoretical model

Path	Hypothesis
Di*S-D	- Psychosomatic diathesis and stress jointly predict depression.
SS-D	- Social support helps to prevent depression.
SS-S	- Social support moderates stress.
C-S	- Active coping reduces stress.
SS-C	- Social support promotes active coping.
P-C	- Personal resources contributes to coping activity.
Site-D	- Site difference (cultural differentiation) adds to the variation in depression.
Age-D	- Aging predicts less depression.
Gender-D	- Gender makes a difference in depression.

5   Multifactorial scaling methods

This chapter aims to shed light on psychosocial measurement by dealing with the issue of multi-item scaling. Traditional statistical approaches to data reduction will be briefly reviewed, while some unresolved and often unattended issues beyond statistical reduction will be revealed. This will open up an important topic of unidimensionalization in psychosocial research. Some theoretical and practical approaches to unidimensionalized scaling will be explored by learning from science, especially engineering mechanics, as well as by summarizing behavioral and social research experience in weighting via multiple regression.

Statistical reduction and beyond: A perspective
on psychosocial measurement

As has been partially discussed in chapter two and will be fully evidenced later, social support, stress and depression are all multidimensional constructs. Torgerson (1958) roughly stated the typical problem to be handled by multi-dimensional-scaling procedures in terms of the determination of a) the minimum dimensionality of a selected domain of the data set, and b) projections of the scale values on each of the dimensions involved. The concept of dimensionality, nevertheless, is complex, particularly because the distinction between "uni-dimensional" and "multidimensional" is contingent upon the specific scaling model (Jacoby, 1991). It is clear, however, that items of a scale are hardly parallel as required by the most orthodox form of the classical measurement theory (DeVellis, 1991). In addition to the possible problem of incomplete coverage of items as well as the potential issue of redundancy, the prerequisite of the classical model for strict unidimensionality in measurement is apparently impractical to most comprehensive studies. Indeed, despite that some argue that social scientists should strive to develop and use unidimensional concepts because they are more susceptible to theory-relevant research (Shively, 1980), most psychosocial phenomena do not meet the requirement for unidimensionality. It is hard even to identify the relevant dimensions, let alone control them. In this regard, "The methods of multidimensional scaling had the advantage of leaving the issue of dimensionality open, it was one of the parameters determined by the data rather than by the researcher" (Michell, 1990:109). Multidimensional scaling methods, therefore, have become a dominating approach to measurement with greater power and flexibility since the late 1960s. "The appeal of multidimensional scaling resides in its reduction of a matrix of data to a simple geometric picture that allows one (after interpretation) to see at a glance, both the dimensions used and the similarities relations involved" (ibid., p.111). In measurement theory, the relaxation of the assumptions in succeeding scaling models have accordingly allowed for not only nonparallel cases but also multidimensional factors (ibid.). Carmines and McIver (1981), Long (1983), and some other authors have discussed the merits of the general factor model. Chief among them is its improved correspondence to real world data.

Strictly speaking, multidimensional scaling is a set of multivariate, statistical methods for estimating the parameters in and assessing the fit of various spatial distance models for proximity data (Davison, 1983). Yet broadly, it encompasses techniques like cluster analysis and factor analysis. Of the various techniques for representing data structure and reducing redundancy, factor analysis more closely resembles the spatial distance models of multidimensional scaling than does any other technique (ibid.). And, most importantly, the factor scores and loadings of factor analysis provide a richer solution than do the stimulus coordinates (in psychometric terms) of the spatial distance models (MacCallum, 1974). In real terms, factor analysis is far more commonly used in social support studies than any other multidimensional scaling technique. Indeed, "multifactorial scaling" is another term pertinent to our purposes; therefore, it is used interchangeably with the terminology of multidimensional scaling in this book.

Factor analysis is used not only to identify all factors or principal components but to extract a smaller number of them in order to most efficiently or parsimoniously represent original data. The utilization of certain criteria for extracting factors, or for reducing the number of dimensions, entails a reflection on statistical reduction. We are fortunate, indeed, having powerful tools like factor analysis performed by the computer with various statistical packages, which automatically aggregate and "condense" the information for us by calculating a few (statistically "minimum") factors from relatively numerous original items. This automated process, with standardized (regression) analysis of variance or correlations based on empirical data, is superior to any blind combination or arbitrary weighting of the items. Based on such results, we can create relatively few subscales that are composite but unidimensional in nature. This notwithstanding, researchers are warned not to abuse factor analysis. Guilford (1978) discussed some common faults in factor analysis. On top of them is that too many factors are often extracted for the number of experimental variables. As a practical guideline, a rule-of-thumb is proposed to have at least three variables for every factor expected; and it is a good policy to select a domain that is not likely to involve more than 15 factors or 50 variables (ibid.). Strategies like such, however, do not lead to a full understanding and final solutions to the major issues involved in scale development. Statistical software is not absolute as to how many factors should be kept, although it offers the "optimal" level of extraction by conventional standards. In other words, it is our responsibility to make the final decision based on both empirical data and theoretical understanding. The utility of statistical techniques, moreover, depends on the plan by which we handle the extracted factors as well as the way in which we score and weight the various subscales. Even if we decide to use multiple measures, we still have a choice as to whether to adopt factor scores or to construct separate summated subscales. We also have a chance to pursue ultimate unidimensionalization (at the most general level). Here, by unidimensionalization, it is meant *to combine measurement items of different dimensions into a single scale.* Conventional factor analysis can only deal with the issue of multidimensionality by extracting a certain number of factors, based on which subscales of social support can be formulated. The issue of how to combine these factors, i.e., the problem of ultimate unidimensionalization, however, demands a clear theoretical understanding. The picture can easily be distorted in blending different dimensions without pondering on their relationships. A review of the current literature indicates that the practical strategy in this regard is generally weak and inadequate: Either the opportunity for further unidimensionalization is simply given up (e.g., Lin, Dean, & Ensel, 1979; Barrera & Ainlay, 1983), or it is accomplished on a basis that is not fully justified (e.g., Donald & Ware, 1984;

Stokes & Wilson, 1983). In other cases, factor analysis or any other multidimensional scaling procedure is not performed (e.g., Vaux et al., 1986; McFarlane et al.,1981), which leaves the scales far from established assessment tools as the goodness of fit of a dimensionality model accounts for a primary source of errors.

It no longer helps to lament on the myriad of particular ways of conceptualizing social support nor on the profusion of idiosyncratic measures. What seems needed by the research community is to set up certain norms to help bring social support study up to a new scientific standing. The key point here is the manner in which dimensions of social support are reduced in order to facilitate its assessment. In other words, the central theme is unidimensionalization at various levels. In order for the reduction process to be scientific in the interest of appropriate generalization, some primitive requirements for unidimensionalized measurement at all levels could be explored. First, any combination of measurement items must have some theoretical or empirical grounds showing their interrelationships as well as their relative importance to the resulting composite measure. It should further be based on some premises or facts about the relationships among all significant constructs involved in the study. The articulation of the theoretical assumptions or provision of empirical evidence in this regard as a norm will help the scientific community avoid many of the confusions and mistakes. Second, those assumptions and facts should have a knowledge basis and theoretical foundation as integral as possible. This requirement helps to prevent unnecessary and counterproductive variations and inconsistencies in research results due to unmindful designs. It may appear to be too stringent, though, as a notorious fact in this field is that theory has been far behind. However, we should at least be aware that there are such assumptions underlying the operations, and the assumptions should have some rationale to show their plausibility in one way or another. This discussion not only applies to the study of social support but also to the subjects of stress, depression, as well as many other topics. In fact, these are the basic principles for scaling any complex theoretical construct, in which the methodological crux is how to reduce the complexity of data by unifying different dimensions represented by various items and subscales.

Theoretical approach to unidimensionalization:
Learning from science

For the "pure" purpose of research, investigators from all fields may well be satisfied with the results of factor analysis, which involves both the clarification and the reduction of dimensionality among all the original variables involved. They can stay with a few dimensions by proceeding with the development of the subscales and looking at the relationships among these constructs as well as between the constructs and other interested variables. Based on findings of such research, recommendations for prevention of psychosocial disorders in various aspects can be made. In professional practice where a clear-cut diagnosis or an overall assessment of the domain is needed, however, these are not enough, as scores on various dimensions or subscales being simply pooled together could give just the same messy presentation as scores on original variables. The remaining dimensions as represented by the extracted factors might still be too many, though statistically reduced to "the minimum." And more importantly, they vary both in number and in direction (structure), from case to case and from population to population, which also leaves their comparisons with each other and with other studies an all too complicated business.

On the other hand, those who have tried to construct a global scale by combining different subscales or original items have often been trapped in a theoretical pitfall or dilemma: they have somehow related factors that do not show meaningful relationships, or in a way that does not reflect discernable or reasonable affinities. It is, indeed, all too arbitrary: there is no rationale seen in this field that would justify the seemingly violation of mathematical laws. This is, of course, a practical issue; its solution, however, demands some sort of theorization. As is the case of science, most of the theoretical stipulations should eventually take into account the complications of the real world and the needs of practice. Indeed, to establish a pragmatic approach to measurement for the purpose of "social engineering," there is much to learn from engineering mechanics, an applied science that centers around the idea of stress and has much to do with the scaling of support.

Readers may find it interesting how mechanical theories of engineering would contribute to our knowledge of scale development in social, behavioral, as well as biomedical research and practice. Yet as a matter of fact, not only the history of psychometrics was in large portion a history of psychophysics, but a great share of the major ideas in the psychosocial branches of learning came from various theoretical and applied fields of science. Especially, concepts such as "stress," "support," "functioning," and "mechanism" all find their roots in engineering mechanics (Hobfoll, 1988). However, when these terms were grafted to psychosocial studies, their theoretical groundworks were not all taken along with them. It is understandable because it is no ease for behavioral and social scientists to grasp all the fundamentals of the fields other than their own. However, it leaves substantial gaps in knowledge as well as confusions in nomenclature. Here, the most important theoretical foundation that needs to be reviewed is the measurement-related theories in engineering mechanics.

Engineering mechanics, especially its basic component material mechanics, can be regarded as a science of stress of structural parts connected together in such a way as to perform a useful function and to withstand externally applied loads. The kinds of loads include press, pull, and shear, which subject different parts and structures of various materials to tension, compression, bending, and torsion, which results in a balance represented by various external forces that cause the strain and stress in the material. Stress is defined as the intensity of internally distributed force, which, marked by the strain in the material, is a re-action to the external force. The study of strength of materials is aimed at predicting how the geometric and physical properties of a structural part will influence its behavior under service conditions (Timoshenko & Young, 1962). Whether the structure is strong enough to withstand the loads and stiff enough to avoid excessive deformations and deflections, however, also depends on the amount of loads as well as the ways in which they are applied to the structural part. Although its object is materials and structures other than human subjects and relationships, mechanical theories may help advance social stress and support studies with not just the terminology but also the ways of thinking and modes of study. Especially, for our concern with the practical issue of unidimen-sionalization in constructing composite measures of social support, life stress, affective functioning, as well as many other psychosocial or even biomedical constructs, there are so-called strength theories that would render very useful insights.

In predicting the "well-being" state or measuring the relative strength of structural parts of various materials, strength theories specifically deal with the issue of unidimensionalization. The mechanical properties of structural materials are normally determined by tests which subject the specimen to comparatively simple stress conditions, whereas the strength of materials under more complicated cases has only been investigated in a few exceptional cases

(Timoshenko & Young, 1962). Various strength theories therefore have been concerned with relating the simple criteria of allowable stresses to the complicated conditions which occur in practical design. As Timoshenko and Young (ibid., p.314) states, "The purpose of these theories is to predict failure conditions under combined stresses, assuming that the behavior in a simple tension or compression test is known."

The first theory is called the maximum stress theory, considering the maximum (in terms of absolute value) principal stress as the criterion for strength. This is the simplest form of theoretical assumptions underlying the process of unidimensionalization of the measurement because all other dimensions next in importance are simply omitted. There are many examples that are not amenable to or even contradict the maximum stress theory (Timoshenko & Young, 1962). However, this theory served as a milestone indicating an effort of scientific reduction based on a thorough analysis or "factorization" of complicated stress conditions as well as an explicit theoretical assumption that lends itself to empirical falsification. It was a momentous departure from arbitrarily choosing one or more individual indicators, which brought the art of measurement to a scientific standing.

The second theory is the maximum strain theory. The hypothesis is that a material fails when the maximum (in terms of absolute value) equals the failure point strain in simple stress test. As there are well-established theories like Hooke's Law relating strain with stress while stresses of all directions can contribute to the strain along one specific dimension, this theory represents a better case of unidimensionalization. Nevertheless, there are also many cases in which the maximum strain theory may also be shown to be invalid. Especially, experiments show that homogeneous materials under uniform compression can withstand much higher stresses and remain elastic (ibid.).

Being there all the failure cases of the first two theories, there came the third, the maximum shear theory. "This theory assumes that yielding begins when the maximum shear stress in the material becomes equal to the maximum shear stress at the yield point in a simple tension test" (ibid., p.315). Since the maximum shear stress in the material is known equal to half the difference between the maximum and minimum principal stresses, and since the maximum shear stress is equal to half the normal stress in a tension test, the total difference between the maximum and minimum principal stresses becomes the criterion for strength (ibid., p.316). This turns out to be a better example of unidimensionalizing measurement, as the theory is in good agreement with experiments and is widely used in machine design, especially for ductile materials (ibid.).

In addition to these classical strength theories, succeeding development has included some newer theoretical approaches to strength of materials, such as the distortion energy theory which considers the strain energy of deformation per unit volume of the material as a basis of selecting working stresses in machine design (Peterson, 1953). Timoshenko and Young (1962) compared some different strength theories. It is noticeable that the difference between results of different theories is considerable. This indicates the significance of theory in scaling in general and in unidimensionalization in particular.

The most general state of stress which can exist in a body in mechanics is always completely determined by specifying three principal stresses. In behavioral and social sciences, however, the situation can be far more complicated: The number of dimensions we have to deal with are too often more than three, which do not lend themselves to spatial visualization and thus usually can only exist in our abstract reasoning. Besides, human body and mind are distinct from the material part studied in mechanics. However, as we have borrowed the ideas of stress, support, and so forth from the mechanical world, there are a number of useful lessons and inspirations we can draw from the above review. First, and foremost, it shows that there is real possibility to unidimensionalize the results of multidimensional scaling in a scientific fashion. And there are different pathways to achieve this objective by means of alternative theoretical models. Second, appropriate theoretical assumptions are the key to unidimensionalization. The appropriateness of theory can be directly tested by observational data. Third, specificity is the basis for pursuing generality. Before scales can be unidimensionalized individual items must be analyzed by clarifying their dimensionality. The role of principal stresses in strength theory points to the necessity of factor analysis and/or other methods for multidimensional scaling. Fourth, the task of diagnosis is two-fold, requiring the assessment of social stress and social support on the one hand and the establishment of the criteria (critical points of individual and group failure) on the other. It can be told that in behavioral and social sciences, the latter is both a scientific and a political matter. Methodologically, however, it can be done by relatively simple methods provided that there are appropriate theories linking the results to more complicated cases. Finally, it is not necessary for the mathematical representations of such theories to be very simple, especially when researchers are no longer legitimated for hand calculation of routine quantitative transformations in the computer times.

All in all, learning from science could be instrumental to the advancement of psychosocial enterprises. In many aspects mechanical theories have direct relevance to stress study in human sciences. Ideas such as "stress concentration design" may have special implications to social stress as well as network study and intervention. Social support research can also draw from such theories by means of its conceptual connection with social stress as well as by comparing its formats and functional pathways with the ideas of mechanical support. The most significant contribution of the scientific expertise to our inquiry here, however, is a theoretical approach to the general issue of measurement and diagnosis, i.e., unidimensionalization in scaling theoretical constructs.

Weighting and multiple regression:
A practical strategy

Complemental to the theoretical reflection in the above, I shall turn to explore a practical approach to the issue of unidimensionalization in this section by summarizing behavioral and social research experience in weighting different items of a scale. Notwithstanding the fact that we had to resort to scientific/ engineering ideas and methods, psychosociometrists are not to blame for totally failing to provide psychosocial research workers and practitioners with a way out. Theoretically they have predicted the possibility of higher level abstraction; technically they have derived numerous statistical means and passageways based on which a practical approach to the issue of ultimate unidimensionalization could be figured out. Indeed, behavioral and social scientists have the advantage of including samples of study objects (subjects) large enough in most single studies that make such an approach not only feasible but also expedient. A knowledge of unidimensional scaling is fundamental in understanding this, of which one important task is to determine the relative importance of component items or subscales, namely, the weights they carry in the composite scale.

There are two kinds of weights. The nominal weights are those we deliberately assign to components; the effective weights are those the components actually carry in the composite (Ghiselli, 1964). The two may or may not be the same. The point is, "In order for the effective weights to correspond to the nominal weights, we have to be sure that the components carry equal weight to begin with" (ibid., 298). The means by which to achieve this is a procedure of transmuting the scores on the components to standard-score form to equalize the weights they originally carry. When this is done, we can establish the relative role of individual components exactly by differential weighting according to our theoretical understanding and/or based on some empirical grounds. Taking a look at either social support or stress literature, however, one can get surprised that few, if any, studies have emphasized on weighting in the development of needed scales. And this situation appears to have been justified in practical terms. The main grounds can be summarized as follows: a) The problem of assigning weights to items in a scale is one which is rather annoying (Sewell, 1941); b) It is difficult to defend other arbitrary systems of weighting in comparison to an equal-weighting scheme (Nunnally, 1978); c) The problem of assigning weights to items in a scale is not of great practical significance in light of the roughness of most sociometric devices at certain times (Sewell, 1941); and d) Studies have shown that essentially the same final results are obtained with arbitrary common sense weighting as with more complicated, but still arbitrary, statistical techniques (ibid.). These reasons, however, do not warrant desirable results and are no longer tenable in face of the demand for more accurate measurement nowadays. For example, McIver and Carmines (1981) indicate that the interpretation of Likert-Scale scores falling between the extremes is problematic except in relative terms. Indeed, the results obtained in such a manner cannot fully meet the needs of practice, which often requires a cutoff point as a criterion for diagnosis, classification, and differential treatment. As a matter of fact, the function of differential weighting is "to make the composite more precise or reliable, more meaningful, or more predictive of some other variable" (Ghiselli, 1964:293). The question, thus, is not whether or not differential weighting, where applicable, is desirable but whether or not it should be done arbitrarily. According to the new norms we set in the preceding pages, a theoretical/ empirical basis has become necessary to maintain a scale as a more precise and meaningful composite measure.

If unidimensionalization is done mainly through combining different factors or aspects rather than simply dropping some of them, the issue of multidimensional scale development (as unidimensionalized scaling) would eventually lead to more refined mathematical consideration of weighting. However, it is a problem of weighting different factors or components instead of individual items. Here research and theory may complement each other. We could make the scale more reliable or more predictive of some other variable via empirical means. Specifically, the latter can be done by using multiple regression when appropriate scaling models are applied to the data (usually in the linear or linearized situation, or ideally, additive assumption applies). In the study of the relationship between social support and affective functioning, for example, this is feasible by taking one as an outside variable in scaling the other. After comparing the regression coefficients with other possible weights, Ghiselli (1964) concludes that the beta coefficients are the best weights for the predictor variables as components of the composite measure in relation to an outside criterion variable. As the regression model especially accommodates variables of different dimensions that are orthogonal to (independent of) one another, it represents a convenient, practical approach (in contrast to the theoretical approach discussed in the preceding section) to the issue of unidimensionalization. Here regression serves the purpose of reconciling the results of factor analysis, which represent different dimensions, rather than individual items, which often obscure the issue of dimensionality. As a matter of fact, factor analysis has long been used to derive a set of uncorrelated variables when the use of highly intercorrelated variables may yield misleading results in regression analysis (Kim & Mueller, 1978). This method actually makes the weighting of individual items unreasonable or unnecessary.

Multiple regression has special utility in this study, not just because its logic underlies factor analysis itself. It aims at the maximum correlation of the composite variable (to be scaled with a few factors) with a specific criterion variable. This is usually the ultimate purpose of scale development, which will be further discussed later. The application of a linear regression model also makes explicit the fundamental requirement of linearity for the scales that are usually simply summated. Moreover, it not only stimulates awareness about the all-sidedness of item coverage (item sampling adequacy) but also raises the issue of redundancy if items are directly used in the regression equation in place of independent factor scores. It is, therefore, essential to explore the application of such an approach in the interest of both advancing the art of assessment and substantiating the relationships among variables.

To recapitulate, the optimal weights obtained by regression methods are characterized by their specific data base in place of theoretical application. They are also featured by specific objectives and corresponding techniques (Horst, 1966). Yet, the results obtained from individual data sets are subject to explanation, evaluation, and modification from the perspective of established theories. Without appropriate empirical basis *and* adequate theoretical preparation, it is a real danger to use any computational procedures for scaling purpose. By presuming every indicator to be equal, which is the usual case in

94

summated scaling, for example, it is very likely that we will lose important information on items (factors) that have relatively small variations but that in real terms mean a lot to human conditions. Even standardization of the individual items will not guarantee the suitability and utility of a scale, since the role of each item is determined by complicated considerations, including, for example, the degree of sampling adequacy. And, most significant to our concern here, the psychosocial domain to be measured tends to be multidimensional rather than unidimensional, thus the application of unidimensional scaling techniques could be very problematic here.

6　Empirical data and analysis plan

This chapter first describes the empirical data that will be used to demonstrate the use of different approaches to the measurement and analysis issues discussed in preceding chapters. Showing novice readers a way to deal with specific data sets, I will streamline the variables and measures contained in the original data for further scaling treatment and substantive analysis. The appropriateness of the data for the specific research objectives will be addressed, and some measurement consideration and operationalization of the causal model created in chapter four will also be made. With certain limitation of the data sets, a working path model as well as some reduced individual hypotheses will be formulated for empirical examination and demonstration. An integral and optimal approach to data analysis incorporating both scale development and hypothesis testing is discussed by acknowledging the strengths of the FASEM and LISREL techniques. Nevertheless, it is stressed again that confirmatory factor analysis does not promise any breakthrough in scaling multidimensional constructs. It suggests that such approaches cannot be simply followed by the present study, which aims at surmounting the "ultimate limit" of a set of factor or factor-based scores for each of the constructs, which are "too broad" while theoretically may make very good sense.

Before concentrating on the scaling of the major theoretical constructs, necessary preparation in measurement theory will be made by rendering a perspective in psychosocial measurement extending beyond conventional statistical reduction. By reviewing the general status of scientific inquiry in this regard, the chapter holds out a theme of unidimensionalization and considers it central to multi-item scale development. To clarify its meaning and see how it can be reasonably accomplished, a further methodological and theoretical reflection on scaling multidimensional constructs is made, and some basic requirements for unidimensionalized measurement at all levels are speculated. Under these guidelines, a theoretical approach to unidimensionalization is proposed by learning from science, specifically from engineering mechanics where major constructs such as stress and support all find their roots. In addition, another approach is formed by summarizing the strategy of combining factor analysis and regression analysis in scaling practice.

The data sets

The empirical data to be used in the analysis were collected by a research team consisting of investigators from the UCLA School of Social Welfare and School of Public Health, University of Hong Kong, Beijing Medical University, and Sun Yat-Sen University of Medical Science. The project, headed by UCLA professor Harry Kitano, was also co-sponsored by the National Research Center on Asian American Mental Health and supported by UCLA Center for Pacific Rim Studies. Beginning with a cross-national study on elderly Chinese and Chinese Americans conducted during 1990-91, the inter-school and inter-university research team has been accumulating considerable empirical information on Asian and Asian-American elderly. A database has now included survey data on the Chinese elderly living in Beijing, Shanghai, Guangzhou (Canton), and Hong Kong, the Chinese-American elderly living in Los Angeles, as well as the L.A. Japanese-American elderly. As part of an exchange program, survey data on the elderly living in Tawa-Cho, Japan are also imported into the database. Another survey on Korean-American elderly has been on schedule; and a proposal has ever been made to survey the elderly in Taiwan. As subsequent research projects keep going, still more data sets will be made available and added to the database. I have been responsible for managing the database under the direction of Dr. James E. Lubben, Associate Dean of the former School of Social Welfare and one of the principal investigators.

The Asian and Asian-American elderly database is currently combined from six individual data sets named BEIJING.SPSS, SHANGHAI.SPSS, CANTON.SPSS, HONGKONG.SPSS, LOSANGEL.SPSS, and JAPAN.SPSS, respectively. Different research sites are indicated by the names of the data files except for LOSANGEL.SPSS referring to the Chinese-American elderly in Los

Angeles and JAPAN.SPSS to the Japanese-American elderly from the same site. The original versions of BEIJING.SPSS (containing a sample of 500 elderly individuals) and CANTON.SPSS (sized 504) were created in August 1991, accommodating exactly the same 393 user-defined variables for each data set. For SHANGHAI.SPSS (sized 500), it was created in September 1992 with the same data structure. The LOSANGEL.SPSS (sized 204) data set contains more (446) variables than the above three Chinese data sets. Its original version was of the same date as BEIJING.SPSS and CANTON.SPSS. The HONG-KONG.SPSS is a data set borrowed from the 1988 Hong Kong Elderly Health Survey conducted by one of the team members with her Hong Kong colleagues (Chi & Lee, 1989), which holds only a portion of the variables (149 out of the original 363) that could be made compatible with the other data sets. This has limited its use in the joint data analysis.

Only a subset of data on the elderly living in mainland China and the Chinese-American elderly living in Los Angeles will be extracted for analysis in the present study, partly because the measurement tools employed at the four sites were uniquely consistent, and consequently the information obtained was excellently compatible. The special ground for including the group of Chinese-American elderly is that there are common features of Chinese culture shared by all ethnic Chinese, whether in the homeland or overseas (cf. chapter three). Yet it is also intriguing to deal with some potential sociocultural differentiation in various settings (cf. chapter four). It should be noted that the time frame for the Shanghai data set is not the same as that for the other three sites, i.e., it is about one year later than the data from Beijing, Guangzhou, and Los Angeles. Although the rapid change in mainland China in the past few years should be heeded in pursuing site differences, however, a time period of one year would not count much in considering the effect of secular trend on domains such as social support.

The surveys were cross-sectional in nature. The data were obtained by questionnaire interviews performed by trained interviewers. They were mainly based on self-reports of the elderly respondents. All the data sets were representative by virtue of the random sampling design of the surveys, which has been described in detail elsewhere (e.g., Chen, 1991). Basically, in the three survey sites in China which included 88% of the total sample, a multi-stage cluster sampling strategy was used, with stratification of the elderly individuals by sex (ibid.). For the analysis to be performed, results will be reported for 1,708 elder people 60 years of age and over from the four metropolitan sites. The total sample had a sex ratio of 53.3 (with only 1 case missing in the data). Maximum age was 97, with a mean of 69.19 years (SD=6.69) for the whole sample (3 cases missing for this variable). In terms of marital status, 1,166 elderly respondents (accounting for 68.4% of the total sample) were married and 507 (29.7%) widowed; only 32 (1.9%) were divorced/separated, never married, or of other situation (3 cases missing). Slightly over a half (932, or 56.5%) of the sample answered "yes" to the question if they had ever received formal education, while only 38.2% answered "yes" to the question if they were able to read (another 15.6% "read a little," with a total of 52 cases missing). A more accurate measure, i.e., years of education, indicates that 28.8% of the surveyed elderly had only primary schooling (1-6 years), 18.3% reached the secondary level (7-12 years), 10.3% went beyond senior high (13 years and above), whereas 42.6% never entered school (6 cases missing). More description of the sample characteristics will be included in Chapter Six. To see how much the data are appropriate and sound to address the research objectives, however, an overhaul of all the variables contained and measures involved should be made here.

Variables and original scales

The questionnaire was standardized across all the four sites. Questions fell into twelve categories: a) demographics (background information); b) family and social support; c) health status and health behavior; d) functional status; e) life events and daily strains; f) mental health; g) living conditions; h) employment history; i) financial status; j) role in family and society; k) memory; and l) knowledge of Alzheimer's disease. Besides, the LOSANGEL.SPSS data set had an additional part taping the information on ethnic background, immigration history, and acculturation of the Chinese-American elderly. The measures and scales utilized in collecting the data were originally devised in the English language. They were translated into Chinese by bilingual experts and confirmed in meetings with Chinese scholars. I personally helped finalize the Chinese version of the questionnaire by performing some back translations and using Chinese word processors to produce the original questionnaire. In the inception of the survey in 1990, I was doing research in Hong Kong and acted as a volunteer assistant to the principal investigators. Due to this involvement in the original study, I am fairly confident about the high correspondence between the two languages of the scales used.

Family and social support was one major area of the inquiry. The whole category included eighteen questions, with more than half having multiple entries forming several hierarchical structures. The major hierarchical pattern typically tapped different levels of informal relationships, ranging from immediate family, extended family, friends and neighbors, through others. The questions probed into two broad aspects of the metaconstruct social support, namely, social network (and family) composition and mutual care and help. There were additional items that belonged to other portions while were relevant to the measurement of social support, such as marital status (as part of demographic background), living arrangements (as one of the living conditions), help received when ill or having difficulties in performing activities of daily living (in health and functional status sections), as well as some relevant items in mental health section. Family and social support was scaled in terms of social support networks with the use of the Lubben Social Network Scale (LSNS), which was modified from the Berkman-Syme Social Network Index (BSNI) especially for use with older populations (Lubben, 1988). The LSNS is an equally weighted sum of ten aspects of an old person's social networks; response patterns to individual items were carefully weighted in a specific way. The ten items fell into three groups, namely, family networks, friends networks, and interdependent social supports. More specifically, there were three items dealing with family relationships (size of active family network, size of intimate family network, and frequency of contact with a family member). Three similar items dealt with relationships with friends. The four remaining items addressed interdependent relationships (e.g., having a confidant, and the reciprocity of giving help). The English version of the LSNS used in the collection of the present data (see Appendix Ia) differed slightly in wording from its first published, standard format (Lubben, 1988). Modification was made in the interest of accuracy in specifying network members, such as "family members/relative (not include spouse)" instead of mere "relative," and "friends or neighbors" in place of "friends" only. Those dealing with frequencies of interaction were now asked particularly by "How often do you...?" rather than generally "Do you...?" The most notable change was made to the first question, which in the first publication of the scale was phrased "How many relatives do you see or hear from at least once a month," whereas in this survey the activity was switched to "talk to or write to" and kinship was divided into six categories, namely, parents, siblings, children, children-in-law, grand-children, and other relatives. Similar change in format was also made to the last item, namely, living

100

arrangements.

Strictly speaking, there was only one major scale tapping only the emotional aspect of mental functioning of the respondents. Although there was another separate category assessing their memory with two additional questions, on the whole the items used did not seem quite enough to evaluate both cognitive and affective states and status. The Center for Epidemiologic Studies Depression Scale (CES-D) was applied to the assessment of affective functioning of the Chinese and Chinese-American elderly. This scale was developed by the Center for Epidemiologic Studies at the National Institute of Mental Health in the United States, specifically to meet the need for a brief, inexpensive measure of depression suitable for use in community surveys (Marsella, Hirschfeld, & Katz, 1987). "Such an instrument could serve either as the initial screen in a two-stage assessment procedure..., or, more ambitiously, as a basis for generating prevalence rates in its own right" (ibid., p.76). The CES-D was made of 20 items that were culled from other depression scales such as the Beck Depression Inventory (BDI; Beck et al., 1961), the Zung Self-Rating Depression Scale (SDS; Zung, 1965), and Minnesota Multiphasic Personality Inventory (MMPI) Depression (D) scale (Hathaway & McKinley, 1942). The questionnaire used to survey the Chinese and Chinese-American elderly, however, included only 17 items of the scale (see Appendix IIIa). According to the experience of a previous survey of health and living status of the elderly in Taiwan (Taiwan Provincial Institute of Family Planning & University of Michigan Population Studies Center & Institute of Gerontology, 1989), three items of the CES-D were found hard to translate and performed poorly in the pretest. Therefore, they were dropped from the formal questionnaire for that survey. Informed of this practice, a decision was made to adopt the same item structure in the original survey for this study.

In contrast to the part of mental health, physical health and functioning as well as health behavior took up a large portion of the questionnaire. Health status alone was assessed with sixteen questions, with two of them having over ten sub-items, each of which tapped more than one levels or aspects. Functional status was less weighted, being touched in only three major entries, one of which in fact had to do with health practice (exercise). On the other hand, health habits, health-seeking behavior, and preventive service utilization had even more entries than health status category, amounting to as many as twenty-nine major questions that included even more sub-items. Besides, there was a whole section gauging respondents' knowledge of Alzheimer's disease. Of all the physical variables, however, only functional status was scaled in terms of a multi-item measure. The operational components of physical functioning in the most narrow meaning include solely basic care or activities of daily living (ADL). A broader definition also includes mobility; and a still broader one encompasses the other set of more complex activities that are associated with independent life, that is, instrumental activities of daily living (IADL). The questionnaire included thirteen functioning items all together, which were grouped under two major entries. The items were chosen based on the judgment of the principal investigators as to their relevance to the particular research setting.

In addition to the variables mentioned above assessing the elderly by areas of functioning, there were global indicators of life events and daily strains showing all the positive and negative impacts exerted by environmental forces upon the well-being of the elderly. The few life events listed on the questionnaire were some of those that were frequently used to construct stress(or) scales. The selection of the life events as well as some indicators of daily strains was largely based on previous work on elderly population (Lubben, 1983). With the drawbacks of pooling together positive and negative events being recognized, however, the selected items were not intended to constitute a global scale in the original survey. Closely related to the measures of life stress, there were several major categories and individual items that fell within a broad conception of socioeconomic status (SES), including educational background (part of the demographic information), employment history, financial status, living conditions, as well as role in family and society.

The measurement of life satisfaction was placed in the broad category of mental health in the questionnaire while is separated from the latter in this review. Strictly speaking, life satisfaction is also a global measure in terms of the elders' overall functioning, not just an indicator of their mental health. The reason is that the overall measure of satisfaction, though closely related with mental status, would have to do with all areas of life, including its physical and social aspects. Therefore, like the non-specific concept of (life) stress, life satisfaction will be regarded as a global or general measure in contrast to more specific assessments like work satisfaction, leisure satisfaction, or satisfaction with social support. Overall life satisfaction of the Chinese and Chinese-American elderly was gauged by indicators taken from the Life Satisfaction Index developed by Wood, Wylie, and Shaefer (1969). The indicators used, if all together taken as a scale, were a shortened version of the original Life Satisfaction Index drawn with a systematic, split-half strategy (pulling out every other item starting from the first one of the original Index). This short scale seemed to perform fairly well in some preliminary data analysis. Yet, to construct a reliable and valid scale that has good utility in research on the basis of a practical approach like such, further confirmation of its psychosociometric property is demanded. This book, however, will not pursue this line of study. Rather, under the research framework I have built, life stress and life satisfaction will be integrated into the broader conception and measurement of quality of life. Nevertheless, some of the life satisfaction indicators, especially those with a negative tone (dissatisfaction), can be exploited to enhance the discriminating power of depression measures. Those items will be sorted out later in the development of a new depression scale. The point is, when I allow dissatisfaction to be a symptom presentation of depression, the corresponding items should not at the same time serve as an overall subjective indication of stress (quality of life), so that a clear demarcation line between the two constructs could be maintained.

Finally, at the beginning of the questionnaire there was an item indicating the language used during interview, which had two implications. In the first place, the information, along with the indicator of different survey sites, not only helps cross-national study but also useful in marking cultural variations within a nationally, geographically, and socioeconomically heterogeneous country like China. In the second place, it poses a question of comparability of data to our research conclusions. Although the problem of different dialects, such as the difference between Mandarin and Cantonese, would not be so serious as that of different languages, such as the discrepancy between Chinese and English, we need to heed any potential influence caused by the variation of communication tools in the substantive study.

On the whole, although the data sets do not appear very strong in mental health information, they rank among the top ones by providing comprehensive social and health data on the Chinese and Chinese-American elderly. They are selected for the present study not only because they are the only quality data sets on Chinese and Chinese-American elderly readily accessible to me but the weakness mentioned above is highly compensated by the richness of social support material and comprehensiveness of information. They also excel in large sample sizes and in representing different geographic areas. In addition, as they serve as part of a more ambitious project, they are a valuable basis for further cross-national inquiry and cross-cultural comparison.

Some consideration of measures and operationalization of the path model

While the data sets largely address the objectives of the present study, some information is missing while required for the full representation and testing of the theoretical model derived in last chapter. That model is relatively complete, and thus is essential in providing an adequate theoretical understanding about the real world and the analytic task bound to be performed. However, some compromises have to be made to apply the model to the specific data sets. First, measures of a diathesis were not included in the original questionnaire. The role of the diathesis is traditionally defined as "a nervous system so sensitively constituted, and ill adjusted to its surroundings, that when brought in contact with unusually exciting influences, there may occur deranged instead of natural mental action, and it becomes more or less continuous instead of evanescent" (Stearns, 1883, cited from Grob, 1983:40). This representing the important role of the biological aspect, many psychosocial studies could be criticized for ignoring that factor, especially from the point of view of an "endogenous" type of depression. However, it is usually impractical to expect a community health survey to obtain direct information on the nervous system. And since the original survey did not inquire into family history or the genetic aspect of depression due to its emphasis on some other aspects, the role of a diathesis cannot be reproduced in the subsequent analysis. Note that it is helpless to introduce instead some cognitive or social components under the name of a diathesis, since this would potentially confound with the constructs of coping, social support, and stress itself. The theoretical model is instructive, however, reminding us of the limitation of a simple stress-depression connection, which, missing the role of a diathesis, not only contains some spurious proportion in itself but more or less obscures the "stress-buffering" effect of social support.

Second, similar cases are found with the constructs of coping strategy and personality traits. There was neither an established coping scale nor a test of personality traits (e.g., a personality inventory) employed in the original survey. Nevertheless, there was some information provided by the questionnaire that might be made use of by reforming our measurement and analysis ideas. In the first place, some items in the questionnaire were relevant to the concept of coping, though they were not phrased in terms of some general choices as did some regular scales (e.g., Jalowiec & Powers, 1981). Here the idea of coping could be regarded as specifically operationalized in the questionnaire in the light of health- or illness-related behaviors. For example, when one was sick, the choice between "going to see a doctor right away" and "rather avoiding going to the doctor for as long as possible" can be viewed as an indication of different coping strategies in face of the specific kind of life stress. In the second, although there was obviously no idea of personality traits like hardiness underlying the original questionnaire design, there were some items probing into the attitudes of the elderly respondents toward a few things that were relevant to what we call personal resources. Since attitudes constitute an important aspect of personal resources per definition (Moos & Billings, 1982) while they have been typically neglected in previous studies, it is worthwhile to construct a scale emphasizing on this dimension. For example, those who believed that old people may still be able to do something useful would more likely assume an active approach coping style. All these can be used as some measurement proxies of the general construct "personal coping" encompassing personal resources and coping strategy.

With all such specific considerations, a working path model is finally formulated for empirical examination which is shown in diagram 6.1. It should be stressed, however, that the theoretical model derived in last chapter is important in guiding the research. While some of the pathways and meanings of some constructs are reduced to the present format, it is under that framework that the working model and hypotheses are made available. On the other hand, when we draw conclusions from the findings we must note these specific limits. This, in fact, is a general issue in empirical studies where operationalization of theoretical constructs are required yet the item sampling adequacy is not necessarily accomplished. In such cases, the issues of conceptualization, measurement (scaling) and analysis are closely tied together. With an appropriate understanding of all these issues, the use of the theoretical model can be fruitful and versatile. For example, under the rubric of cultural differentiation, we may not only try the variable of research site but also examine how different dialects would make a difference.

Table 6.1 displays the accordingly reduced individual hypotheses. Since some conventional bivariate and multivariate analyses will also be performed with foci on specific pathways, these hypotheses are phrased with less causal intonation to suit such preliminary tests.

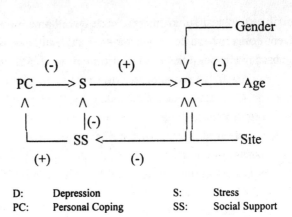

Diagram 6.1 Psychosocial determinants of depression: The working model

Table 6.1 Summary of the loosened individual hypotheses to be tested

Path	Hypothesis
S-D	- Stress is positively related to depression.
SS-D	- Social support is negatively related to depression.
SS-S	- Social support is negatively associated with stress.
PC-S	- Positive personal coping is negatively related with stress.
SS-PC	- Social support is positively associated with positive coping.
Site-D	- Site difference (cultural differentiation) more or less accounts for the variation in depression.
Age-D	- The older the age, the less likely the depression.
Gender-D	- Gender makes a difference in depression.

Scale development and hypothesis testing: An integral and optimal approach to data analysis

The three core constructs in this inquiry, namely, social support, stress, and depression, will be given elaborate measurement treatment. The data analysis,

106

therefore, involves two basic tasks, that is, scale development and hypothesis testing. Conventionally, investigators would either concentrate on scaling issues or focus on substantive hypothesis or model testing using existing measures. In this study, however, I will try to combine the two research modes into an integral approach to data analysis. Scale development and substantive model testing are viewed as two aspects of an inseparable process. The best substantive results must be the best measurement results. In other words, substantive findings depend on the measures used, whereas the development of measurement tools are tested by substantive results, and ultimately serves the specific purposes of the research.

Generally speaking, the simultaneous analysis of measurement and statistical models has been a central feature of the optimal scaling strategy as well as the optimal approach to data analysis. Jacoby (1991) described such an approach, named "Alternating Least Squares, Optimal Scaling (ALSOS)," to data analysis. It is based upon the idea that the measurement characteristics of the data can be regarded as parameters to be estimated during the course of an analysis. As Jacoby (ibid., p.74) wrote,

> The ALSOS approach holds that empirical statistical analyses involve two different models of the observations. The first represents the structural relationships between the variables. The second involves the measurement characteristics of the variables.

Notably, "This approach, based on data theory notions, holds out promise for regression estimation in the face of ordinal independent variables" (ibid., p.1). As a most powerful tool for performing statistical control over variables, regression is not only the fundamental technique in path analysis but also a major means of developing needed scales. With a root in this technique, factor analysis is also crucial to multidimensional scaling for the purpose of psychosocial study and practice. And there are now more advanced statistical packages incorporating both programs, such as the LISREL (Jöreskog & Sörbom, 1989) and the EQS (Bentler, 1985), which provide a truly integral and optimal approach to data analysis by simultaneously handling the measurement and substantive model testing issues. This kind of methods, generally called Factor Analytic Simultaneous Equation Model (FASEM) (Bentler, 1986), have been developing rapidly in recent years. Taking LISREL for example, "it is a very versatile approach that may be used for the analysis of causal models with multiple indicators of latent variables, reciprocal causation, measurement errors, correlated errors, and correlated residuals to name but a few" (Pedhazur, 1982:637-38). The major idea underlying such methods is to take confirmatory factor analysis (CFA) "as a submodel of the more general Structural Equation Modeling (SEM) approach" (Pedhazur & Schmelkin, 1991:632).

Nonetheless, as a measurement model of relations of indicators ("manifest variables") to factors ("latent variables") as well as relations among the latter, confirmatory factor analysis does not promise any breakthrough in scaling multidimensional constructs. Rather, it seems to serve the contrary view that concepts like social support, stress, and depression are actually unscalable in terms of a general measure in each case where more than one factor is identified. This is the focal-point issue I ended up with in reviewing the state of the art of scale development by exemplifying the field of social support. It suggests that the FASEM approach cannot be followed as-is by the present study, which aims at surmounting the "ultimate limit" of a set of factor or factor-based scores for each of the constructs that are "too broad" while truly or theoretically make sense.

Analysis procedures and a caveat about causation

The goal of the study provides the tasks of data analysis both in scale development and substantive hypothesis testing. The next chapter will center on the scaling of three major theoretical constructs, that is, social support, stress, and depression. Before we enter that topic, some preparation in measurement theory is essential. This will be done in the next section by proposing some ideas based on which certain general multifactorial scaling methods will be developed. In the following, I shall give a brief account of the analytic procedures to be followed in the rest of the book.

At the first step of scale construction, I will focus on selecting items from the original survey instruments for those key measures according to the qualitative criteria of item relevance, item sampling adequacy, mutual exclusiveness of measures, as well as logical relationships among the constructs to be scaled. These criteria are corresponding to the ideas of content and construct validity of measurement. However, they can only be attained to the extent that the employed data sets would allow for. After the item pools are decided, exploratory factor analysis (EFA) will be performed to uncover different dimensions as well as obtain resultant subscales such as component scores. While the common factor model is more in line with the spirit of dimensional analysis, principal components analysis is favored in this study. For similar reasons that will be given for the above choice, confirmatory factor analysis will not be performed as refined pursuit of dimensionality is not the ultimate objective. Instead, based on the components and component scores obtained (customarily also called factors and factor scores), I shall focus on the development of a general scale in each domain by advancing a theme of unidimensionalization as well as different approaches to its accomplishment. Different scales derived by different approaches will be compared via multiple means, conclusively in light of criterion-related validity, for the purpose of examining different scaling models.

Once such general measures of the key constructs are obtained, substantive analysis ranging from univariate statistics to complex model testing can be made empirically more succinct and theoretically more relevant. Some univariate statistics will be obtained first to show the parameters of the distributions of some major variables. Then, some bivariate analyses will be performed, as well as certain moderator or suppressor variables introduced in order to achieve the effect of some preliminary statistical control. Such analyses would highlight different portions of the structural model. The full test of the substantive model, however, requires truly multivariate analyses. A single-equation multiple regression will be conducted to show the results of the common practice, though it is a path analysis or a set of structured regression equations that would give the most accurate findings. Path analysis can be handled by some structural equation modeling (SEM) procedures. Since the statistical program EQS has the merit of simplicity in contrast to the more popular yet more complex package LISREL, it will be utilized in this study. The EQS computer software can deal with a series of regression equations simultaneously and generate an estimated covariance matrix of the hypothesized relationships between the variables contained in the model (Bentler, 1985). Analyses other than the test of the path model will be performed with SPSS-X. All the "runs" will be completed on the mainframe managed by the Office of Academic Computing (OAC) at UCLA. A more detailed discussion of the advantages and limitations of the techniques involved will be given along with a report of the major findings upon the completion of all the analyses.

Some notes are needed in concluding this section. Path analysis "is nothing but a repeated application of multiple regression analysis (applied to each variable in succession, with the prior variables as its determiners)" (Van de Geer, 1971:86). However, since "the term path analysis has been used to refer to the analysis of causal models when single indicators are employed for each of the variables in the model" (Pedhazur & Schmelkin, 1991:695), conditions for causal inference should be borne in mind. James, Mulaik and Brett (1982) stated the logical foundation; a major principle reads:

A structural model is confirmed if the predictions regarding correlations (variances/covariances) among manifest variables are consistent with the observed (i.e., empirically derived) correlations (variances/covariances) among manifest variables. A structural model is disconfirmed if predictions and observed correlations (variances/covariances) are inconsistent. (ibid., p.59)

The notion of causation, however, should be clarified because it is central to the inquiry. Pedhazur and Schmelkin (1991) point out that the scientist *qua* scientist seems to find a causal framework indispensable for central concepts and principles of design, analysis, and interpretation of scientific research. Even in the modest claims of "descriptive" findings we see various causal allusions in euphemisms such as: independent and dependent variables; mediating or moderating variables; proportion of variance accounted by; effect; influence; risk factors (ibid.). Especially, any single regression may be referred to as an analysis of "multiple causation" (Li, 1988). Nevertheless, as "a notorious philosophical tar pit" (Davis, 1985:8) and "a logical labyrinth" (Hanson, 1969:275), causation is one of the most controversial topics in philosophy and science (Pedhazur & Schmelkin, 1991). Generally, "the design type has important implications for the validity of conclusions, inferences, and generalizations from research," and various authors have asserted that it is only through variable manipulation that one may hope to study causation (ibid., p.697). Indicating problems of internal validity in experimental and quasi-experimental designs, however, Pedhazur and Schmelkin (ibid., p.698) point to the fact that

Inability or unwillingness to manipulate variables has led many to make causal inferences from nonexperimental research. This in turn has led to conferring the status of cause on variables that are not manipulable in principle (e.g., race, sex) or in practice (e.g., religious affiliation, marital status).

Indeed, one can hardly imagine the popularity of modern structural equation modeling techniques without the idea of causation applied in nonexperimental settings. Saris and Stronkhorst (1984:2) contend that "Although this non-experimental research may seem to be less convincing or conclusive, it can still be used in tests of causal hypotheses." Historically, Simon (1954) and Blalock's (1962) work laid the foundation of such causal analysis. The Simon-Blalock approach is based on statistical control, which is considered more efficient than experimental design (Saris & Stronkhorst, 1984). Path analysis, also called analysis of dependence, is a somewhat different procedure suggested by Boudon (1965) and Duncan (1966) based on the work of Wright (1934). "In this approach causal theories are specified including all important variables. Furthermore, procedures have been developed to establish the relationship between the causal effects specified in the theory and the measures for covariation between the variables" (Saris & Stronkhorst, 1984:4). Most importantly, since 1973 the program LISREL has been available which not only provides an efficient estimation procedure for the causal effects but also a test of causal theories (ibid.). As Saris and Stronkhorst (ibid., pp.4-5) write,

> This test is based on the relationship between the measures of co-variation between variables (covariance and correlation) and the causal effects. If the theory is correct, the measures for the covariation derived from the estimated effects should be the same as the measures of covariation obtained from the data, apart from sampling fluctuations. If they are not the same, the causal theory on which the computations are based has to be rejected.

All this illustrates that there are certainly possibilities to test causal hypotheses on nonexperimental data, including those obtained from cross-sectional surveys. In fact, many explanatory studies are cross-sectional (Babbie, 1992). However, explanatory cross-sectional studies have an inherent problem. "Typically, their aim is to understand causal processes that occur over time, yet their conclusions

111

are based on observations made at only one time" (Babbie, 1992:99). Nevertheless, there are ways in which the problem can be dealt with (ibid.). Especially, due to the difference between experimental and nonexperimental designs, one has to pay more attention to theory formation in nonexperimental research than in experimental research. "If important variables have been omitted in a nonexperimental study the conclusions from the analyses of the data are questionable, while this is not necessarily true in experimental studies" (ibid., p.5).

7 Scale development

As the first step of scale construction, this chapter focuses on selecting items from the original survey instruments for those key measures according to the qualitative criteria of item relevance, item sampling adequacy, mutual exclusiveness of measures, as well as logical relationship among the constructs to be scaled. These criteria are corresponding to the ideas of content and construct validity of measurement. However, they can only be attained to the extent that the employed data sets would allow for. After the items pools are decided, exploratory factor analysis is performed to uncover different dimensions as well as obtain such resultant subscales as component scores. The development of a general scale in each domain as well as the approaches to its accomplishment is the focus of this chapter under the central theme of unidimensionalization. Different scales derived by different approaches are then compared with one another via multiple means, conclusively in light of criterion-related validity, for the purpose of examining different scaling models. In this relative and relational context, the validity of the scales is expressed more adequately in terms of measurement power or scaling effectiveness.

Item selection and content and construct validity

The following requirements serve as the major criteria for developing the needed multi-item scales in this study: a) Good item coverage of the content area, or item sampling adequacy (representativeness of selected items); b) Parsimony; c) Relevance and good characteristics of individual items (e.g., suitable for the specific population, appropriate item wording, etc.); and d) Mutual exclusiveness between the measures of different constructs. Psychosociometric tests like reliability analysis as well as some other statistical trials provide additional criteria for the selection of measurement items for particular scaling purposes (e.g., summated subscale buildups).

The first requirement corresponds to the concept of content validity - "that is, the extent to which a specific set of items reflects a content domain" (DeVellis, 1991:43). As long as item sampling adequacy is achieved, the comparability of scaling results of a construct based on different sets of items can be regarded as being basically attained, provided that the scaling procedures are also standardized. The latter concern will be detailed later. The issue of item sampling adequacy, however, is very subtle as the contents of the constructs to be scaled are noted for intricacy. There are both theoretical and practical strategies dealing with such issue (DeVellis, 1991). The discussions made in the preceding chapters have indicated our theoretical understanding of social support and stress specifically as health- or more definitely depression-related constructs, which will operate as an aid to clarity. The issue, however, also depends on the exhaustiveness of consideration as well as the capacity of measurement tools in the initial research design. In a secondary data analysis, obviously, any manoeuvre for better item coverage is strictly limited to the initial choices.

The requirement for parsimony has to do with the issue of redundancy, which is not in itself a problem in scale development (DeVellis, 1991) and can be resolved anyway by the joint function of dimensional (factor) analysis and optimal (regression) weighting after data are collected. In view of the richness and complexity of the content domain as well as the practical demand for economy and efficacy, nevertheless, a stingy control over redundant items needs to be applied. The rules-of-thumb of involving no more than 50 variables and 15 factors as well as ensuring at least 3 variables for each factor are advisable (ibid.; Guilford, 1978), though these are not absolute requirements. Since sometimes we have much more items than such a suitable number, a careful selection should be carried out. Rather than a random choice, however, some special reasons for excluding certain variables need to be considered. These include not only the validity of content but also the fit of format.

The requirement for good item characteristics exhibits the importance of suitable format. In terms of statistical properties, however, it should be noted that the usual item scaling procedures are not necessary until factor analysis is performed and factor scales obtained. Moreover, at the components level, advanced statistical techniques like residual analysis in the regression procedure will provide more comprehensive and powerful means for examining scaling conditions, which are superior to the conventional item scaling procedures. Nonetheless, certain precaution should be taken regarding the format of items and the status of data. For example, dichotomously precoded variables may unnecessarily complicate factor analysis when models requiring multinormal distributions are used. Variables with too many missing values should also be excluded (in certain cases, this can be remedied by way of mean substitution or some other treatments) to ensure the soundness of statistics as well as the applicability of the scale to a specific population, from which the empirical data were gathered. In addition, care should be taken to recode any highly doubtful responses into either missing or other more likely categories.

The idea of construct validity views each concept as well as its measurement not only on its own but in relation to other concepts and measures. It dictates our emphasis and focus on certain part of the content domain in order to highlight some reasonable connection and/or to avoid some undesired confounding. This book will pay more attention to the latter since the problem of confounding is posing a deadly threat to research findings regarding social support, stress, and depression. Theoretically, we should first draw some clear-cut boundary lines between the constructs, even though the requirement for mutual exclusiveness may not be necessary in certain circumstances and for certain research purposes. Secondly, in operationalizing these constructs, such boundary lines must be observed and maintained to serve specific research purposes and ensure analytic meaningfulness. Chapter Three has addressed the theoretical concern, whereas the guideline for measurement will be followed in the empirical operations that will be performed in the following.

The domain of social support

The data to be used in this study were originally generated by social support and health experts, which is a vantage point from which we can construct a scale with confidence of both theoretical and empirical quality. Fortunate indeed, almost a hundred items/sub-items in the original questionnaire are found relevant to the measurement of social support. The questions went far beyond a single intended scale of social support (i.e., the Lubben Social Network Scale), which left much room for further scaling manipulation. In reexamining the domain, thus, a more inclusive and comprehensive view is possible by taking into consideration all the available information.

It is noticed that answers to some questions were collapsed at the time they were recorded. Although this might have been necessary to facilitate data collection, such precoding is fatal from the viewpoint of item scaling (Donald & Ware, 1984). For the purpose of factor analysis which transcends the scaling issues at individual item level, the original raw scores instead of categorized responses are also more desirable. Item characteristics like such, if "bad" enough, may constitute grounds for avoiding inclusion of certain variables in the new Social Support Scale (SSS). Another typical treatment is done towards responses to questions regarding numbers of family members in order to combine differentiated categories to form a meaningful indicator of size of the family network, which is also to reduce the number of individual items to be put in factor analysis. Responses over 30 for siblings and individual categories of offspring are deemed intolerable (based on inspection of their distributions) and thus recoded as missing values. For responses between 11 and 30, however, a possibility is taken into consideration that the respondents might have somehow exaggerated the numbers but they did have large numbers of those family members, and therefore they are recoded as 10 (a maximum value much likely as indicated by the distributions of the responses). For another category "other relatives," the same treatment is applied except that the tolerance limit is extended to 50.

In addition to such general treatments, some variables crave special concerns. Marital status has significant implications to one's life, though it does not give exact indication of social support all by itself. In this detailed study of social support where more direct measures are used, different marital status categories mainly serve as a logical control for calculating one's family network. Similarly, living arrangements are an important part of one's social networks, yet they are not necessarily indicative of support or even mere normal interaction. Therefore, numbers of persons lived with are mainly counted as one basis for (double-check of) measures of support acts and relationships, which are indeed the high points of social network studies. The last item of the Lubben Social Network Scale, nevertheless, makes sense by placing values on the joint function of marital status and living arrangements as a potential of support (i.e., 0 for living alone, 1 for living with other unrelated individuals, 4 for living with relatives other than spouse or friends, and 5 for living with spouse) (Lubben, 1988). Although whether these assignments have been optimal is still a question, the present study will adopt this item in the new scale since the multidimensional scaling strategies will take care of the weights on an empirical basis. And as mentioned earlier, social support and social stress in the "informal" sense can be unified in a scale by assigning opposite codings. Therefore, it does not defy the possibility of life stress stemming from this aspect of a "support network."

Later in discussing the measurement of life stress, I shall indicate that there is a lasting theoretical disagreement on whether positive and negative life events should be included in a single scale. In general, the operationalization of theoretical constructs of social well-being, mental health, and quality of life is full of pitfalls in that their positive and negative elements can hardly be distinguished from each other. On the other hand, when some questions are purposively reversed in applying a scale as a legitimate, desired, and usual practice of research methodology, the possibility for a very strict measure of social support that does not allow for any negative item seems very slim. In other words, the problem does not seem to be that whether a social support, life stress, or depression scale should allow for both negative and positive items, but that how these items should be assigned weights and valences, including negative and positive signs, to form a unified scale. In short, appropriate weighting is central to reconciling all such negative and positive elements, which will be tackled later with the advancement of some feasible approaches to a more general theme of unidimensionalization in psychosocial scaling.

Through an examinations on both contents and formats, 29 individual indicators are secured for further dimensional analysis, including all 10 LSNS items and 19 additional variables. Among them, 13 are aggregated measures, each summarizing information from all different levels (subitems) of the major hierarchical entries on social support, which have been mentioned in last chapter. The original items as well as the methods to derive all the composite indicators are exhibited in Appendix Ib. Content analysis shows that they fall in three major categories: a) network composition/resources, including living arrangements, sizes of family and friends/neighbors networks, and frequencies of contacts (network interaction); b) support acts, consisting of financial aid, task help, advice/information, and emotional support; and c) support appraisal, comprising satisfaction with living arrangements, feeling of close network members, and perception of the quality and reliability of relationship in terms of financial, task-oriented, and emotional help.

There are some features of this items pool. First and foremost, the part of support acts and behaviors is emphasized by inclusion of as many as 12 relevant

117

items. The content validity for the whole domain of social support is therefore greatly improved by relatively complete item coverage as compared with many measures used in previous research. Second, among the rest 17 items, more objective facts of network resources (7 items) are combined with more subjective indicators of support appraisal (10 items). The third is that it evaluates not only the support received but also that provided by the elderly, which clearly indicates that social support is a reciprocal phenomenon. Fourth, the codings of some original items are reversed when being pooled together, which demonstrates the close relationship between social support and social stress (in the "informal" network sense). More specifically, the items are coded in a manner in which possibly neutral situations are assigned the value of 0, whereas potentially stressful cases are given negative valences. These help to keep all the nominal weights positive, though this is not imperative. The fifth is that three items are taken from the depression scale (codings being reversed, too), which would reduce the confounding effect on the one hand and enhance the measurement of social support on the other. And the last, through careful selection and control, inappropriate formats are avoided and missing values are reduced to minimum. The maximum number of missing values is for item 8, i.e. financial assistance received, which accounts for 377 cases or 22.07% of the total sample. Since this is the only variable whose missing values appear to be still too many, pairwise deletion in statistical treatment is desired.

The measurement of life stress

Skodol and colleagues (1990) provide a fairly comprehensive review in terms of the assessment of psychosocial stressors. They bear in mind the nature of stress and, from a historic point of view, point to the relationship of extreme stressors to adverse health changes. However, as they narrate,

> Because most people do not experience such extreme stressors, the relatively high rates of mental disorders found in community populations, if they are in fact related to environmentally induced stress, must be in response to stressors that occur more frequently in the general population ... Such more common stressful life events might include divorce, loss of a job, or death of a loved one (Skodol et al., 1990:9)

118

They proceed with the topic of assessing stress according to DSM-III Axis IV, Severity of Psychosocial Stressors Scale, and its revision into rating scales focusing separately on acute events *and* enduring circumstances (American Psychiatric Association, 1987). However, with a conventional emphasis on life events, they fail to pursue the line leading to a thorough consideration of long-term and latent strains, such situations as "being a single mother" or "chronic unemployment," probably because "systems for rating the severity of stressful life events have evolved more rapidly than have systems for rating the severity of ongoing stressful life circumstances" (Skodol et al., 1990:5).

Indeed, too often stress has been equated with life events in measurement. Although this is taken for granted by many and the approach is in line with my "stimulus-oriented" definition, this study cannot afford to loose sight of other sources of life stress by simply subscribing to the idea of major events. A more exhaustive consideration is needed for the test of the general theoretical model. The problems is, however, the inclusion of chronic strains will most likely cause a measure not to correspond exactly with those elicited by the life events approach. As Skodol et al. (1990) indicate,

> Current theoretical models in stress research generally consider these as ongoing social situations that may contribute to the development of mental disorders quite independently from life events; indeed, most researchers assume that their effects are quite different. (p.7)

An overall scaling approach, therefore, is deemed particularly problematic for the assumption is that all psychosocial stressors differ from one another only quantitatively, while the evidence suggests that chronic, ongoing stressors exert an effect that is quite different from that of a single, stressful life event. Especially, the value of making a single global rating on Axis IV has been questioned (Kendell, 1983; Rutter & Shaffer, 1980).

This notwithstanding, it is my belief that the role of enduring circumstances should not be simply ignored. And stress as a general construct with universal etiological significance is scalable, and this scalability should not be confined to merely some subscales. It is because qualitatively different stressors all have their quantitative representation that their role may possibly be integrated in a general measure. In fact, it is due to the difference between acute events and enduring circumstances that a comprehensive scale is more adequate than a one-sided measure of stress. The conventional life events approach, in contrast, is insufficient and inappropriate especially when we are not even certain whether the symptomatology under study is induced more by acute happenings or more by chronic situations. Hence, in this study, I shall take into account both conventionally recognized life events and more enduring situations such as chronic ill health, poor socioeconomic status, as well as other major everyday strains. This would hopefully open the door to the incorporation of various bio-psychosocial factors influencing affective functioning with the general stress models, which are co-existing but not well-consolidated in current theoretical and research literature.

It is noticeable that when Skodol and colleagues (1990) expanded from extreme stressors to more common and frequent stressful life events, they warned that "the magnitude of such events is less clear-cut, their relationship to adverse health changes is much weaker, and its interpretation is more problematic than that for extreme situations" (ibid., p.5). Such a statement might even be more pertinent as research further extends to enduring circumstances. However, as long as we adhere to the general idea of stress as well as persist in achieving item sampling adequacy and weighting appropriateness in scale building, its function should be able to be faithfully represented in our results. Moreover, Chapter Three has provided a proper understanding of life stress by integrating the idea with other broad and related concepts. As long as the logical requirement for mutual exclusiveness of the key measures is well observed, a general scale is possible to make best sense out of the mental health-related theoretical construct. Here a specific condition is to set the social support-social stress construct apart from the general field of life stress/well-being (quality of life). On the other hand, the stress scale should not be confounded with a depression measure. For example, since there is a need to consider dissatisfaction as a symptom presentation of depression in order to enhance its assessment, the related items should no longer be contained in the stress scale.

In considering the rating of stress, a problem arises that is similar to the issue of objectivity vs. subjectivity in scaling social support. "One approach to measuring the magnitude of these more usual stressful events has been to get subjective ratings of the events" (Skodol et al., 1990:10). However, the use of subjective ratings may be confounding with regard to the relationship between stressful events and psychopathology. Therefore, historically two major objective measures of life event stress were used: ratings by judges in terms of the severity of lists of life events (Holmes & Rahe, 1967) and by researchers in terms of the contextual threats attributed to particular events (Brown & Harris,

120

1978). Nonetheless, the latter still has a confounding problem, whereas the former is somewhat arbitrary with regard to their magnitude ratings. Recent development in measuring life event stress included assessing variability within life event categories (independence from the health outcomes and from the predispositions to such outcomes; the positive vs. negative valence; the amount of change resulting; the degree of anticipation possible; and the degree of control over the occurrence of the event), and the concept that the co-occurrence of certain kinds of events may be critical to life event stress process (Skodol et al., 1990). Generally, according to the instructions of DSM-III-R,

> The rating of the severity of the stressor should be based on the clinician's judgment of the stress an "average" person in similar circumstances and with similar sociocultural values would experience from the particular psychosocial stressor(s). (American Psychiatric Association, 1987:19)

However, it is argued that this decision is questionable, as the patient's state would be more clinically meaningful (Frances & Cooper, 1981; Roth, 1983). Yet it is not meant that a stress rating should echo the psychiatric diagnosis. Rather, it is the particular meaning of the stressor to a specific individual that should be considered by probing into the subjective ratings of the respondent.

For all the above reasons, both objective and subjective indicators will be included in a proposed Life Stress Scale (LSS) in the present study. As discussed earlier, the manner in which the ratings of individual stressors are combined into a composite score re-presents a certain approach to weighting. While giving a few clues to deal specifically with multiple stressors, DSM-III-R did not provide a final and definite guideline. A vague language was used instead by merely saying that "in the case of multiple severe or extreme stressors, a higher rating should be considered" (American Psychiatric Association, 1987:19). In research practice, although the term "a pathogenic triad" indicates a special combination of three specific kinds of events that may approximate the stress conditions of extreme situations (Skodol et al., 1990), it is evident that a straightforward additivity presumption is favored by investigators, especially by those endorsing the life events approach (e.g., Holmes & Rahe, 1967). However, as is the case of scaling social support (cf. Chapter Two and Chapter Four), this practice of simple summation is typically unjustified, with various more or less arbitrary weighting schemes being used. Empirical studies evaluating the practical use

121

and usefulness of DSM-III Axis IV suggested that Axis IV ratings had limited reliability and uncertain validity (Skodol et al., 1990). When a multi-item scale is used in research rather than clinical diagnosis, it can be even more problematic in terms of these psychosociometric properties. For any multidimensional scale, as is the case of a social support measure, the concept of reliability in terms of internal consistency is not applicable, though stressful events and conditions cannot be required to be independent of one another and the alpha coefficient is not necessarily equal to zero as suggested (Cleary, 1980). More on this later. For the new Life Stress Scale (LSS) to be developed in this study, the items are coded in a manner in which possibly neutral situations are assigned the value of 0, whereas potentially positive or supportive other than stressful cases are given negative valences. More detailed considerations can be made by considering the amount of change in the person's life caused by the stressor, the degree to which the event is desired and under the person's control, and the number of stressors (American Psychiatric Association, 1987). However, these speculations at various levels are arbitrary in nature, and they are not necessary when advanced statistical procedures are to be utilized. In applying those multivariate analytic techniques, the key is not the weighting of individual items, but the integration of the results of dimensional analysis on an empirical basis. I shall deal with this core issue in multidimensional scaling later.

DSM-III-R provided a rather complete listing of the types or areas of "etiologically significant psychosocial stressors" to be considered in research. These include conjugal (marital and nonmarital; e.g., engagement, marriage, discord, separation, death of spouse), parenting (e.g., becoming a parent, friction with child, illness of child), other interpersonal (problems with one's friends, neighbors, associates, or nonconjugal family members; e.g., illness of best friend, discordant relationship with boss), occupational (including work, school, and homemaking; e.g., unemployment, retirement, school problems), living circumstances (e.g., change in residence, threat to personal safety, immigration), financial (e.g., inadequate finances, change in financial status), legal (e.g., arrest, imprisonment, lawsuit, or trial), developmental (phases of the life cycle; e.g., puberty, transition to adult status, menopause, "becoming 50"), physical illness or injury (e.g., illness, accident, surgery, abortion), and other psychosocial stressors (e.g., natural or manmade disaster, persecution, unwanted pregnancy, out-of-wedlock birth, rape). Such an exhaustive view-point is now endorsed by many authors. For example, acknowledging that the role of stress reactions is of primary importance to modern psychiatric thinking, Noshpitz and Coddington

(1990) presented a book reviewing all types of stressors in terms of stress arising from object loss (death of relatives or parental divorce), illness (acute, chronic, and surgical; accidents and toxic ingestions; pain), developmental sources, natural disasters, human violence, and social trauma (prejudice and exclusion; malfeasance; forced displacement; geographic change; loss of an ideal; economic trauma).

The DSM-III-R listing is impressive indeed. With such a broad conception of stress embodied in all kinds of stressors, it seems no longer necessary to separate the functions of health, socioeconomic status, and so forth to explain mental disorders, given the general stress-(diathesis)-disease model. It should be pointed out that the inclusion of Axis IV in the multiaxial diagnostic system in DSM-III-R has etiological implications. As Skodol and colleagues (1990:19) wrote,

> The rationale for including in DSM-III an axis for assessing psychosocial stressors was to try to add predictive validity to the Axis I diagnosis. It was assumed that an individual's prognosis might be better if a disorder developed from severe stress rather than after no-or only minimal-stress.

However, these etiological inferences are more suited for research as hypotheses to be tested than for clinical diagnosis as criteria, which has been criticized as craving further study based on the Axis IV assessment.

With the understanding clarified in the above, the items on the original questionnaire are sorted for the purpose of developing an appropriate stress scale. In addition to the criteria similar to those employed in scaling social support, the logical requirement for mutual exclusiveness is added since the content of social support (with its reversed portion indicative of "informal social" stress) has been determined. This clearly demonstrates that the expansion from theoretical constructs to empirical measures counts on specific objectives and analytic plans so that the confounding problems could be avoided or reduced. Altogether, 44 individual indicators are obtained from the available data for the construction of the LSS. They fall in seven major categories, namely, physical health conditions and events (including major events, chronic conditions, stressful symptoms, functional status, and subjective ratings), physical build (over- and underweight), cognitive functioning (memory), socioeconomic status (education, unemployment/retirement, income, ethnic/regional issue), living circumstances (changes and events, home conditions), work stress, and development (aging) stress. The individual items and their time frames are displayed in Appendix II. It is noticeable that some significant sources of stress such as marital discord and friction with children are emphasized neither in the special social support-social stress scale nor in the broad quality of life (life stress/well-being) measure since detailed information on these aspects is not available. This will certainly blunt the discriminating power of both scales in detecting the relationship between social support and stress as well as their association with depression and other constructs. On the whole, however, necessary content and construct validity is ensured by the thorough theoretical understanding while the empirical data are largely capable of affording the relatively complete scaling scheme.

Symptoms of depression

DSM-III-R provides depressed mood as the essential feature of depression (American Psychiatric Association, 1987). In the case of major depression, loss of interest or pleasure is also given special attention. Strictly speaking, only these core features would be counted as always essential. Nevertheless, there are a number of associated symptoms that are deemed important, including appetite disturbance, change in weight, sleep disturbance (insomnia or hypersomnia), psychomotor agitation or retardation, decreased energy (fatigue), feelings of worthlessness or excessive or inappropriate guilt (low self-esteem in the case of dysthymia), difficulty thinking or concentrating, and recurrent thoughts of death or suicidal ideation or attempts (feelings of hopelessness in the case of dysthymia). Advocating a symptom approach to depression, Costello (1993) organizes a more detailed book around the following specific symptoms: dysphoria, loss of interest, anhedonia, social dysfunction, problems of memory and concentration, low self-esteem, shame and guilt, hopelessness, psychomotor agitation and retardation, eating problems, sleeping problems, and suicide attempts. Kantor (1992) further points out that in some patients the depressed mood is either well hidden or expressed only in derivative form as attitudinal, behavioral/acting-out, existential, and/or physical mood equivalents. Especially, a detailed description of mood equivalent behaviors is given encompassing disability (loss of interest, inability to enjoy oneself, inability to function), upset (dissatisfaction, crying, agitation), self-destructiveness (vicious cycling, suicidal behavior), other-destructiveness, regressivity (regression, dependence, isolation), addition (alcohol and drug addiction, smoking), eating disorders (paranoid, hypomanic, obsessive, hysteric), obsessive-compulsive states, narcissism, and psychopathic-impulsive states (manipulation, stealing, gambling, promiscuity, infidelity) (ibid.). On the other hand, physical manifestations of depression are also recognized by identifying the underlying mechanism. Kantor (ibid.) lists the following physical symptoms for the diagnosis of depression: fatigue and hypersomnia, insomnia (lying awake, middle awakening), pain, diarrhea and constipation.

It is seen from the above that the symptoms of depression can be so inclusive as to contain nearly the whole "human dimension" (ibid.). Such extensive consideration is certainly needed in clinical practice. And all these render a valuable framework for the scaling enterprise. However, pathological attitudes, behaviors, existential positions, and physical symptoms are not always depressive in origin (ibid.). Especially, in a research dealing with the relationships of depression with other psychosocial variables, the boundaries between the theoretical constructs must be made definite and their measures must not confound with one another. Since social functioning/dysfunction has been conceptualized in this study in terms of social support/stress, the measurement of depression as a mental status should not involve such "social" items. On the other hand, physical symptoms like pain may be included in the measurement of general life stress rather than depression for the purpose of examining its impact on affective functioning. In addition, some indicators of depression, such as weight loss, are not available in the existing data sets even if a broader scope of its conception is desired.

It is worth mentioning that the symptom approach is a general one, which is especially useful for the development of a survey instrument. Under the guidance of the above frameworks, 25 items are garnered from the available data sets, which can be classified into mood disturbance, loss of interest, psychomotor disturbance, decreased energy (fatigue), sleep disturbance, decreased appetite/constipation, concentration problem, dissatisfaction, and hopelessness. Specifically, the Depression Scale (DS) to be pursued includes 14 out of the 17 original CES-D items (excluding 3 "social" items), and 6 originally life satisfaction indicators (LSI) (some are aggregated in constructing the new scale items). The time frame is specified "during the past week" for the CES-D items while remains very general for the LSI indicators. There are 5 additional symptom items selected from the physical health section, for which the time frame is "in the past year." The methods used to derive the new scale items as well as all the original indicators are exhibited in Appendix IIIb.

It is noticeable that like a usual life events scale, a depression scale is often treated as unidimensional, built up by simple summation without any differential weighting. This study attempts to prove that as a multidimensional construct it demands more reasonable and feasible approaches to unidimensionalization in measurement. Generally speaking, such approaches would not require much refined scaling of the individual items. Nevertheless, the selected items are treated with care in the interest of better intuitive sense as well as consistent signs of individual weights. The codings of some original items are reversed when they are pooled together, which demonstrates the close relationship between positive and negative mental health. Specifically, those items are coded in a manner in which possibly neutral situations are assigned the value of 0, whereas potentially positive cases are given opposite signs in order to contrast them with the straightforward indications of depression.

Personal coping: Health behaviors
and social attitudes

Owing to the limitation of available data as mentioned in last chapter, personal coping can only be operationalized in terms of some health- and illness-related behaviors as well as respondents' attitudes toward a number of social arrangements. Theoretically, the focus on these aspects may be of special significance since health is usually the premier concern in old age while attitudes have been typically overlooked in previous research. Therefore, this study will focus on these variables as some proxy measures of personal coping and explore their role in effecting depression. After careful selection, 11 individual items are obtained for a Health Behaviors and Beliefs (HBB) measure (see Appendix IVa), 9 items for an Attitudes Toward Social Support (ATSS) measure (see Appendix IVb), and 4 items for an Attitudes Toward Elderly (ATE) measure (see Appendix IVc). For all these measures, higher scores are expected to reflect more desirable (or positive) categories of personal coping in relation to social support, stress, and depression.

8 Factor analysis: Dimensionality and subscales

This chapter carries out dimensional analysis of the items pool for scaling each theoretical construct domain. Traditional factor analysis procedures are used to provide guidance for constructing subscales with the calculation of factor scores or via some conventional unidimensional treatments. The major purpose, however, is to provide needed material for demonstrating how to perform ultimate unidimensionalization, a central theme of this volume. The various approaches to its accomplishment will be explored immediately after this chapter.

Descriptive statistics and factor analysis procedures

Table 8.1 shows some statistics of the various items pools. In performing dimensional analysis using factor analysis procedure, principal components analysis rather than more accurate common-factor model is specified for extraction. There are three reasons for this. One, the theme of the book is unidimensionalization; that is, the purpose is to explore some viable approaches to the general measurement of social support, stress, depression, and other psychosocial constructs instead of elaborating on the latent factor structures of the specific data sets. Two, without requiring imposing "what some may consider a questionable causal model" (Kim & Mueller, 1978:20), principal components analysis is the only means by which exact factor scores can be obtained (Norusis, 1988). And three, some factor models entail multinormal distribution of the variables, which has been usually violated in practice, whereas principal com-

Table 8.1 Descriptive statistics of the items for major scales development

VARIABLE	MEAN	STD DEV	MINIMUM	MAXIMUM	VALID N
SSS1	4.38	1.25	.00	5.00	1686
SSS2	8.79	6.32	.00	35.00	1672
SSS3	3.71	3.62	.00	12.00	1701
SSS4	4.63	1.08	.00	5.00	1702
SSS5	3.00	2.01	.00	5.00	1644
SSS6	3.11	1.57	.00	5.00	1704
SSS7	2.33	1.60	.00	5.00	1706
SSS8	2.66	1.44	.00	4.00	1331
SSS9	2.29	2.15	.00	5.00	1445
SSS10	1.36	1.23	.00	4.00	1658
SSS11	2.06	.90	1.00	3.00	1620
SSS12	1.03	1.95	.00	9.00	1708
SSS13	2.95	1.78	.00	5.00	1707
SSS14	.94	1.18	.00	4.00	1361
SSS15	1.96	.22	.00	2.00	1563
SSS16	1.96	.96	-1.00	3.00	1692
SSS17	1.88	.91	-1.00	3.00	1689
SSS18	-1.77	1.09	-3.00	1.00	1687
SSS19	2.70	1.16	.00	4.00	1676
SSS20	.72	1.10	-2.00	2.00	1704
SSS21	5.13	3.50	.00	36.00	1699
SSS22	4.03	3.69	.00	14.00	1698
SSS23	1.66	.64	-2.00	2.00	1588
SSS24	2.60	1.27	.00	4.00	1626
SSS25	3.29	.90	.00	4.00	1698
SSS26	2.20	.72	-1.00	3.00	1684
SSS27	-.29	.72	-3.00	.00	1577
SSS28	-.09	.41	-3.00	.00	1569
SSS29	-.08	.38	-3.00	.00	1569
LSS1	.19	.40	.00	1.00	1704
LSS2	1.69	4.67	.00	50.00	1569
LSS3	1.93	1.32	.00	12.00	1286
LSS4	.61	1.27	.00	5.00	1651
LSS5	.64	1.39	.00	5.00	1645
LSS6	.40	1.05	.00	5.00	1653
LSS7	.59	1.25	.00	5.00	1653
LSS8	.46	1.07	.00	5.00	1652
LSS9	2.66	4.87	.00	27.00	1701
LSS10	.41	.49	.00	1.00	1659
LSS11	.45	.63	.00	2.00	1652
LSS12	20.25	62.55	.00	365.00	1647
LSS13	2.25	.64	1.00	4.00	1231
LSS14	.84	.95	-1.00	3.00	1659
LSS15	.48	.95	-1.00	3.00	1659
LSS16	.35	.48	.00	1.00	1232
LSS17	.44	.57	.00	2.00	1638
LSS18	.85	1.00	-1.00	3.00	1704
LSS19	-.19	.98	-2.00	2.00	1696
LSS20	2.04	1.01	.00	3.00	1702
LSS21	1.08	.92	.00	2.00	1656
LSS22	.03	.16	.00	1.00	1706
LSS23	2.58	.90	.00	4.00	1701
LSS24	.33	.47	.00	1.00	1391
LSS25	-.03	.55	-1.00	2.00	1704
LSS26	.67	.93	.00	3.00	1703
LSS27	.36	.82	.00	5.00	1708
LSS28	.17	.46	.00	3.00	1708
LSS29	.06	.24	.00	1.00	1704
LSS30	.06	.25	.00	1.00	1614
LSS31	.01	.12	.00	1.00	1593
LSS32	.37	.70	.00	4.00	1677
LSS33	.00	.05	.00	1.00	1675

Table 8.1 Descriptive statistics of the items for major scales development (continued)

VARIABLE	MEAN	STD DEV	MINIMUM	MAXIMUM	VALID N
LSS34	.00	.05	.00	1.00	1670
LSS35	.06	.31	.00	4.00	1688
LSS36	1.56	.80	.00	2.00	1551
LSS37	.77	.88	.00	2.00	1706
LSS38	.09	.29	.00	1.00	1702
LSS39	.53	.92	.00	4.00	1706
LSS40	.37	.48	.00	6.33	1184
LSS41	.27	.75	.00	3.00	1701
LSS42	.07	.75	-2.00	3.00	1697
LSS43	.44	.70	-1.00	1.00	1678
LSS44	.88	1.03	.00	3.00	1706
DS1	.31	.71	.00	3.00	1596
DS2	.23	.64	.00	3.00	1581
DS3	.14	.51	.00	3.00	1567
DS4	.17	.58	.00	3.00	1577
DS5	1.76	1.29	.00	3.00	1612
DS6	.21	.41	.00	1.00	1697
DS7	1.79	1.31	.00	3.00	1631
DS8	.28	.72	.00	3.00	1641
DS9	.33	1.01	.00	5.00	1655
DS10	.15	.54	.00	3.00	1571
DS11	.24	.65	.00	3.00	1576
DS12	.22	.60	.00	3.00	1611
DS13	.58	1.41	.00	5.00	1626
DS14	1.19	1.72	.00	5.00	1660
DS15	.50	1.28	.00	5.00	1649
DS16	.45	.89	.00	3.00	1621
DS17	1.33	1.88	.00	5.00	1635
DS18	.32	.74	.00	3.00	1632
DS19	.81	1.43	.00	5.00	1674
DS20	.59	1.34	.00	5.00	1618
DS21	.19	.58	.00	3.00	1584
DS22	1.11	1.69	.00	5.00	1626
DS23	.12	.52	.00	3.00	1571
DS24	1.06	.74	.00	3.00	1704
DS25	.24	.44	.00	2.00	1706
HBB1	1.84	1.10	.00	3.00	1653
HBB2	.78	.98	.00	3.00	1655
HBB3	-.95	1.10	-3.00	.00	1651
HBB4	.54	.50	.00	1.00	1584
HBB5	1.55	.69	1.00	3.00	1657
HBB6	1.72	.60	1.00	3.00	1657
HBB7	1.42	.52	1.00	3.00	1653
HBB8	2.31	2.36	.00	5.00	1703
HBB9	4.24	8.10	.00	60.00	1701
HBB10	3.25	.59	1.00	4.00	1649
HBB11	3.03	.75	1.00	4.00	1618
ATSS1	1.17	.81	.00	2.00	1706
ATSS2	1.16	.80	.00	2.00	1706
ATSS3	1.55	1.43	.00	3.00	1705
ATSS4	1.96	1.83	.00	4.00	1669
ATSS5	2.26	1.71	.00	4.00	1708
ATSS6	1.86	1.55	.00	4.00	1708
ATSS7	2.02	1.54	.00	4.00	1705
ATSS8	2.01	1.51	.00	4.00	1706
ATSS9	1.89	1.86	.00	4.00	1704
ATE1	1.00	.98	-2.00	2.00	1702
ATE2	1.16	.99	-2.00	2.00	1692
ATE3	.98	1.23	-2.00	2.00	1700
ATE4	.97	1.13	-2.00	2.00	1698

ponents analysis does not hold such stringent requirements (Morrison, 1990). As Kim and Mueller (1978:72) write, "if the objective is some simple summary of information contained in the raw data without recourse to factor analytic assumptions, the use of component scores has a definite advantage over factor scaling." Especially, when the real data do not possess a plain common factor structure or coincides with some priori conceptual scheme, this approach is most practical to summarize the empirical information by a unidimensionalized scaling. This is in fact the case of the present study. Although some conceptual schemes are given in the above, they do not imply any necessary or "ideal" common factor patterns. In real terms, the correlation matrix for each items pool suggests that it is unlikely that the selected items will fall in the few theoretical categories for any of the scales. Table 8.2 exemplifies this by displaying the zero-order correlation coefficients among the Social Support Scale items.

The Social Support Scale (SSS)

The final statistics for each factor and each item variable contained in Table 8.3a confirm the above observation; the 9 factors extracted by principal axis factoring (a common factor model) explain only 40.2% of the total variance, with the first four whose eigenvalues are greater than 1 representing only 29.4% (note the commonalities for many of the variables are pretty low). This in general indicates that the unidimensionalization of measurement in this field is not an easy task that can be accomplished in any way with good chance, especially by some simply but arbitrarily summated scaling. In particular, contrasted with Table 8.3b, it shows principal components analysis has a higher goodness of fit, or better representation of data in terms of measurement (57.1% vs. 40.2% of the total variance explained). The factor matrix extracted by principle components (PC) analysis is given by Table 8.4a.

To achieve a simpler structure of the relationship between the components and the individual items, rotation of the initial factor matrix is necessary. Different methods for rotation are used for different approaches to unidimensionalization, which will be handled in the next large section. For the purpose of the practical approach discussed earlier, orthogonal components are desired so that the interaction effects in a multiple regression model would be eliminated. The algorithm used for orthogonal rotation is the varimax method, which attempts to minimize the number of variables that have high loadings on a factor   and

Table 8.2 Correlation matrix of the Social Support Scale (SSS) items

	SSS1	SSS2	SSS3	SSS4	SSS5	SSS6	SSS7
SSS1	1.00000						
SSS2	.06516	1.00000					
SSS3	.02391	.16082	1.00000				
SSS4	.28709	.12236	.00655	1.00000			
SSS5	-.04444	.10311	.28379	.05262	1.00000		
SSS6	.17694	.20146	.19772	.09086	.08712	1.00000	
SSS7	.11264	.17114	.28670	.06001	.11579	.62810	1.00000
SSS8	-.00219	.11447	.02832	.20450	.03162	.20919	.19496
SSS9	-.09179	-.03377	-.03605	.09399	-.05853	-.05611	-.08058
SSS10	.15645	.02169	.22103	.08594	-.04278	.23604	.28204
SSS11	.02320	.12398	.09303	.10431	.13229	.18980	.14991
SSS12	-.06196	.05612	-.04283	.00233	-.00089	-.00312	.00426
SSS13	.10557	.15288	.13584	.13376	.12571	.32379	.29997
SSS14	.12362	.03462	.08869	.02151	-.05770	.12901	.17017
SSS15	.05820	.03029	.03610	.04350	.03728	.03269	.04071
SSS16	.14643	.00180	.07681	.03023	.06457	.26727	.26768
SSS17	.21157	.09509	.18358	.05382	.07119	.35124	.31567
SSS18	.14255	-.00351	.08010	.00994	-.11178	.07315	.12092
SSS19	.15110	.13462	.22287	.03193	.09355	.39806	.42354
SSS20	.00844	.04655	.05602	-.03691	.02529	.11438	.13025
SSS21	.12598	.39506	.35653	.09783	.06110	.26908	.24915
SSS22	.02146	.15702	.84981	-.01303	.24833	.26329	.35024
SSS23	.21516	.10557	.12426	.04815	.09422	.22379	.17455
SSS24	.07804	.17111	.05024	.19449	.04106	.32488	.27316
SSS25	.24704	.13853	.10081	.13766	.04836	.33868	.26045
SSS26	.04623	.04424	.09097	.01739	.12089	.15286	.13626
SSS27	.21305	.07961	.08862	.08747	.07912	.11719	.10226
SSS28	.08291	.01411	.06501	-.00518	.05739	.07072	.04343
SSS29	.07692	.04062	.03316	.01608	.05836	.06085	.02098

	SSS8	SSS9	SSS10	SSS11	SSS12	SSS13	SSS14
SSS8	1.00000						
SSS9	.36548	1.00000					
SSS10	.10675	-.02850	1.00000				
SSS11	.18605	-.00117	-.04107	1.00000			
SSS12	.03249	.03672	-.13148	.13378	1.00000		
SSS13	.19788	-.08055	.22665	.10481	-.13254	1.00000	
SSS14	.05585	.02652	.22978	.03724	-.02039	.03296	1.00000
SSS15	.08119	.00441	.03343	.09656	-.04822	.01730	-.05746
SSS16	.06424	-.06104	.15763	.08959	-.14564	.07348	.17508
SSS17	.14039	-.01255	.24759	.10771	-.05777	.17054	.21979
SSS18	-.03203	.03627	.20261	-.05085	.00994	.04979	.16777
SSS19	.18064	-.05552	.32595	.07339	-.09022	.29429	.17037
SSS20	.01465	.03229	.02292	.09322	.05260	.04131	.13009
SSS21	.11257	-.01459	.14031	.10685	-.04535	.10455	.10321
SSS22	.01052	-.08452	.24471	.08682	-.03841	.17234	.10057
SSS23	.13035	-.03110	.11926	.13057	-.01244	.07907	.07813
SSS24	.60736	-.14374	.15538	.21779	.00205	.21512	.11370
SSS25	.26307	-.00570	.17608	.21847	-.00481	.17321	.18260
SSS26	.08856	-.04822	.04645	.12779	-.07351	.08977	.10575
SSS27	-.00526	-.02142	.05895	.06006	-.16275	.07412	.04997
SSS28	.02596	-.03036	-.00731	.04112	-.10067	.04806	-.01715
SSS29	-.02756	-.02938	.00109	.08725	-.01466	.01075	-.01548

	SSS15	SSS16	SSS17	SSS18	SSS19	SSS20	SSS21
SSS15	1.00000						
SSS16	.11821	1.00000					
SSS17	.05323	.24321	1.00000				
SSS18	.00813	-.01943	.08077	1.00000			
SSS19	.06379	.29046	.38117	.11195	1.00000		
SSS20	.02561	.12742	.13461	.00976	.09860	1.00000	
SSS21	.03980	.11596	.16811	.07748	.20349	.06764	1.00000
SSS22	.03814	.11192	.20778	.09415	.26343	.07790	.39670

131

Table 8.2 Correlation matrix of the Social Support Scale (SSS) items (continued)

	SSS15	SSS16	SSS17	SSS18	SSS19	SSS20	SSS21
SSS23	.10764	.21771	.30621	-.00914	.21693	.14583	.15698
SSS24	.08396	.13831	.30916	-.04401	.24834	.05946	.15344
SSS25	.07884	.21389	.49603	.05884	.27790	.09981	.17505
SSS26	.08374	.59734	.22544	-.06431	.19581	.18068	.11478
SSS27	.10932	.13911	.12295	-.00259	.11720	.02879	.10767
SSS28	.11196	.15038	.08826	-.06315	.03154	.04623	.05581
SSS29	.01919	.02890	.03167	-.02661	.00212	.03548	.04801

	SSS22	SSS23	SSS24	SSS25	SSS26	SSS27	SSS28	SSS29
SSS22	1.00000							
SSS23	.13866	1.00000						
SSS24	.06153	.25159	1.00000					
SSS25	.11704	.30426	.46051	1.00000				
SSS26	.12012	.23289	.18388	.23092	1.00000			
SSS27	.07891	.12207	.08732	.17239	.10772	1.00000		
SSS28	.07880	.12527	.05712	.08184	.13209	.33682	1.00000	
SSS29	.04784	.04003	.03252	.07765	.05058	.19268	.33512	1.0000

Table 8.3a SSS: Final statistics for factors extracted by principal axis factoring (PA)

VARIABLE	COMMUNALITY	*	FACTOR	EIGENVALUE	PCT OF VAR	CUM PCT
SSS1	.38402	*	1	4.34806	15.0	15.0
SSS2	.31655	*	2	1.76386	6.1	21.1
SSS3	.86655	*	3	1.36017	4.7	25.8
SSS4	.24058	*	4	1.06554	3.7	29.4
SSS5	.22157	*	5	.89680	3.1	32.5
SSS6	.59481	*	6	.67689	2.3	34.9
SSS7	.60842	*	7	.61562	2.1	37.0
SSS8	.89358	*	8	.51011	1.8	38.7
SSS9	.22466	*	9	.42666	1.5	40.2
SSS10	.36115	*				
SSS11	.18267	*				
SSS12	.15283	*				
SSS13	.29186	*				
SSS14	.20343	*				
SSS15	.04636	*				
SSS16	.69254	*				
SSS17	.46330	*				
SSS18	.18009	*				
SSS19	.38736	*				
SSS20	.09825	*				
SSS21	.46797	*				
SSS22	.83400	*				
SSS23	.23310	*				
SSS24	.55273	*				
SSS25	.54885	*				
SSS26	.56761	*				
SSS27	.27637	*				
SSS28	.57841	*				
SSS29	.19408	*				

Table 8.3b SSS: Final statistics for factors extracted by principal components analysis (PC)

VARIABLE	COMMUNALITY	*	FACTOR	EIGENVALUE	PCT OF VAR	CUM PCT
SSS1	.65152	*	1	4.82737	16.6	16.6
SSS2	.67070	*	2	2.06305	7.1	23.8
SSS3	.85747	*	3	1.82751	6.3	30.1
SSS4	.52408	*	4	1.68078	5.8	35.9
SSS5	.48035	*	5	1.47899	5.1	41.0
SSS6	.63150	*	6	1.25989	4.3	45.3
SSS7	.62070	*	7	1.23292	4.3	49.6
SSS8	.76211	*	8	1.13966	3.9	53.5
SSS9	.65099	*	9	1.03600	3.6	57.1
SSS10	.50389	*				
SSS11	.40906	*				
SSS12	.57259	*				
SSS13	.52449	*				
SSS14	.43004	*				
SSS15	.23584	*				
SSS16	.70453	*				
SSS17	.50403	*				
SSS18	.43431	*				
SSS19	.49734	*				
SSS20	.34797	*				
SSS21	.66454	*				
SSS22	.85324	*				
SSS23	.39852	*				
SSS24	.66499	*				
SSS25	.54962	*				
SSS26	.70446	*				
SSS27	.49185	*				
SSS28	.63447	*				
SSS29	.57096	*				

thus, "should enhance the interpretability of the factors" (Norusis, 1988:208). For the theoretical approach, on the other hand, all the concern is how the data could be better represented by the factors (components)[1] as it is more flexible in dealing with the component scores. Therefore, oblique rotation is used that gives a better model-data fit. "An oblique rotation is more general than an orthogonal rotation in that it does not arbitrarily impose the restriction that factors be uncorrelated" (Kim & Mueller, 1978:37). The specific method used is the direct oblimin rotation. Tables 8.4b through 8.4d contain the rotated matrices that display the sorted factor loadings; the factor correlation matrix for factors resulted from oblique rotation is also given in Table 8.4e.

133

Table 8.4a SSS: Factor matrix extracted by principle components analysis (PC)

	FACTOR 1	FACTOR 2	FACTOR 3	FACTOR 4	FACTOR 5	FACTOR 6	FACTOR 7	FACTOR 8	FACTOR 9
SSS6	.67172	.00893	-.12235	-.06399	-.02250	.08139	-.28440	.24694	-.11024
SSS7	.65794	-.12858	-.17111	-.10272	-.08015	.01092	-.22793	.25871	-.07752
SSS19	.61605	-.05572	-.05476	-.23663	-.08187	-.12639	-.15859	.08846	-.00885
SSS17	.60907	.11341	.05624	-.20572	-.07543	.09758	.05949	.06355	.22788
SSS25	.59988	.32948	.03122	-.04348	.02513	.17936	.03621	.02186	.20917
SSS24	.54118	.51342	-.23011	.17974	-.01111	-.13830	.01733	.05856	.01640
SSS21	.47194	-.27641	-.14486	.18967	.15371	.17026	.17612	-.23264	-.41316
SSS16	.46616	.09031	.43788	-.17917	-.38517	-.11542	.00044	-.22938	-.18878
SSS23	.45746	.14445	.19516	.03131	-.09361	.18916	.08070	-.14728	.23784
SSS22	.52012	-.66916	-.14006	.19206	-.03421	-.10819	.20684	-.04599	.14375
SSS3	.47476	-.65496	-.15439	.23732	-.01018	-.13127	.24910	-.09140	.18765
SSS8	.37523	.53169	-.38741	.25344	-.00179	-.32202	.13282	.03833	-.03663
SSS28	.19661	.01370	.55773	.25051	.26607	-.13776	.15166	.32395	-.06402
SSS27	.28481	.01574	.46374	.10627	.40507	-.07520	.08738	.06738	-.04715
SSS18	.12582	-.14162	-.19678	-.44645	.23044	.12421	.28072	.07809	.08336
SSS5	.22011	-.24848	.06137	.44338	-.13676	-.10533	-.19135	-.10813	.30283
SSS10	.43290	-.13115	-.14603	-.43497	.15244	-.23186	-.06246	.04164	.07828
SSS14	.30089	.01867	-.05004	-.39928	-.07062	.14645	.36767	.05560	-.11190
SSS11	.29719	.18033	-.04090	.38717	-.12048	.28588	-.07100	.07410	.17283
SSS26	.41028	.12028	.43106	.01644	-.47873	-.06468	.05229	-.26290	-.17424
SSS1	.32016	.12182	.19486	-.27325	.47094	.29754	-.03709	-.29344	.15410
SSS20	.21753	.02496	.11328	-.00572	-.33376	.25889	.24296	.17141	-.14260
SSS12	-.10204	.08727	-.28360	.21022	-.18226	.56240	.08269	.18982	.19381
SSS9	-.03438	.35955	-.30205	.15261	.01613	-.32011	.54522	.02018	-.07486
SSS13	.43110	-.01080	-.15026	-.02868	.14047	-.23773	-.46952	.11787	-.06736
SSS29	.11914	-.00949	.39412	.25732	.31186	.07618	.12269	.46217	-.05844
SSS4	.20936	.27836	-.13089	.09856	.42403	.05521	-.07350	-.43099	.04378
SSS2	.32684	-.08286	-.19568	.31420	.17930	.30952	-.09087	-.18192	-.50069
SSS15	.15261	.09882	.19445	.14398	.05177	-.13368	.05636	-.22504	.26134

Table 8.4b SSS: Rotated factor matrix (varimax)

	FACTOR 1	FACTOR 2	FACTOR 3	FACTOR 4	FACTOR 5	FACTOR 6	FACTOR 7	FACTOR 8	FACTOR 9
SSS6	.73327	.05560	.12008	.03132	.08340	.02082	.07255	.16763	.18592
SSS7	.72179	.18535	.10729	.01262	.03030	-.06805	.12362	.11520	.13997
SSS13	.66470	.03032	-.08112	.05014	-.01605	.07921	-.16977	-.17534	.08098
SSS19	.61759	.16037	.23174	.04052	-.01074	.06102	.16672	-.05659	.00415
SSS10	.42718	.20631	.00855	.06998	-.03243	.13127	.42198	-.26134	-.09607
SSS17	.42155	.14141	.29423	.07756	.07106	.25534	.27865	.22248	-.12787
SSS3	.14103	.89783	.01728	.00230	.03696	-.00658	.08602	-.00160	.14959
SSS22	.21603	.87080	.04743	-.03947	.04702	-.04291	.11057	.00380	.16789
SSS5	.11357	.47674	.07139	-.04396	.02281	.09064	.45112	.13091	-.06128
SSS26	.08002	.04905	.82434	.03845	.03486	.02990	-.09594	-.00608	.05733
SSS16	.20553	.00699	.79697	-.02771	.04929	.06732	.02851	-.13482	.01882
SSS23	.14153	.14415	.36478	.03748	.08460	.35843	.06180	.28542	-.04820
SSS20	.02084	.01083	.35666	.01390	.09382	-.22242	.21136	.32882	.09460
SSS8	.26541	-.02837	.02025	.81503	-.03557	.09777	-.08008	.07151	.06190
SSS9	-.24550	-.01399	-.04929	.74248	.00259	-.08477	.16468	-.04980	-.00583
SSS24	.40923	-.05213	.14057	.62020	.03970	.21095	-.04886	.19610	.05896
SSS28	.01470	.05255	.12673	.03631	.77773	.00648	-.07201	-.05447	-.03260
SSS29	.03037	-.00821	-.07710	-.02883	.73469	-.06099	-.00579	.13651	.03229
SSS27	.06447	-.05216	.10475	-.01673	.61119	.27223	.01601	-.14300	.07315
SSS1	.11926	-.08447	-.03209	-.19768	.13230	.69812	.27419	.00021	.10002
SSS4	.03548	-.05717	-.10435	.20436	-.06061	.62487	-.06719	-.05800	.25474
SSS25	.37570	.00953	.24288	.20902	.11847	.38936	.16564	.33363	-.03621
SSS15	-.06412	.17038	.16281	.11232	.09654	.33023	-.14741	-.02391	-.15134
SSS18	.07689	.09183	-.17780	-.04976	-.04236	.09567	.61089	-.03316	-.02544
SSS14	.10206	.01340	.22953	.07133	-.01558	-.01508	.59450	.06135	.06336
SSS12	-.11361	-.03169	-.18684	-.01470	-.15225	-.08987	.03752	.69933	.04268
SSS11	.15278	.08409	.08251	.13010	.07541	.13326	-.21828	.52688	.07880
SSS2	.15427	.04375	-.00167	.02937	.02246	.08316	-.07928	.11820	.78514
SSS21	.11849	.33194	.12198	.05903	.06039	.08701	.15157	-.00586	.69838

135

Table 8.4c SSS: Pattern matrix (oblimin rotation)

	FACTOR 1	FACTOR 2	FACTOR 3	FACTOR 4	FACTOR 5	FACTOR 6	FACTOR 7	FACTOR 8	FACTOR 9
SSS6	.71027	.00108	.07317	-.04697	-.06094	.15492	.00241	.03705	-.13302
SSS13	.70871	.00976	.01171	.19049	.09989	-.17448	.03341	-.04178	-.03791
SSS7	.69408	-.13849	.01960	-.09719	-.04611	.10207	-.00807	.13096	-.08966
SSS19	.56980	-.11841	-.03307	-.14566	.19151	-.06346	.02221	.00279	.04095
SSS17	.31463	-.10572	.04626	-.27221	-.21389	.22948	.05058	-.18202	.17664
SSS3	.00072	-.91954	.01042	-.06896	.06172	-.01806	.00558	.06530	-.11923
SSS22	.08185	-.84498	.02031	-.09047	.03125	-.01478	-.03819	.10378	-.13534
SSS5	.07362	-.47989	-.00453	.46125	-.03062	.13522	-.06116	-.03831	.08588
SSS28	-.02258	-.01990	.78772	.06418	-.04691	-.08808	.04216	.07199	.04339
SSS29	.02133	.03527	.76195	-.00439	.17137	.11254	-.02336	.11617	-.02151
SSS27	.00165	-.02252	.60775	-.02018	-.04742	-.16073	-.02312	-.22635	-.05369
SSS18	.02666	-.10467	-.02951	.61847	.21925	-.01473	-.03916	-.11022	.03714
SSS14	.00904	-.00111	-.02205	.59120	-.20331	.04704	.07274	-.03058	-.05481
SSS10	.37440	-.19349	-.03987	-.41523	.03312	-.25339	.07306	-.09184	.13079
SSS26	-.02719	-.00695	-.02311	.11692	-.85680	-.04735	.01306	.02957	-.05276
SSS16	.10929	.04180	-.00638	-.00729	-.82969	-.16918	-.05161	-.00954	-.00844
SSS20	-.04604	.01057	.08467	-.20352	-.32873	.29774	.00711	.25710	-.09500
SSS23	.01775	-.11959	.04886	-.05822	-.30971	.29020	.00376	-.30653	.08259
SSS12	-.11749	.01699	-.13510	-.04441	.23564	.71680	-.02795	.06997	-.04051
SSS11	.10152	-.06413	-.06490	.22376	-.01709	.52529	.09901	-.09140	-.04865
SSS25	.26812	.03105	.09713	-.16190	-.15976	.33956	.17302	-.32370	.08802
SSS8	.21821	.04870	-.03413	.08650	.02313	.04183	.81153	-.02719	-.03047
SSS9	-.30252	-.03402	.01966	-.17530	.07155	-.08473	.77169	.12035	-.00386
SSS24	.34453	.09149	.03048	.05854	-.08030	.17554	.59853	-.13308	-.01342
SSS1	.03150	.10268	.11196	-.27946	-.00658	.03464	-.23190	-.72455	-.06738
SSS4	-.02539	.06017	-.07753	.06826	-.09700	-.04246	.17735	-.65705	-.22995
SSS15	-.13538	-.17055	.07228	.14211	-.13751	-.01580	.09998	-.29227	.16731
SSS2	.10607	-.02238	.01085	.10823	-.02104	.07799	.00493	-.12650	-.77473
SSS21	-.00309	-.32091	.03710	-.12326	-.11981	-.05261	.04532	-.10041	-.68398

136

Table 8.4d SSS: Structure matrix (oblimin rotation)

	FACTOR 1	FACTOR 2	FACTOR 3	FACTOR 4	FACTOR 5	FACTOR 6	FACTOR 7	FACTOR 8	FACTOR 9
SSS6	.75498	-.19536	.15251	-.14877	-.24449	.23846	.10653	-.11328	-.22111
SSS7	.74216	-.30912	.09247	-.19882	-.22443	.18124	.07757	-.02237	-.18224
SSS13	.66343	-.13281	.05130	.10836	-.01531	-.12669	.09907	-.16769	-.09160
SSS19	.64637	-.28190	.06107	-.23576	-.33050	.01716	.10345	-.14168	-.01877
SSS17	.46479	-.25555	.15992	-.32719	-.39741	.29000	.15091	-.29851	.11770
SSS3	.21203	-.91039	.08776	-.10114	-.09030	.02873	.02371	-.02920	-.16905
SSS22	.28452	-.89708	.10142	-.13502	-.12666	.03964	-.01293	-.00117	-.19179
SSS5	.13563	-.49045	.07436	.43455	-.11362	.15285	-.01639	-.10305	.06754
SSS28	.03187	-.09131	.78299	.07359	-.17880	-.03696	.03816	-.04355	.04048
SSS29	.03036	-.01439	.71710	.01357	.02200	.12894	-.03166	.03760	-.05100
SSS27	.10513	-.11573	.64107	-.02003	-.17154	-.11358	.00889	-.31137	-.04450
SSS14	.13817	-.06063	.01350	.61107	-.25695	.09436	.09225	-.00227	-.08102
SSS18	.09275	-.10027	-.05276	.60712	.14395	-.04367	-.04555	-.09291	.00194
SSS10	.45412	-.27986	-.00062	-.45961	-.08736	-.22032	.10265	-.18775	.08546
SSS26	.13582	-.13882	.13964	.05025	-.82711	.08675	.08763	-.06679	-.01535
SSS16	.25768	-.11763	.15299	-.08481	-.81446	-.03766	.02708	-.11750	.02387
SSS23	.19718	-.22891	.18019	-.08824	-.43344	.34404	.10517	-.37138	.06526
SSS20	.04047	-.04214	.12650	-.22879	-.36281	.35831	.02965	.21556	-.12028
SSS12	-.13064	.06950	-.16194	-.01964	.18766	.66273	-.01049	.14217	-.09405
SSS11	.17468	-.13160	.13102	.20149	-.14540	.55464	.17855	-.14292	-.09704
SSS8	.29549	-.02554	-.00502	.06440	-.08921	.12763	.84175	-.16332	-.07598
SSS9	-.22394	.03254	-.02808	-.12712	.06415	-.04643	.70587	.07782	-.00515
SSS24	.44711	-.04846	.10450	.01251	-.24017	.26941	.67891	-.28247	-.07030
SSS1	.17484	-.00566	.19901	-.28460	-.10816	.03003	-.12898	-.70293	-.05648
SSS4	.09097	.00518	.01243	.07124	.05026	-.02955	.25300	-.64094	-.20930
SSS25	.42480	-.12970	.21127	-.20558	-.35465	.40213	.29108	-.43081	.03323
SSS15	-.02927	-.19229	.14441	.15061	-.18925	.00251	.13710	-.32906	.18754
SSS2	.21191	-.10375	.06158	.05870	-.04443	.15507	.06985	-.13492	-.78507
SSS21	.20714	-.39226	.11539	-.17164	-.17842	.04518	.09790	-.14413	-.69587

The theoretical treatment of the multifactorial outcome is based on factor solutions shown in Tables 8.4c and 8.4d, which give the grouping of items corresponding to each factor. On the whole, the results of factor analysis do not exactly confirm the initial conceptual scheme which conforms to the typical understanding of the field. Specifically, network resources, support acts and support appraisal are not clearly distinguished from one another, which makes it difficult to derive specific sets of subscales under such theories as the social isolation hypothesis and the quality of relationship (in terms of appraisal of support) hypothesis mentioned earlier. Although our emphasis is not on a confirmatory factor analysis (otherwise a common factor model rather than principal components analysis would be preferred), this outcome has significant implications to scaling strategies. It is clear that although substantive studies of social support have developed numerous scaling schemes, they have susceptible utility in dealing with the real world. This is because empirical analysis will not necessarily come up with the factor structure as specified beforehand (see also Donald & Ware, 1984), and therefore the substantive classification schemes may not be applicable. In fact, as social support can be classified with multiple criteria, the specific factor structure of a data set depends on a number of considerations in designing the measurement tool used to obtain the data. In other words, it is usually a result of a particular way of mingling those multiple criteria, which can hardly be made standardized or comparable to other designs. One of my objectives is to obtain factor (component) scores, which can be used in subsequent analyses to represent the values of the components as subscales of social support. Tables 8.5a and 8.5b give the factor score coefficients used to calculate regression method factor scores for the data. Both sets of factor scores based on different methods of rotation are saved as the composite measures resulted from factor analysis. Conventionally, only the first 9 factors extracted by default settings are considered for the purpose of constructing factor scales or component scores. This book, however, will proceed with the issue of unidimensionalization emphasizing on a standardized multifactorial scaling procedure for weighting at the components (factors) level. Instead of using these subscales as final products of multidimensional scaling, it will explore two different approaches discussed in the methodology chapter. For this purpose, scores for some other factor sets using different criteria in extraction are also saved for later use (e.g., minimum or 1 factor solution, maximum number factor solution, etc.).

Table 8.4e SSS: Factor correlation matrix (oblimin rotation)

	FACTOR 1	FACTOR 2	FACTOR 3	FACTOR 4	FACTOR 5	FACTOR 6	FACTOR 7	FACTOR 8	FACTOR 9
FACTOR 1	1.00000								
FACTOR 2	-.23446	1.00000							
FACTOR 3	-.08705	-.10654	1.00000						
FACTOR 4	-.12783	.03515	.01016	1.00000					
FACTOR 5	-.21114	.17210	-.19707	.07933	1.00000				
FACTOR 6	.08250	-.04912	.05757	-.00892	-.15526	1.00000			
FACTOR 7	.11808	-.03347	.01532	-.00528	-.09784	.09106	1.00000		
FACTOR 8	.19065	.11163	-.13426	.00132	.12117	-.00483	-.13310	1.00000	
FACTOR 9	-.10315	.04829	-.01589	.04232	-.03141	-.08163	-.03215	-.02478	1.00000

Table 8.5a SSS: Factor score coefficient matrix (oblimin rotation)

	FACTOR 1	FACTOR 2	FACTOR 3	FACTOR 4	FACTOR 5	FACTOR 6	FACTOR 7	FACTOR 8	FACTOR 9
SSS1	-.08971	.06746	.00582	-.14967	.05091	.03961	-.20391	-.51489	-.03266
SSS2	-.01294	.11535	-.01592	.08401	-.04418	-.01372	-.04733	-.04911	-.62194
SSS3	-.14745	-.49246	-.02185	-.02817	.07975	-.01478	.04102	-.02487	.02398
SSS4	-.10633	-.02085	-.11091	.07332	.06128	-.06967	.05073	-.47788	-.16101
SSS5	.01246	-.28030	-.05650	.32884	.02013	.09783	-.05171	-.06706	.15735
SSS6	.35993	.12965	-.03995	.03436	-.06056	.07281	-.07303	.12159	-.05506
SSS7	.34710	.04524	.01220	.00127	.06439	.04167	-.05908	.17751	.01129
SSS8	.04297	.01709	-.01337	.06745	.05130	-.05650	.46465	.05729	-.01005
SSS9	-.24778	-.09110	-.05605	-.16635	.01924	-.11108	.52009	.12098	-.01036
SSS10	.13444	-.07567	.02717	-.22046	.08225	.19126	.04846	-.02188	.14514
SSS11	.00763	-.02319	.01857	.14616	.01888	.37074	-.00933	-.04608	.02413
SSS12	-.06452	-.00909	-.05279	-.07185	.16104	.55967	.06855	.02894	.00682
SSS13	-.43008	.09750	-.00401	.20498	.12571	-.16914	-.02917	.02998	.01077
SSS14	-.10946	.03104	-.00213	.39188	-.10190	.02898	.04744	.07105	-.05462
SSS15	-.14928	.15123	-.00992	.10250	-.05472	.01587	.05556	-.22979	.17082
SSS16	-.04695	.07731	-.08465	.03850	.49710	-.17502	-.04567	.03788	-.04338
SSS17	.05311	.03234	-.00567	-.13895	-.02476	.16224	-.02251	-.07739	.20249
SSS18	-.05157	-.05678	.01175	-.40690	.16460	.02243	-.01172	-.06705	.05002
SSS19	.25309	-.01697	-.04532	-.02577	-.03820	-.07841	-.02521	.06858	-.07662
SSS20	-.09221	.04877	.06134	-.15786	-.18222	.20837	-.00361	.22955	-.08697
SSS21	-.15225	-.07001	-.00757	-.06957	-.09219	-.10174	.01696	-.03473	-.52732
SSS22	-.09556	.45331	-.01309	-.03593	.06726	-.01397	.00874	.06383	-.00717
SSS23	-.12464	-.07120	.03450	-.01878	-.11988	.20541	-.05081	-.20498	.11581
SSS24	.09931	.07073	.00562	.06641	.02451	.05332	.30143	-.00824	.03453
SSS25	.02258	.03680	.02151	-.07552	.00906	.22715	.02662	-.17043	.12967
SSS26	-.13147	.03372	-.09894	.10275	.52739	-.09095	-.00649	.05282	-.07413
SSS27	-.05313	.01737	.36605	-.01559	.03911	-.12642	-.00572	-.10509	-.03081
SSS28	-.02330	.01524	.51430	.01322	.05123	-.06727	.05835	.12752	.04293
SSS29	.03193	.05911	.52781	-.04367	.18980	.09722	.00130	.15866	-.00043

Table 8.5b SSS: Factor score coefficient matrix (varimax rotation)

	FACTOR 1	FACTOR 2	FACTOR 3	FACTOR 4	FACTOR 5	FACTOR 6	FACTOR 7	FACTOR 8	FACTOR 9
SSS1	-.04502	-.06842	-.04813	-.18335	.01715	.47638	.14204	.00772	.04549
SSS2	-.00702	-.10504	-.00635	-.03504	-.01239	-.00926	-.06453	.01863	.61264
SSS3	-.07989	.46666	-.04291	.03219	-.01208	-.00079	.02932	-.01281	-.01723
SSS4	-.07091	-.02812	-.08452	.06747	-.09693	.43884	-.07399	-.08535	.16992
SSS5	.02244	.27134	.00123	-.04144	-.04059	.09481	-.32752	.08287	-.14405
SSS6	.31429	-.10503	-.04894	-.06513	.03132	-.11290	-.02490	.07520	.06892
SSS7	.30661	-.02635	-.04922	-.05646	.00397	-.16226	.00806	.04444	.02418
SSS8	.05053	-.01534	-.03823	.45646	-.02016	-.02420	-.06719	-.03838	-.00327
SSS9	-.19489	.07546	-.00093	.49562	.04577	-.09103	.15944	-.08144	.00154
SSS10	.13998	.07300	-.06791	.03837	-.03054	.03719	.21809	.20103	-.13507
SSS11	.01867	.02721	-.01435	.00742	.01983	.06000	-.14755	.36227	-.01163
SSS12	-.05057	.00188	-.11176	-.05609	-.06363	-.03560	.06599	.54385	-.00029
SSS13	.35424	-.07775	-.13510	-.02492	-.01005	-.02301	-.19524	.17451	-.00492
SSS14	-.06087	.03136	.10922	.03971	-.00456	-.07388	.39020	-.04055	.04844
SSS15	-.10446	.14141	.06793	.06171	.06651	.24871	-.10947	-.02990	-.16282
SSS16	-.01513	-.05919	.44400	-.03845	-.05452	-.02847	-.02726	-.15347	.03318
SSS17	.08457	.03687	.06303	-.01479	-.00092	.10252	.13356	.14572	-.18709
SSS18	-.01912	.04458	-.13357	-.02095	-.00002	.05698	.39808	.00950	-.04596
SSS19	.23466	-.00341	.03991	-.02360	-.04287	-.05128	.03208	-.08041	-.06569
SSS20	-.06189	-.03958	.19391	-.00444	.06235	-.21787	.16069	.23088	.07797
SSS21	-.10030	.06925	.05581	.01883	.00126	-.00627	.08501	-.06682	.51638
SSS22	-.03783	.43227	-.03304	.00044	-.00477	-.04071	.03892	-.01016	-.00060
SSS23	-.06614	.07027	.14249	-.03482	-.01714	.21722	.01394	.19038	-.10549
SSS24	.10441	-.06096	-.00529	.30394	.00230	.03698	-.06618	.06093	-.02237
SSS25	.05613	-.02983	.02961	.04040	-.02499	.18784	-.06924	.21104	-.11253
SSS26	-.08608	-.01920	.47642	.00273	-.06570	-.04081	-.09114	-.06490	.06166
SSS27	-.03404	-.00680	-.01238	-.00843	.36051	.12125	.00965	-.11701	.03474
SSS28	-.02027	.00068	-.00011	.04669	.49767	-.08153	-.02101	-.04509	-.04161
SSS29	.01961'	-.04298	-.12192	-.00805	.49968	-.12363	.03471	.11352	.00456

The Life Stress Scale (LSS)

The life stress variables seem more independent of one another than the items pool of social support per an inspection of the correlation matrix. Principal components analysis extracted as many as 16 factors out of the 44 life stress items, explaining 57.1% of the total variance (see Table 8.6). Tables 8.7a and 8.7b contain the rotated matrices that display the sorted factor loadings; the factor correlation matrix for factors resulted from oblique rotation is also given in Table 8.7c. The results of factor analysis reflect the initial conceptual scheme which conforms to the comprehensive understanding of life stress. However, similar to the scaling of social support, they do not particularly confirm the categorization of the sources of stress. Specifically, major life events do not distinguish themselves from more enduring stressful conditions. This has similar implications to scaling as mentioned in dealing with social support.

Tables 8.8a and 8.8b contain the factor score coefficients used to calculate regression method factor scores for the life stress items. The two as well as some other sets of factor scores based on different methods of extraction and rotation are saved as the composite measures (subscales) resulted from factor analysis.

Table 8.6 LSS: Final statistics for factors extracted by principal components analysis (PC)

VARIABLE	COMMUNALITY	*	FACTOR	EIGENVALUE	PCT OF VAR	CUM PCT
LSS1	.44653	*	1	4.39474	10.0	10.0
LSS2	.42804	*	2	2.36657	5.4	15.4
LSS3	.47357	*	3	1.89056	4.3	19.7
LSS4	.60619	*	4	1.67800	3.8	23.5
LSS5	.61196	*	5	1.58419	3.6	27.1
LSS6	.50897	*	6	1.47818	3.4	30.4
LSS7	.52504	*	7	1.38224	3.1	33.6
LSS8	.45520	*	8	1.36302	3.1	36.7
LSS9	.62509	*	9	1.32361	3.0	39.7
LSS10	.43959	*	10	1.17292	2.7	42.4
LSS11	.66099	*	11	1.14407	2.6	45.0
LSS12	.66493	*	12	1.12889	2.6	47.5
LSS13	.37515	*	13	1.11854	2.5	50.1
LSS14	.44078	*	14	1.05717	2.4	52.5
LSS15	.51958	*	15	1.03780	2.4	54.8
LSS16	.67998	*	16	1.01037	2.3	57.1
LSS17	.68953	*				
LSS18	.76022	*				
LSS19	.77623	*				
LSS20	.60052	*				
LSS21	.61699	*				
LSS22	.50244	*				
LSS23	.73852	*				
LSS24	.52810	*				
LSS25	.60796	*				
LSS26	.60520	*				
LSS27	.68225	*				
LSS28	.51511	*				
LSS29	.56171	*				
LSS30	.60765	*				
LSS31	.46331	*				
LSS32	.42905	*				
LSS33	.58939	*				
LSS34	.62516	*				
LSS35	.38795	*				
LSS36	.58447	*				
LSS37	.64869	*				
LSS38	.50426	*				
LSS39	.60482	*				
LSS40	.60861	*				
LSS41	.75621	*				
LSS42	.65821	*				
LSS43	.57876	*				
LSS44	.43796	*				

Table 8.7a LSS: Rotated factor matrix (varimax)

	FACTOR 1	FACTOR 2	FACTOR 3	FACTOR 4	FACTOR 5	FACTOR 6	FACTOR 7	FACTOR 8
LSS12	.80171	.00401	.01757	.10153	.01764	.01884	-.035R8	.01595
LSS11	.75700	.04004	.05031	.21521	-.03183	.00043	.12942	.07525
LSS9	.63908	-.03594	.14922	.13641	.04568	.14246	.00947	.29429
LSS1	.50841	-.02288	.09099	-.04446	.04511	-.10793	.14383	.07601
LSS13	.35633	.05642	.14886	.31557	.05296	.19386	.22939	-.01762
LSS44	.31041	.12070	.25202	.11582	.05560	.30370	.02302	.07250
LSS27	.06344	.70638	-.03890	.00590	.01840	.17888	.00374	-.08529
LSS2R	.01918	.65907	.04791	.08759	.03550	.04959	-.06138	-.09468
LSS20	.06204	-.63950	.16614	.06581	.17491	.15176	-.03968	.03674
LSS37	.01990	-.60820	.06584	.04715	.06372	-.06863	-.07365	-.04114
LSS19	.12050	-.05534	.85089	.03478	.03332	.07983	.11950	.08172
LSS1R	.09946	-.03145	.84222	.08938	.06964	.03959	.06624	.11604
LSS5	.16567	.00696	.03449	.74619	-.00279	.08551	.09861	.02275
LSS4	.11602	-.02892	.06713	.72909	-.02283	-.08327	.18930	.05636
LSS3	.14740	.16615	.0092R	.45591	.09461	-.14625	.25897	.04494
LSS41	-.05345	.15436	-.07349	-.06165	-.83888	-.01474	.00883	-.06337
LSS23	-.06596	.09603	.01824	-.04034	.79895	-.11940	.00056	-.08229
LSS24	-.12727	.04960	-.05809	-.00003	-.53699	-.08301	-.06857	-.25315
LSS25	.03672	-.01017	.07440	.00139	.03410	.72262	-.00447	.16822
LSS26	.01767	.14106	.01975	-.04275	-.10427	.71492	.14745	-.00197
LSS32	-.01311	-.13986	-.08965	-.02596	-.03942	-.33313	.11358	.25511
LSS6	.05972	-.02604	.04517	.05880	-.00101	.07910	.67728	-.07390
LSS7	.02503	.03412	.10011	.19480	.03550	.02077	.65520	.15666
LSS8	.10893	-.04412	.03300	.24203	.01933	.03131	.54890	.20104
LSS2	.32632	-.15524	.06370	-.04576	.01162	-.09411	.33230	-.19904
LSS15	.09449	-.10015	.34771	.10841	.02203	.01543	.02146	.57533
LSS10	.13337	-.02602	-.05498	-.06246	.05190	.14451	.14991	.56293
LSS14	.10013	-.15679	.33374	.15803	.07659	.00787	.02948	.48012
LSS21	.01514	-.08091	-.01293	-.06493	.09170	-.02867	.06879	.05558
LSS36	-.03391	-.04710	.02585	.18883	-.03580	.04741	-.12399	-.01981
LSS17	.09383	.06516	.05830	.05834	-.07820	-.00556	.07271	-.00352
LSS16	-.03727	-.11693	.00434	.05815	.08088	.06348	-.04322	.01244
LSS42	.10816	-.08635	.05171	.08395	.00141	.23436	-.08440	.09297
LSS43	-.02271	.05415	.02248	-.00088	-.04123	-.15882	.16236	-.13750

143

Table 8.7a LSS: Rotated factor matrix (varimax) (continued)

	FACTOR 1	FACTOR 2	FACTOR 3	FACTOR 4	FACTOR 5	FACTOR 6	FACTOR 7	FACTOR 8
LSS29	.00186	.02659	.03788	-.00773	.03876	.01013	.01733	-.05011
LSS39	-.04347	.11945	.03559	.09784	-.04653	.12355	-.05970	.14483
LSS38	-.12159	-.19366	-.00042	.12488	.01689	.13435	.00538	.09117
LSS22	.26743	.03844	.06796	-.08923	.00774	.14745	-.04642	-.21027
LSS34	-.03524	-.10480	.06818	.06398	-.04044	.12838	-.01460	-.10806
LSS35	.07067	.01493	.15140	.13242	.06460	.09977	-.03875	.04815
LSS31	-.03704	.11820	.11071	-.14816	-.01817	-.14238	.03024	.19974
LSS10	.00916	-.07523	-.03829	.00854	.06500	.07656	-.04604	.03926
LSS33	.01556	-.01408	.03772	-.02811	-.07432	-.00748	.01190	-.08397
LSS40	-.01187	.10039	.05248	-.02503	.01112	.06577	-.03149	.07355

	FACTOR 9	FACTOR 10	FACTOR 11	FACTOR 12	FACTOR 13	FACTOR 14	FACTOR 15	FACTOR 16
LSS12	.02707	-.03438	.01223	-.01327	-.01093	-.06050	-.00525	-.05358
LSS11	.04276	.01540	-.08062	-.00977	.02164	.05765	.03595	-.01786
LSS9	-.18830	.03474	.06367	-.07176	-.09970	-.07647	-.01223	-.06024
LSS1	.05939	.08429	.16292	.06744	.21118	.08731	.00666	.20768
LSS13	-.11155	.03568	.04767	-.10252	-.03814	-.02493	-.01035	-.03544
LSS44	-.00123	.10262	.23955	.02406	-.00119	.06575	.09102	-.26056
LSS27	-.36427	-.02916	-.00752	.00917	-.01260	-.01015	-.05869	.02613
LSS28	-.17539	-.06642	.09449	-.02025	.01448	-.04335	-.03481	.07839
LSS20	-.26882	-.07095	-.00291	-.09504	-.00630	-.03483	.02761	.10428
LSS37	-.23238	.02268	.22235	-.17189	.30210	-.02037	-.06371	-.16342
LSS19	-.01857	.04082	.03505	.03393	-.00918	-.00395	.00484	.02153
LSS18	-.00050	.03137	.03994	.05458	.01960	-.00186	-.00383	.04232
LSS5	-.02816	.05039	.04023	.02506	.05256	.02073	.00268	-.01188
LSS4	.03701	.04206	-.01682	.01277	-.02244	.07149	-.01255	-.00035
LSS3	.17504	.06317	.12264	.15952	-.07400	.15719	-.02982	-.03003
LSS41	.04460	-.00578	-.08192	.05638	-.00798	.01104	.00509	.01308
LSS23	.17424	.04545	-.01129	.06867	.15131	.03485	.04272	-.02075
LSS24	.10098	.08637	.23304	-.00236	.23833	.01935	.09189	-.06667
LSS25	-.04637	-.01082	.12305	-.06190	.09834	.08181	-.00455	.10807
LSS26	.01594	.07060	-.07260	.07463	.11203	.06570	-.07805	.00097
LSS32	-.09689	.04371	.27586	.08036	.30358	.11501	.02628	.10077

144

Table 8.7a LSS: Rotated factor matrix (varimax) (continued)

	FACTOR 9	FACTOR 10	FACTOR 11	FACTOR 12	FACTOR 13	FACTOR 14	FACTOR 15	FACTOR 16
LSS6	-.06372	-.01609	.03776	-.03302	-.09952	.07916	-.05589	-.05162
LSS7	.02320	.07133	.06437	-.02372	.04878	-.05071	.05131	-.04287
LSS8	.02573	-.02812	-.03735	.02526	.09838	-.13535	-.02485	.08095
LSS2	.04779	-.00619	-.12668	.30437	-.07687	.12123	-.00641	.02479
LSS15	.06394	-.03949	-.03172	.01521	.08745	-.06503	-.07445	-.10709
LSS10	-.01428	.05721	-.05644	.05207	-.14217	.05371	-.01814	.12974
LSS14	.07901	-.02746	.10197	.02981	.07054	.07954	.02274	.04895
LSS21	.72378	.02813	.04556	-.01893	.04998	-.02680	.02587	-.24044
LSS36	.63086	-.06490	-.04924	-.06890	-.16966	-.00895	-.02139	.29459
LSS17	.03681	.80187	-.06242	-.04718	.05683	.03218	-.05614	-.01847
LSS16	-.04913	.78713	.03715	.08996	-.08969	-.09141	.02873	-.01536
LSS42	-.04906	-.03502	.71884	.00017	-.10688	-.03739	-.00387	-.15951
LSS43	.06935	-.01660	.65595	.06822	.06936	.03801	-.08977	.21976
LSS29	-.07207	.03263	-.00301	.73616	-.00991	-.04874	-.00402	.06636
LSS39	.02110	.00358	.08907	.70957	.01898	.03225	-.00222	-.15021
LSS18	-.17259	-.03394	-.05294	.03143	.60979	-.03506	.01919	-.03916
LSS22	.14297	-.02577	-.00319	-.06984	.54701	.03680	-.11973	.08829
LSS34	-.08313	-.04317	-.00577	-.00134	-.18137	.72621	-.02893	.06525
LSS35	.12781	-.02488	.02570	.08248	.17205	.51770	.03057	.03692
LSS31	-.09798	.00550	-.00368	-.16416	.06497	.50234	.11555	-.21410
LSS30	-.04333	-.04926	.04881	.02343	-.12551	.07022	.74084	.09926
LSS33	.05538	-.07397	-.10625	-.03050	.07222	-.06029	.73730	-.02728
LSS40	-.04854	-.02205	.03851	-.04817	.02982	-.00571	.07873	.75524

145

Table 8.7b LSS: Pattern matrix (oblimin rotation)

	FACTOR 1	FACTOR 2	FACTOR 3	FACTOR 4	FACTOR 5	FACTOR 6	FACTOR 7	FACTOR 8
LSS5	.74780	.03627	.03584	.00372	-.08671	.02744	-.04519	-.04189
LSS4	.72812	-.00910	.12572	.03251	-.03485	-.03803	-.03670	.01370
LSS3	.42260	.15966	-.17395	-.09074	-.06569	.09571	-.05043	.16552
LSS27	.00281	.73124	.15551	-.03350	-.05584	-.02771	.02380	-.32666
LSS28	.08938	.64417	.02465	-.04890	-.00429	.07445	.06285	-.14191
LSS20	.05424	.59550	.12710	.14214	.02119	.02512	.06869	-.30013
LSS37	.04305	.56534	-.08799	-.05471	-.01538	.23305	-.02300	-.23487
LSS26	-.07410	.13328	.73447	.09813	.03559	-.06197	-.06886	.04772
LSS25	-.02845	-.00186	.71889	-.02919	.02543	.13759	.01249	.01848
LSS12	-.03835	.12238	-.34056	.03354	-.00135	.22648	-.03751	-.07947
LSS44	.06009	.14302	.26299	-.04846	-.24098	.23962	-.08782	.03586
LSS41	-.03909	.08612	.00523	.84323	-.00346	-.08899	.00356	.03933
LSS23	-.05543	.13667	-.10676	.82043	.09915	-.02282	-.04355	.18604
LSS24	.01978	.00815	-.06737	.52446	.09380	.22634	-.08577	.11178
LSS12	.05900	.00707	-.01710	-.00088	.82610	.01135	.04030	.01673
LSS11	.16327	.03704	-.03369	.04967	.75271	-.09740	-.00863	.02762
LSS9	.08433	-.00761	.08359	-.01853	.61757	.05955	-.02704	.18323
LSS1	-.10596	.00616	-.11972	-.03497	.50175	.13020	-.08016	.05195
LSS2	-.09779	-.18996	-.08549	-.00113	.30927	-.13001	-.01486	-.00608
LSS11	.27090	-.03355	.15772	-.04027	-.28362	.05026	-.03062	-.11201
LSS42	.05388	.07947	.19167	.00227	-.06347	.74416	.05259	-.01153
LSS43	-.03526	.02737	-.16215	.01482	.05832	.64645	.02454	.07730
LSS17	.02454	-.04590	-.00186	.07619	-.05066	-.10781	-.81131	.03291
LSS16	.04147	-.13115	.05708	-.08341	.07929	.01458	-.79219	-.06275
LSS21	-.08781	.11347	.01896	-.10004	-.01065	.05595	-.01448	.74548
LSS36	.20838	-.08070	.07449	.04077	.04465	-.03187	.05939	.60096
LSS19	-.04654	-.00521	-.03178	-.00443	.00973	.02262	-.03166	-.01351
LSS18	.01564	.02111	.01232	-.01238	.02888	.02264	-.02261	.00327
LSS34	.06640	-.12278	.11657	.04867	.07655	-.00506	.03426	-.11572
LSS35	.13627	-.00990	.10575	-.07054	-.06346	.00635	.02197	.11978
LSS31	-.15888	.12483	-.15391	.01831	.04380	-.03072	-.00429	-.07168
LSS40	-.01923	.09020	.06647	-.00504	.01874	.02297	.00532	-.07879
LSS29	-.02586	-.01582	.00271	-.01365	.00662	-.01615	-.01864	-.10404
LSS39	.08411	.07844	.10615	.05120	.06311	.07431	.01772	.01896

146

Table 8.7b LSS: Pattern matrix (oblimin rotation) (continued)

	FACTOR 1	FACTOR 2	FACTOR 3	FACTOR 4	FACTOR 5	FACTOR 6	FACTOR 7	FACTOR 8
LSS30	.02744	-.08289	.05658	-.07539	-.01689	.06395	-.04047	-.05030
LSS33	-.00987	.01500	-.01082	.06042	-.04123	-.09364	.08419	.06267
LSS10	-.09588	-.04546	.13568	-.03590	-.12079	.04325	-.04974	-.00580
LSS15	.07186	-.06939	-.01697	.00835	-.04381	-.05182	.05136	.08658
LSS14	.12837	-.13486	-.02217	-.04743	-.04447	-.12369	.03484	.07692
LSS3R	.13258	-.15900	.13653	-.02143	.13032	-.07306	.03341	-.15333
LSS22	-.11687	-.04788	.17072	-.01363	-.27808	-.01984	.01784	.15817
LSS6	-.00660	-.02861	.09205	.00171	.02591	.03793	.02678	-.05719
LSS7	.12952	.04154	.02347	-.03469	.07396	.04511	-.05529	.04505
LSS8R	.19269	-.04121	.03451	.02717	-.04046	-.05422	.03987	.02984

	FACTOR 9	FACTOR 10	FACTOR 11	FACTOR 12	FACTOR 13	FACTOR 14	FACTOR 15	FACTOR 16
LSS5	.01755	-.01381	-.01009	.01749	-.01273	-.04081	.06561	-.03067
LSS4	-.02720	.07717	.00312	.00196	.00473	-.00902	.03321	-.11799
LSS3	-.07050	.14670	-.02593	.13965	.02354	-.00349	-.08946	-.19575
LSS27	.03964	-.01251	.00981	.00572	.05498	-.05924	-.01281	-.01829
LSS28	-.05851	-.04680	.07334	-.02335	.02903	-.08722	.00217	.05854
LSS20	-.13548	-.01939	.10026	-.08427	-.03185	-.01822	.01499	-.02909
LSS37	-.04113	-.00823	-.15308	-.15656	.06149	-.09229	.30942	.07467
LSS26	.00112	.06072	-.00298	.06148	-.07152	-.00891	.11578	-.16908
LSS25	-.04777	.08045	.10197	.05421	.00807	.14845	.10271	-.00043
LSS32	.08069	.09317	.10577	.07289	-.02678	.26357	.30109	-.09806
LSS44	-.21651	.05585	-.25462	.01729	-.09059	.01149	-.02003	.01131
LSS41	.02009	.01251	.01354	.06248	.00349	-.00111	.00394	-.01919
LSS23	.00788	.02289	-.01333	.05711	-.04840	-.13124	.14227	.00053
LSS24	.02503	.01765	.04572	.00054	-.08949	-.22899	.21637	.05346
LSS12	.03729	-.07051	-.06109	-.01731	-.00301	.01111	-.03757	.10275
LSS11	.00443	.04499	-.02422	-.00325	-.04179	.03442	.00083	-.05076
LSS9	-.09661	-.08235	-.07084	-.07416	.00859	.25319	-.10229	.05439
LSS1	-.06761	.06565	.21403	.04844	-.01104	.04525	.17473	-.08591
LSS2	-.04345	.10983	.01605	.29477	.00208	-.21992	-.09538	-.29537
LSS13	-.09585	-.02359	-.03687	-.11345	.00357	-.07436	-.04427	-.19198
LSS42	-.01782	-.04394	.15324	.00266	-.00332	.08468	-.12921	.08461
LSS43	-.02524	.02330	.23533	.05380	.07926	-.12893	.02156	-.16296

147

Table 8.7b LSS: Pattern matrix (oblimin rotation) (continued)

	FACTOR 9	FACTOR 10	FACTOR 11	FACTOR 12	FACTOR 13	FACTOR 14	FACTOR 15	FACTOR 16
LSS17	-.04654	.03358	.01036	-.08128	.06769	-.01479	.03994	-.02350
LSS16	.01662	-.08674	.00892	.06662	-.02128	.00959	-.08836	.08474
LSS21	.01689	-.04462	-.22038	-.03202	-.02015	.04129	.02181	-.07594
LSS36	-.04054	-.00404	.30954	-.08268	.02044	-.01753	-.19681	.14509
LSS19	-.88155	-.00510	.03614	.03461	-.00025	-.05536	-.03244	-.05763
LSS18	-.87447	-.00290	.05724	.05631	.00774	-.02423	-.00144	.00348
LSS34	-.06640	.74336	.05984	-.01278	.03391	-.11713	-.19853	.03293
LSS35	.17253	.51573	.03476	.06771	.03323	.04326	.16027	.06497
LSS31	-.12563	.49768	-.21153	-.16908	-.10387	.18230	.06147	-.03372
LSS40	-.07463	-.00653	.75921	-.06354	-.08420	.08916	.01909	.04809
LSS29	-.04629	-.06308	.05103	.74456	.00001	-.05527	.00003	.03034
LSS39	-.04154	.01550	-.16489	.72055	.00321	.13370	.03482	.10802
LSS30	.05589	.05717	.10897	.02208	-.74427	.03405	-.10722	.04583
LSS33	-.03973	-.07667	-.01470	-.02348	-.73949	-.10624	.08775	-.02686
LSS10	.07530	.03881	.11745	.03857	.02340	.58184	-.12580	-.13028
LSS15	-.35432	-.07313	-.10818	-.00933	.08883	.50452	.10621	.02548
LSS14	-.33686	-.07376	.04920	.02965	-.01630	.40428	.08631	.03013
LSS38	.00908	-.03660	-.03675	.04225	-.01738	.03958	.64076	-.00603
LSS22	-.06254	.03071	.09972	-.07666	.11929	-.25028	.51198	.05643
LSS6	-.01129	.06866	-.05742	-.05500	.05283	-.09062	-.10628	-.69798
LSS7	-.06772	-.07076	-.03954	-.04726	-.05306	.11477	.05424	-.65478
LSS8	-.00157	-.15147	.07643	.00904	.02101	.16806	.11197	-.53479

148

Table 8.7c LSS: Factor correlation matrix (oblimin rotation)

	FACTOR 1	FACTOR 2	FACTOR 3	FACTOR 4	FACTOR 5	FACTOR 6	FACTOR 7	FACTOR 8	FACTOR 9
FACTOR 1	1.00000								
FACTOR 2	-.04120	1.00000							
FACTOR 3	.09239	-.00676	1.00000						
FACTOR 4	-.05579	.09639	-.02357	1.00000					
FACTOR 5	-.18783	-.00224	-.10412	.08909	1.00000				
FACTOR 6	.05508	.04850	.00235	.00339	-.06571	1.00000			
FACTOR 7	-.05287	-.02717	.00043	-.00021	.06740	-.07087	1.00000		
FACTOR 8	.02773	.00606	-.09398	.01992	-.01350	-.04400	-.01722	1.00000	
FACTOR 9	-.17551	.09113	-.11079	.12489	.22553	-.05199	.04433	.02963	1.00000
FACTOR 10	.00160	.04918	-.00515	-.00661	-.05349	.04835	-.00323	-.03923	-.01144
FACTOR 11	-.01236	.03798	-.01408	-.00379	-.00739	-.00310	.05315	.03825	.04779
FACTOR 12	.03645	.08214	.00546	-.01076	-.03221	.02812	-.06799	.06249	-.00806
FACTOR 13	.03485	-.00255	-.02161	-.02637	-.02975	.02479	.02375	-.00504	.01041
FACTOR 14	.09999	-.02921	.04293	-.09020	-.05578	.03300	-.02103	-.03133	-.17146
FACTOR 15	-.01162	-.00545	-.02898	.01464	-.02405	.09678	-.01627	.00516	-.02845
FACTOR 16	-.18804	-.00319	.03513	.02339	.20141	-.02705	.08390	-.00338	.13888

	FACTOR 10	FACTOR 11	FACTOR 12	FACTOR 13	FACTOR 14	FACTOR 15	FACTOR 16
FACTOR 10	1.00000						
FACTOR 11	.00564	1.00000					
FACTOR 12	.05197	.04906	1.00000				
FACTOR 13	-.02907	.02810	.00845	1.00000			
FACTOR 14	.03211	-.02094	.00678	-.03092	1.00000		
FACTOR 15	.04461	.00298	-.01516	.02038	.01754	1.00000	
FACTOR 16	-.06226	-.02838	-.10244	-.01936	-.06154	-.01058	1.00000

149

Table 8.8a LSS: Factor score coefficient matrix (oblimin rotation)

	FACTOR 1	FACTOR 2	FACTOR 3	FACTOR 4	FACTOR 5	FACTOR 6	FACTOR 7	FACTOR 8
LSS1	.24213	.00276	-.01185	.15554	.00648	-.11465	.04601	.01528
LSS2	.17474	-.13796	.02394	.14911	-.00713	-.06696	.21690	-.22339
LSS3	-.02220	-.08725	.01570	.23266	.05057	-.11120	.05961	-.01975
LSS4	-.06626	-.00465	-.02007	.47036	-.02823	-.07628	-.03256	-.01826
LSS5	-.04427	.00906	-.05027	.49620	-.00345	.02701	-.09632	-.04800
LSS6	.01951	-.02865	.01573	.10529	.00603	.06764	.4866R	-.12199
LSS7	-.09702	.04228	-.02022	.01257	.01582	.01308	.42990	.06365
LSS8	-.03864	-.01487	-.07479	.04108	-.02823	.01785	.33617	.10775
LSS9	.26179	-.00473	-.03636	-.01669	-.01373	.01539	-.08913	.15298
LSS10	.03173	-.01236	.17176	-.13439	-.00596	.05686	.08221	.43899
LSS11	.33746	.01153	-.06175	.01588	-.04344	-.05338	-.02110	-.00857
LSS12	.39336	-.00827	-.06388	-.03499	.01134	.03334	.11161	-.04436
LSS13	-.08858	-.02335	.01611	.12537	.01981	.09522	.07893	-.11034
LSS14	-.02920	-.03047	.10558	.05251	-.01777	-.04837	.06827	.30336
LSS15	-.01724	.01879	.10765	.01087	-.05141	-.04061	-.06280	.39248
LSS16	-.03657	-.06669	-.03265	.01535	.04444	.02944	-.06139	-.00246
LSS17	.01720	.04064	.01731	-.02426	-.04503	-.01790	.00575	-.00956
LSS18	-.05522	.03874	.50492	-.01677	-.01629	-.04919	-.04024	.07585
LSS19	-.04092	.02129	.51215	.06941	-.03636	-.02071	.01252	-.10843
LSS20	.00411	-.32705	.02853	.03026	.05758	.07953	.01553	-.07035
LSS21	.00611	.00215	-.02117	-.10061	.04846	.05666	.06754	.04696
LSS22	.14312	.03062	.05254	-.09045	.01712	.10252	-.03166	-.19079
LSS23	-.04098	.10649	.00113	.02525	.48738	-.04563	.01473	-.10048
LSS24	-.03369	.00074	.04963	.03679	-.28857	-.04215	-.03251	.13721
LSS25	-.04340	-.02023	-.04586	-.03440	-.02086	.44306	-.00554	.07326
LSS26	-.04066	.04914	-.03448	.07797	-.03725	.45691	.12855	-.04073
LSS27	-.01135	.35263	.01144	.02040	.06315	.07197	.00197	-.03994
LSS28	.01887	.34566	.07920	.09071	-.06475	-.00069	-.06518	-.05402
LSS29	.01779	-.06440	.01590	-.02800	.01711	-.02820	-.01898	-.06416
LSS30	.00482	-.03791	-.05041	.02529	-.04389	-.00827	-.02720	.02339
LSS31	-.02721	.10606	.06879	-.12206	-.01702	-.13176	-.03060	.16732
LSS32	-.01326	.08522	-.09012	-.05288	-.02593	-.25230	.05738	.25261
LSS33	-.01602	.03066	.04676	.00358	-.03044	-.02894	-.03066	-.06605
LSS34	-.02726	-.09770	.05363	.04581	.02671	.06047	-.03348	-.12707
LSS35	.02184	-.01068	-.13086	.08206	.04465	.05846	-.07056	.04141
LSS36	-.02642	-.02968	.02976	.15230	-.03282	.08651	-.12516	.02192
LSS37	-.00513	-.28289	.00287	.04202	.00907	-.04809	-.05688	-.07623
LSS38	-.09723	-.06740	-.04267	.11307	.00595	.07132	-.01376	.06095
LSS39	-.04002	.00991	-.01284	.05067	-.03406	.03832	-.09852	.10292
LSS40	-.00650	.01994	.02109	-.00153	.00047	.01271	-.03458	.05445
LSS41	.01387	.02040	.03003	.02716	.48416	-.01646	.01971	.03152
LSS42	-.00653	-.04540	-.03505	.01929	-.00033	.12943	-.08374	.03915
LSS43	-.02403	-.00098	.02391	-.05322	-.00932	-.09711	-.11208	-.10961
LSS44	.07773	.08721	.09118	-.00489	.02848	.14801	-.04342	-.02604

Table 8.8a LSS: Factor score coefficient matrix (oblimin rotation) (continued)

	FACTOR 9	FACTOR 10	FACTOR 11	FACTOR 12	FACTOR 13	FACTOR 14	FACTOR 15	FACTOR 16
LSS1	.04040	.06465	.08992	.04882	.15628	.06177	.01776	.19677
LSS2	.00119	.02604	.11187	.25947	-.06766	.10067	-.01453	.03301
LSS3	.09019	.01002	.06653	.07131	-.06038	.10835	-.00266	-.02875
LSS4	-.01196	-.00816	-.05539	-.01724	.01996	.04465	.00941	.01349
LSS5	-.03837	-.00655	-.01578	-.01007	.04152	-.03757	.02211	.00152
LSS6	-.03867	-.03739	.02412	-.05797	-.10066	-.04858	-.04281	-.05656
LSS7	.01914	.01972	.03667	-.06867	.03691	-.06961	.06429	-.05017
LSS8	.01561	-.05046	-.04877	-.00422	.08185	-.13639	-.00681	.06706
LSS9	-.11285	.00540	-.02438	-.05273	-.10117	-.07026	-.00998	-.04101
LSS10	.00516	.04950	.04982	.02036	-.12124	.03167	-.02845	.11765
LSS11	.02174	-.01267	-.09800	.00878	.01753	.03743	.03258	-.00700
LSS12	.02225	.04661	-.01454	-.00733	-.01974	-.05614	-.00128	-.03670
LSS13	-.06508	-.00125	.00927	.09655	-.05060	-.03348	-.00512	-.02452
LSS14	.04492	-.02981	.10320	.02106	.06359	.05883	.01292	.04914
LSS15	.05444	-.04849	-.04824	-.02015	.07321	-.06339	.05910	.09470
LSS16	-.04299	.58786	.02405	-.04394	-.07772	-.05139	.01881	-.04009
LSS17	-.02038	.60439	-.07325	-.08234	.05247	.05090	-.05014	.02899
LSS18	.00959	-.00228	-.00771	.02037	.00189	-.00796	-.00421	.03670
LSS19	.00250	-.00425	-.00797	-.00561	-.02563	-.00902	-.00092	.01819
LSS20	.18645	-.05285	-.00863	-.00953	-.04590	-.01548	.00628	.12767
LSS21	.50992	-.00250	.06461	-.04114	.05175	-.03716	.02198	-.22152
LSS22	.13239	-.01193	-.05362	-.04957	.44503	.02355	-.09679	.07731
LSS23	.10878	.03688	-.00206	.03336	.14772	.02639	.05684	-.03366
LSS24	.07486	.06081	.16335	-.00723	.18042	.00943	.09249	-.05272
LSS25	.03940	-.01275	.06958	.01491	.06343	.03785	-.03318	.08578
LSS26	.07793	.04108	.07717	-.01169	.09980	.02502	.03467	-.02079
LSS27	-.22210	-.02020	-.02800	-.05124	.01430	-.02353	-.03561	-.01981
LSS28	-.10026	-.04977	.05644	-.07600	.03243	-.05411	-.00717	.02921
LSS29	-.07888	-.00713	-.03369	.58450	-.00039	-.05243	-.00248	.06384
LSS30	-.04087	.04166	.07576	.01992	-.08612	.04064	.61907	.07975
LSS31	-.07106	.02283	.01499	-.14652	.05599	.42032	.09933	-.20472
LSS32	-.08336	.04272	.18322	-.04804	.24131	.08331	.06078	-.08960
LSS33	.02961	.06138	-.05220	-.01537	.09507	-.06969	.62624	-.04917
LSS34	-.06912	-.01125	.02315	-.00660	-.17302	.60973	-.05992	.06573
LSS35	-.08390	-.00806	.01522	.04787	.13893	.41879	-.03574	.03390
LSS36	.43217	.03989	-.00400	-.07355	-.12795	-.01461	-.04363	.26365
LSS37	-.16080	.01284	.14248	-.06905	.19293	.00023	-.03768	.10171
LSS38	.10661	-.03265	-.09967	.04819	.50255	-.03798	.03309	-.02878
LSS39	-.00299	.04265	.02963	.53714	.02450	.00030	.00330	-.13980
LSS40	-.02759	.03101	.03344	-.04587	.02638	-.01002	.05037	.67224
LSS41	.03234	-.00350	-.07150	.04403	.01343	-.00768	-.00866	.00976
LSS42	.01170	-.05359	.55230	-.02651	-.15647	-.06104	.01637	-.13674
LSS43	.05610	-.01435	.49664	-.02219	-.00059	.00863	-.04314	.19953
LSS44	.03779	.04071	.15686	-.02568	-.01986	.02933	.08303	-.23985

151

Table 8.8b LSS: Factor score coefficient matrix (varimax rotation)

	FACTOR 1	FACTOR 2	FACTOR 3	FACTOR 4	FACTOR 5	FACTOR 6	FACTOR 7	FACTOR 8
LSS1	-.18302	-.01983	-.10780	-.00473	-.26374	.06316	-.06586	.03181
LSS2	-.18143	-.17005	-.05096	.01253	.17708	-.11068	.03019	-.03325
LSS3	.23261	.08367	-.12350	-.05243	.05390	.05662	-.00545	.08347
LSS4	.50171	.01193	-.10127	.02903	.09477	-.06406	.00602	-.03023
LSS5	.53151	-.03252	-.00187	.00140	.07057	-.01751	.00458	-.05065
LSS6	-.14773	-.03504	.09270	-.01105	.08572	.03383	.04338	-.02957
LSS7	-.04479	.04316	.03233	-.02389	.13997	.03143	-.01071	.04307
LSS8R	.02292	-.01847	.03651	.02624	.05405	-.05440	.05571	.02312
LSS9	-.02321	.00095	-.00770	-.02338	-.28581	.02718	-.00407	-.11074
LSS10	-.14511	-.04139	.06376	-.01258	-.04685	.04092	-.04632	.01190
LSS11	-.00755	.00121	-.06011	.04808	-.36955	-.10344	.01257	.00915
LSS12	-.04326	-.01477	-.04399	.01652	-.43832	.00392	.04757	.01317
LSS13	.11822	-.00623	.08545	.01947	-.06464	-.01949	.00243	-.06600
LSS14	.05633	-.02708	.05827	.03036	.03323	-.11975	.03073	.04778
LSS15	-.00870	.02935	-.05090	.06422	.03730	-.06253	.05397	.07563
LSS16	-.00928	-.01153	-.02758	-.04771	.05710	.00659	.59458	-.05615
LSS17	.04071	.02595	-.00828	.04155	.00278	-.10696	.61586	.01612
LSS18R	-.04346	.06650	-.07112	.03325	.11319	-.01465	-.00300	-.00842
LSS19	-.10358	.04659	.03827	.05335	.10129	-.01073	-.00295	.00269
LSS20	.03334	-.31234	.07005	-.04797	.00707	.00976	.04881	.21370
LSS21	-.12173	-.01942	.09426	-.05759	-.00291	.07519	.00874	.53989
LSS22	-.10762	.03759	.12831	-.02386	.15257	-.06726	.00417	.14281
LSS23	-.03562	.13309	-.03509	.50513	.06264	-.01054	-.03562	.12221
LSS24	.03923	-.01550	-.04032	.28399	.02884	.15752	-.05823	.08346
LSS25	-.04341	-.02371	.45601	-.02312	.06883	.08279	.01158	.05604
LSS26	-.09602	.04200	.48514	-.02875	.06904	-.06589	-.04090	.10043
LSS27	.01996	.37991	.05651	-.07095	-.00185	-.03865	.01660	-.19896
LSS28R	.09559	.37465	-.02004	-.07170	.03407	.04628	.04704	.07877
LSS29	-.03632	.09827	.03327	.01093	-.02533	-.04005	.01690	-.11270
LSS30	.04229	.04512	-.00956	-.05442	.01433	.08520	-.03354	-.04530
LSS31	-.12996	.11029	-.13957	.01567	.02960	-.03850	-.02173	-.04786
LSS32	-.05797	.07131	-.25708	.02167	-.00769	.14524	-.03860	-.06959
LSS33	-.01499	.03711	-.03600	.01759	-.03099	-.04476	.07208	.04054
LSS34	.05043	-.11388	.05167	.03400	.05712	-.02333	.00155	-.10247
LSS35	.09246	.02974	.06512	.04919	-.02444	-.03087	.00324	.07480
LSS36	.16796	-.05080	.10292	.03753	-.03858	.01022	.03348	.41018
LSS37	.04546	.26136	-.05981	-.00768	-.00817	.14608	-.01344	.16117
LSS38	.12663	-.04396	.07667	.01331	.09242	-.12022	.03157	-.09130
LSS39	.05143	.02031	.02687	.03807	.03440	.02324	.05817	-.00422
LSS40	.00621	.00688	.01491	.00567	.00876	.01870	-.04693	.06165
LSS41	-.02301	-.01608	-.00982	.49392	-.03853	-.07798	.00363	.02575
LSS42	.00912	.04687	.10598	-.00214	.01119	.57929	.06669	.04090
LSS43	-.07905	-.02094	-.09728	-.00533	.04882	.49636	.01934	.05972
LSS44	-.02327	.09843	.13406	-.03212	-.05484	.16543	-.03222	.06732

Table 8.8b LSS: Factor score coefficient matrix (varimax rotation) (continued)

	FACTOR 9	FACTOR 10	FACTOR 11	FACTOR 12	FACTOR 13	FACTOR 14	FACTOR 15	FACTOR 16
LSS1	.01386	.04799	.20188	.03768	-.01923	.01813	.13272	-.02376
LSS2	-.01916	.09431	.02454	.25597	.01206	-.22483	-.08372	-.20396
LSS3	-.00832	.10694	-.02601	.06469	-.00050	-.03573	-.06615	-.03596
LSS4	.03295	.05612	.01532	-.01647	-.01419	-.04548	.03516	.06571
LSS5	.07178	-.02514	.00286	-.00662	-.02888	-.07423	.05891	.12642
LSS6	.03249	.04182	-.06114	-.07219	.04176	.11470	-.10755	.53056
LSS7	.03292	-.08358	-.04782	-.08197	-.06412	.06056	.04318	-.46195
LSS8	.08565	-.14700	.06273	-.01171	.00526	.11172	.09579	-.35341
LSS9	.05449	-.07108	-.04888	-.04905	.00891	.16329	-.09779	.10609
LSS10	.18004	.02021	.10757	.01050	.03362	.48562	-.10656	-.08448
LSS11	.07986	.03306	-.01174	.00676	-.03453	-.00776	.00944	.04903
LSS12	.08945	-.05977	-.04229	.01057	-.00302	-.03772	-.03338	.13558
LSS13	.00557	-.02794	-.02496	-.09941	.00108	.12337	.05293	-.07944
LSS14	.12101	.05674	-.04787	.02422	-.00730	.28218	.07850	.09422
LSS15	-.12456	-.06836	.09729	-.01226	.06638	.37593	.09135	.07606
LSS16	.04456	-.04670	.05815	.02566	-.01327	.00685	-.07849	.08910
LSS17	-.01572	.05463	.05138	-.10770	.06018	-.00813	.03988	.02193
LSS18	.54561	-.00373	.04841	.02608	.00694	-.14666	.01567	.06715
LSS19	.55156	-.00533	.02972	.01000	.00414	.17634	-.04592	.00689
LSS20	-.01481	-.00443	.12266	-.00335	-.01059	-.08285	-.03496	-.01475
LSS21	.02505	-.05226	-.20800	-.05047	.01697	.04229	.03073	-.08640
LSS22	.05455	.01982	.07722	-.05477	.09745	-.22116	.41965	-.03385
LSS23	.01465	.01751	-.02716	.02499	-.06052	-.13294	.13995	.01881
LSS24	-.06603	-.00672	-.03665	-.00589	.09142	-.14479	.16483	-.01199
LSS25	.06046	.03786	.08278	.00864	.03560	.07910	.06532	-.03382
LSS26	.04789	.02171	.02154	.00192	-.02971	.03922	.10151	-.15760
LSS27	-.00985	-.02258	-.02756	-.05131	.03369	-.03691	.01785	-.01218
LSS28	.08632	-.05343	.02967	-.07537	-.00337	.06413	.02704	.06374
LSS29	-.02394	-.06145	.05020	.59553	.00134	.06651	.00985	.05679
LSS30	.06469	.02822	.08894	.01876	.62307	.02131	-.07200	-.02720
LSS31	.07946	.41605	.20216	.15141	.08915	.15545	.05361	-.03457
LSS32	.08243	.06583	.09310	.04331	.05992	.26321	.24470	-.04689
LSS33	-.04540	-.08565	-.03773	-.00923	.62917	-.09262	.10842	-.04118
LSS34	-.05450	.62659	.06183	-.01645	.06399	-.13166	-.19014	.05132
LSS35	-.14276	.42005	.03216	.03791	.03907	.04173	.13250	.08902
LSS36	.04030	-.00811	.27495	-.08402	.04240	.01941	-.14896	.14117
LSS37	.01039	.00711	-.09654	-.05977	.03546	-.09921	.19581	.05640
LSS38	.04640	-.04085	-.02779	.05670	.03176	.02657	.52867	.01422
LSS39	.00668	-.01028	.15307	.55178	-.00292	.09918	.04215	.13165
LSS40	-.03850	-.00899	.67803	-.06052	.05517	.07011	.01652	.05429
LSS41	-.06117	.00796	.00988	.04832	.01473	.05263	.01253	.01358
LSS42	.05552	-.06551	-.13191	-.02320	-.02223	.05371	-.17295	.06702
LSS43	.02674	-.00143	.21177	.01133	.03516	-.09890	-.03623	-.11876
LSS44	-.07803	.02501	-.23407	-.02567	.08181	-.04666	-.03128	.04097

The Depression Scale (DS)

In contrast to the life stress items, the proposed depression scale (DS) seems to be more internally consistent, as indicated by more notable correlations among the items. Accordingly, principal components analysis extracted 7 factors out of the 25 items, explaining 56.1% of the total variance (see Table 8.9). Tables 8.10a and 8.10b contain the rotated matrices that display the sorted factor loadings; the factor correlation matrix for factors resulted from oblique rotation is also given in Table 8.10c.

A primary conclusion drawn from the results of factor analysis is, however, that depression is a multidimensional phenomenon. Therefore, just like social support as well as life stress, this field is not amenable to unidimensional scaling treatment when conceptualized under the framework discussed earlier. As the first step of the multidimensional scaling procedures being developed in this book, the two as well as some other sets of factor scores based on different methods of extraction and rotation are obtained and saved as some subscales to be further handled. Tables 8.11a and 8.11b give the factor score coefficients used to calculate regression method factor scores for the depression items.

Table 8.9 DS: Final statistics for factors extracted by principal components
analysis (PC)

VARIABLE	COMMUNALITY	*	FACTOR	EIGENVALUE	PCT OF VAR	CUM PCT
DS1	.64166	*	1	6.11708	24.5	24.5
DS2	.60349	*	2	1.86892	7.5	31.9
DS3	.55486	*	3	1.79899	7.2	39.1
DS4	.49839	*	4	1.17154	4.7	43.8
DS5	.81246	*	5	1.04809	4.2	48.0
DS6	.38095	*	6	1.01241	4.0	52.1
DS7	.82601	*	7	1.00052	4.0	56.1
DS8	.44588	*				
DS9	.51967	*				
DS10	.60639	*				
DS11	.51983	*				
DS12	.33873	*				
DS13	.60760	*				
DS14	.64275	*				
DS15	.61787	*				
DS16	.64340	*				
DS17	.66591	*				
DS18	.65430	*				
DS19	.73765	*				
DS20	.35285	*				
DS21	.53089	*				
DS22	.36388	*				
DS23	.52200	*				
DS24	.65223	*				
DS25	.27791	*				

155

Table 8.10a DS: Rotated factor matrix (varimax)

	FACTOR 1	FACTOR 2	FACTOR 3	FACTOR 4	FACTOR 5	FACTOR 6	FACTOR 7
DS1	.76468	.10091	.02927	.18344	.10629	.00128	-.03056
DS10	.75629	.12730	-.04856	-.02368	-.04387	.09833	.06084
DS3	.70791	.05722	.06303	-.02153	-.00539	.21339	.02119
DS21	.69438	.13623	-.00853	-.10560	.13218	-.00704	-.03762
DS2	.68929	.00085	.04361	.26356	.18564	-.08229	-.12559
DS23	.67421	.07726	.04644	-.14765	-.02856	.16252	.10144
DS4	.62796	.02719	.09756	.25462	-.02090	.05818	-.15859
DS11	.62752	.20299	.04380	.13402	.18048	.16247	-.07742
DS8	.58975	.03788	-.00144	.24694	.04962	-.10940	-.14570
DS12	.51196	.07576	-.08387	.00559	.14341	.04069	.20396
DS15	.11700	.76237	.02812	.04356	.06008	.08522	-.09704
DS14	.10936	.73708	.01589	.05986	.24486	.15265	.02006
DS9	.25702	.57551	.04011	.29074	-.04435	-.17930	.04629
DS7	-.00838	.01413	.90854	-.00573	.01091	.01174	-.00007
DS5	.01552	.03973	.89854	.05411	.00691	.01642	-.00452
DS17	.08345	.13954	.03118	.74132	.20339	.15265	.15581
DS16	.30726	.01992	-.03009	.70892	.16992	.05733	.11383
DS20	.06464	.24644	-.01880	.47002	-.12765	.14770	-.16900
DS19	.08503	.24923	.01323	.05166	.81347	.05832	.01792
DS18	.39119	-.01278	.02384	.20905	.66899	.08203	-.05051
DS13	.03282	.09688	-.09722	.16432	.04133	.74761	-.00749
DS6	.21004	-.05296	.25867	.02006	.07853	.48589	-.15640
DS22	.14640	.33463	-.01786	.17303	.04028	.39687	.20266
DS24	.13732	.02845	.15355	.02951	.01249	-.03390	.77898
DS25	.15463	.07125	.24402	-.05541	.03554	.01094	-.43003

156

Table 8.10b DS: Pattern matrix (oblimin rotation)

	FACTOR 1	FACTOR 2	FACTOR 3	FACTOR 4	FACTOR 5	FACTOR 6	FACTOR 7
DS10	.7947R	.07484	-.07009	.0917R	.05564	.09221	.0502R
DS1	.73903	.02970	.00545	.1197R	-.03366	-.06121	-.05629
DS3	.7285?	-.00449	.03797	.0831?	.02106	.05154	.17066
DS23	.70944	.02998	.02633	.21389	.09822	.01026	.11990
DS21	.670R6	.07R13	-.01525	-.03790	-.04406	-.09468	-.061R0
DS2	.640?7	-.07214	.01789	.21595	-.12894	.15294	-.13349
DS4	.60595	.03R61	.07223	-.21477	-.15223	.064R2	.01711
DS11	.57471	.11270	.02500	.061RR	.07142	-.13703	.10550
DS8	.56645	-.01561	-.0229R	-.20R24	-.14694	-.0172R	-.15134
DS12	.51054	.02725	-.09081	.04250	.19280	-.11582	.00141
DS15	.02563	.77713	.01715	.05741	-.1040R	-.03039	.029R3
DS14	-.0175?	.73311	.0074R	.0445R	.00642	.21971	.09271
DS9	.18413	.56986	.04689	-.22682	.05100	.08611	-.23832
DS7	-.08454	.01014	.920R2	.00772	.05497	.00470	-.01336
DS5	-.069R4	.02986	.91054	-.05032	.05057	.01312	-.01212
DS17	-.084R0	.04R84	.04231	-.74525	.15967	-.16646	.11970
DS16	.174R1	-.07975	.03429	-.71155	.11874	-.12864	.01961
DS20	-.010R9	.21114	-.02636	-.45RR6	-.16313	.16273	.13033
DS24	.14309	-.00192	.20335	-.0367R	.79442	.01784	-.06037
DS25	.12599	.07575	.21314	.08971	-.42186	-.03542	-.00310
DS19	-.10575	.20518	-.00363	.02202	-.01294	.83506	.01046
DS18	.23992	-.09715	-.00266	-.15620	-.07305	-.67086	.03612
DS13	-.027?6	.03046	-.11870	-.1419R	-.01R11	-.01225	.75045
DS6	.16406	-.10713	.23120	.00500	-.14779	-.05745	.47721
DS22	.07997	.2R854	-.01786	-.12756	.19890	-.00074	.36724

Table 8.10c DS: Factor correlation matrix (oblimin rotation)

	FACTOR 1	FACTOR 2	FACTOR 3	FACTOR 4	FACTOR 5	FACTOR 6	FACTOR 7
FACTOR 1	1.00000						
FACTOR 2	.21067	1.00000					
FACTOR 3	.11979	.02867	1.00000				
FACTOR 4	-.25350	-.23673	-.02083	1.00000			
FACTOR 5	-.021R1	.02611	-.12349	.03062	1.00000		
FACTOR 6	-.27120	-.14433	-.06080	.15440	-.05065	1.00000	
FACTOR 7	.13012	.15554	.06620	-.08092	.01702	-.10178	1.00000

157

Table 8.11a DS: Factor score coefficient matrix (oblimin rotation)

	FACTOR 1	FACTOR 2	FACTOR 3	FACTOR 4	FACTOR 5	FACTOR 6	FACTOR 7
DS1	.18013	-.02751	-.01112	-.01736	-.02971	.02778	-.08703
DS2	.12766	-.10501	-.00678	-.10873	-.12374	-.06813	-.15991
DS3	.22149	-.04214	.00617	.13674	.03004	.11028	.15386
DS4	.14620	-.07442	.02117	-.12566	-.14213	.13565	-.00759
DS5	-.06751	.00645	.50687	-.02596	.05330	.02845	-.02927
DS6	.00272	-.15296	.10041	.05676	-.13824	-.01482	.45256
DS7	-.06295	.00021	.51350	.01541	.05923	.00880	-.02399
DS8	.13189	-.04182	-.02646	-.12579	-.13938	.04829	-.17143
DS9	.00034	.39455	.02856	-.11083	.03876	.18230	-.30436
DS10	.25622	.03291	-.04846	.14165	.06310	.15102	.03470
DS11	.11254	.02446	.00063	.05652	.06616	-.03365	.05782
DS12	.13873	-.01504	-.04980	.10433	.18496	-.05627	-.01682
DS13	-.07193	-.09904	-.09328	-.03565	-.02696	.06655	.69562
DS14	-.10672	.47027	-.00935	.17464	-.00815	-.09933	-.00077
DS15	-.05962	.53420	-.00548	.15546	-.10808	.06728	-.05282
DS16	-.07820	.17874	.01562	.50656	.09154	.00176	-.04340
DS17	-.18028	-.10270	.02092	-.52097	.12374	-.02413	.03807
DS18	-.08391	-.18424	-.02358	-.00526	-.08472	-.55612	-.01480
DS19	-.20855	.04463	-.01914	.16451	-.03355	-.71860	-.05936
DS20	-.07189	.08992	-.03001	-.33781	-.16835	.24260	.07478
DS21	.16374	.01682	-.02240	.04894	-.03933	-.01435	-.09096
DS22	-.03350	.12369	-.01622	-.00898	.17921	.09436	.30304
DS23	.23158	.00039	.00587	.24251	.10552	.05526	.11051
DS24	.06078	-.02015	.15671	.00646	.75447	.04929	-.06830
DS25	.01233	.05959	.09134	.08402	-.39535	-.03050	-.01013

Table 8.11b DS: Factor score coefficient matrix (varimax rotation)

	FACTOR 1	FACTOR 2	FACTOR 3	FACTOR 4	FACTOR 5	FACTOR 6	FACTOR 7
DS1	.16735	-.01984	-.00686	.02408	-.02090	-.07821	-.03021
DS2	.13981	-.09215	.00107	.10641	.06594	-.15293	-.12295
DS3	.17756	-.03216	.01379	-.12436	-.09678	.15521	.02843
DS4	.13423	-.06168	.03034	.11977	-.12361	-.00698	-.14903
DS5	-.02732	.00699	.49661	.02192	-.01910	-.01665	.02153
DS6	.01538	-.12262	.12176	-.05428	.02001	.43968	-.14115
DS7	-.02563	-.00088	.50381	-.01754	-.00152	-.01162	.02814
DS8	.12857	-.03757	-.02022	.12282	-.04469	-.16558	-.14119
DS9	.01185	.36454	.01348	.13292	-.16429	-.27868	.03065
DS10	.19954	.03223	-.04557	-.12525	-.13599	.04081	.06322
DS11	.11314	.03585	.00269	-.04068	.04097	.06729	.06855
DS12	.11988	-.00753	-.05554	-.09396	.05952	-.00855	.19058
DS13	-.05987	-.05400	-.07558	.03453	-.04992	.67438	-.02093
DS14	-.06072	.44268	-.00760	-.11698	.10150	.02437	.00080
DS15	-.03730	.49357	-.00106	-.09764	-.05813	-.02852	-.10472
DS16	-.01861	-.13302	.00208	.46550	.01145	-.04295	.08335
DS17	-.09923	-.05651	.00508	.48416	.03831	.03905	.11660
DS18	.00872	-.15216	-.00926	.01540	.52551	-.00738	-.06545
DS19	-.08655	.05493	-.00791	-.12514	.67755	-.04034	-.00630
DS20	-.04877	.10046	-.02671	.32498	-.22183	.07184	-.17701
DS21	.15297	.01809	-.01658	-.03410	.01722	-.08059	-.03675
DS22	-.02623	.13975	-.02190	.02007	-.07394	.30520	.17882
DS23	.18193	.00228	.00983	-.22135	-.04580	.11602	.10676
DS24	.03700	-.00477	.10657	-.02366	-.02779	-.05343	.74079
DS25	.02886	.04479	.11742	-.06324	.02161	-.00830	-.39717

The personal coping proxy scales

Principal components analysis extracted 4 factors out of the 11 items comprising the Health Behaviors and Beliefs (HBB) measure, explaining 56.6% of the total variance (see Table 8.12a). Since the components structure is fairly consistent across different methods of rotation, only the factor loadings obtained by varimax rotation are displayed in Table 8.12b. Table 8.12c is the corresponding factor score coefficients.

For the Attitudes Toward Social Support (ATSS) measure that consisted of 9 individual items, 3 factors were extracted by principle component analysis, explaining 74.2% of the total variance (see Table 8.13a). Tables 8.13b and 8.13c provide the information similar to the kinds that are explicated in the above.

For the Attitudes Toward Elderly (ATE) measure, the 4 items ended up with a reduced 2-factor structure, representing 77.3% of the total variance (see Tables 8.14a through 8.14c).

Different sets of factor scores for each of the three proxy measures are saved for use in further scaling efforts.

Table 8.12a   HBB: Final statistics for factors extracted by principal components analysis (PC)

VARIABLE	COMMUNALITY	*	FACTOR	EIGENVALUE	PCT OF VAR	CUM PCT
HBB1	.74134	*	1	2.35648	21.4	21.4
HBB2	.47773	*	2	1.45331	13.2	34.6
HBB3	.71148	*	3	1.24790	11.3	46.0
HBB4	.42980	*	4	1.16640	10.6	56.6
HBB5	.64922	*				
HBB6	.61824	*				
HBB7	.52166	*				
HBB8	.77298	*				
HBB9	.77163	*				
HBB10	.14337	*				
HBB11	.38664	*				

160

Table 8.12b HBB: Rotated factor matrix (varimax)

	FACTOR 1	FACTOR 2	FACTOR 3	FACTOR 4
HBB5	.78245	.18337	.05075	.02815
HBB6	.77044	.09597	.09747	-.07711
HBB7	.70151	.07188	.10050	.11949
HBB9	.13123	.86843	-.01514	-.00390
HBB8	.15357	.85869	.02494	.10690
HBB1	.04940	-.03569	.83162	.21456
HBB3	.11391	.02074	.80409	-.22697
HBB11	.01700	.07013	-.05936	.61475
HBB4	-.22429	.09168	.21662	.56935
HBB2	.35631	-.15193	-.15231	.55180
HBB10	.13191	.04359	.23954	.25825

Table 8.12c HBB: Factor score coefficient matrix (varimax rotation)

	FACTOR 1	FACTOR 2	FACTOR 3	FACTOR 4
HBB1	-.04855	-.04426	.56020	.15643
HBB2	.20494	-.17779	-.14880	.45534
HBB3	.00672	.00152	.54794	-.22118
HBB4	-.19081	.07307	.15094	.48356
HBB5	.40695	.00445	-.03235	-.02942
HBB6	.41555	-.04921	.00406	-.11546
HBB7	.36891	-.06275	.00655	.05520
HBB8	-.05194	.55530	-.00308	.04744
HBB9	-.05632	.56980	-.02565	-.04403
HBB10	.03291	-.00165	.14577	.20199
HBB11	-.03118	.02149	-.05959	.51661

Table 8.13a ATSS: Final statistics for factors extracted by principal components analysis (PC)

VARIABLE	COMMUNALITY	*	FACTOR	EIGENVALUE	PCT OF VAR	CUM PCT
ATSS1	.96983	*	1	3.13506	34.8	34.8
ATSS2	.96956	*	2	1.94629	21.6	56.5
ATSS3	.85557	*	3	1.59641	17.7	74.2
ATSS4	.85725	*				
ATSS5	.59674	*				
ATSS6	.64073	*				
ATSS7	.60393	*				
ATSS8	.65360	*				
ATSS9	.53055	*				

161

Table 8.13b ATSS: Rotated factor matrix (varimax)

	FACTOR 1	FACTOR 2	FACTOR 3
ATSS8	.80739	.02737	.03109
ATSS6	.79483	.05756	.07529
ATSS7	.77394	-.06381	.02951
ATSS5	.76906	-.02541	.06817
ATSS9	.71775	-.07076	.10186
ATSS1	-.02248	.98446	-.01271
ATSS2	-.02651	.98392	-.02747
ATSS4	.07238	-.02610	.92268
ATSS3	.10955	-.01198	.91838

Table 8.13c ATSS: Factor score coefficient matrix (varimax rotation)

	FACTOR 1	FACTOR 2	FACTOR 3
ATSS1	.00797	.50538	.01435
ATSS2	.00775	.50474	.00578
ATSS3	-.03568	.01432	.54351
ATSS4	-.04901	.00660	.54877
ATSS5	.25846	-.00020	-.02076
ATSS6	.26799	.04298	-.01683
ATSS7	.26265	-.02065	-.04520
ATSS8	.27538	.02674	-.04504
ATSS9	.23747	-.02358	.00266

Table 8.14a ATE: Final statistics for factors extracted by principal components analysis (PC)

VARIABLE	COMMUNALITY	*	FACTOR	EIGENVALUE	PCT OF VAR	CUM PCT
ATE1	.77371	*	1	1.95572	48.9	48.9
ATE2	.71635	*	2	1.13545	28.4	77.3
ATE3	.80760	*				
ATE4	.79351	*				

Table 8.14b ATE: Rotated factor matrix (varimax)

	FACTOR 1	FACTOR 2
ATE3	.89704	.05404
ATE4	.87241	.18003
ATE1	.00392	.87960
ATE2	.23870	.81202

Table 8.14c ATE: Factor score coefficient matrix (varimax rotation)

	FACTOR 1	FACTOR 2
ATE1	-.15696	.64208
ATE2	.01055	.55010
ATE3	.58337	-.12323
ATE4	.54423	-.02669

Note

1. When principal components analysis is performed by the procedure of factor analysis, it is very easy to confuse components with factors because of the unified computer statistical language. The rest of the book focuses on components even though the term "factors" is universally applied as usual.

163

9 The CAUS and the falsification of measurement models

In search of amenable measurement instruments, current multidimensional or multifactorial scaling methods were surveyed in the foregoing chapters. The state of the art mirrors a serious limitation of scaling in behavioral and social studies. Although there could be a variety of ways to deal with the results of a dimensional analysis (i.e., factors and factor scores), the lack of a guideline is a major source of confusion in measurement and incompatibility in substantive results.

In this chapter, methods for scaling multidimensional (multifactorial) constructs such as social support, stress, and depression are explored by elaborating on a central theme of unidimensionalization in psychosocial research. An attempt is made to establish a theoretical approach to unidimensionalization by learning from science, specifically from the strength theories in engineering mechanics, in order to bring a breakthrough to the stalemate or the "ultimate" limit in scale development. A practical strategy of optimal weighting via multiple regression is also explored to extend the scaling effort beyond the factors (components) level. These approaches, articulated as the Chen Approaches to Unidimensionalized Scaling (CAUS), systematize and symbolize a variety of generalized and standardized scaling models based on either theoretical assumptions or practical interests. A few specific scaling hypotheses are articulated to illustrate the theoretical approach, as well as to provide some specific scaling archetypes for empirical inquiry.

Multiple measures are developed based on different models and methods for the key constructs involved in the current study. For each construct, results obtained with different scale instruments are compared, and those proven more

164

powerful or effective in detecting the relationships among the theoretical constructs are recommended. The logical requirements for relational analysis with specific objectives are followed, and the opportunity of achieving effectiveness with multiple scaling procedures is demonstrated. All these show the importance of research purpose, theoretical understanding, and appropriate measurement manipulation in psychosocial research.

Theory-guided unidimensionalization

What is important to practice is to prove theoretical constructs like social support, life stress and depression are scalable, as well as to explore the ways in which meaningful global scales may be derived. By the theoretical approach to unidimensionalization discussed in the methodology chapter, the key point is to articulate appropriate theoretical assumptions underlying various scaling strategies and to validate or falsify them using empirical design. By learning from science, we have got some tips as to how general approaches to global scaling may be formulated. In the following, I shall try to establish some of the measurement hypotheses by unfolding their corresponding scaling programs for the construction of the desired global measures.

Hypothesis 1. The effect of a multidimensional measure is determined by its maximum (in terms of absolute value) component score. This can be called the maximum component (factor) theory for scaling any multidimensional psychosocial construct. If G stands for the score on a global scale and abs(P_i) for the absolute value of the ith component score, then the hypothesis can be expressed by the equation

$$G = \max\{abs(P_i)\} \qquad i=1,2,...,n \qquad (1)$$

in which "max{ }" is a function used to extract the maximum from the assemblage of absolute values of the components that are numbered n.

It should be pointed out that the "maximum component" in this hypothesis is case-specific, considering the relative magnitude of all the components of, for example, social support to each individual, other than its general distribution among the population that distinguishes between the relative importance of

165

components in explaining the total variance. In fact, if the latter is the case, then we have a different hypothesis.

Hypothesis 2. The effect of a multidimensional measure is determined by its first component, which represents a maximum portion of its total variance among a population. This can be called the first principal component (factor) theory. Using the same mathematical denotation as above, we have a general equation to express this hypothesis:

$$G = P_1 \qquad\qquad (2)$$

Compared to the maximum component theory, this hypothesis seems to involve a well-known "ecological fallacy" in methodology (Li, 1988). It emphasizes on the relative magnitude of the first component of a measure in light of the total variance among the population explained rather than on its real importance to the individuals, which are in real terms the analytic unit of most psychosocial studies. Nevertheless, both theories are comparable in that all other components of less importance are simply dropped.

Measures like such, indeed, might not be regarded as "global." The approaches explicated here, however, distinguish themselves by clearly articulating theoretically plausible hypotheses and building firmly on empirical components analysis. In applying the second hypothesis, for example, we secure a truly unidimensional scale that fits the data better than any other arbitrarily chosen variables, that explains or represents the largest portion of the total variance, or measurement information. Also, the first hypothesis introduces a way of unidimensionalization with more theoretical underpinning by learning from science, though the qualitative difference among various psychosocial components may prevent its use in multifactorial scaling from matching its counterpart in engineering mechanics.

Hypothesis 3. The effect of a multidimensional measure is determined by the sum total of its components. This can be called the summated factors (components) theory, which is the simplest additivity hypothesis applied to components. The mathematical expression of this hypothesis is

$$G=\sum P_i \qquad i=1,2,...,n \qquad (3)$$

where $\sum P_i$ represents summation of all the extracted components that are numbered n.

This hypothesis theorizes the usual practice of summated scaling, except that they are based on the results of factor or components analysis rather than on the original items. In theory, this has several advantages. First, component scores are standardized based on the variance and covariance matrices, which make unnecessary any arbitrary treatment of the original items. Second, it makes clear multidimensionality of the psychosocial phenomena and the necessity of supplying appropriate grounds for performing unidimensionalization in measurement. This focal issue is consolidated with the weighting problem in determining the relative importance of various components. As mentioned earlier, it is injurious for a simple summation strategy to completely ignore this issue even in unidimensional scaling. The matter has doubled significance in multifactorial scaling.

The pursuit of an appropriate weighting scheme, however, is extremely difficult in the psychosocial field where the subject matter is highly complicated while the state of the art is yet premature. For example, we do not yet have a theory in life stress or social support studies that has the potential comparable to Hooke's Law in science and engineering, by which we can go some distance beyond the crude and inaccurate hypotheses explicated above. We do not have any other established transformation formula to relate different components as simple as the maximum share stress theory or as complex as the distortion energy theory in engineering mechanics either (Timoshenko & Young, 1962). Indeed, in psychosocial studies we are uncertain about the relationship between different components of a specific phenomenon, like stress or social support, in terms of their various effects on human life. Without such knowledge, although we can conceive of some mathematically more elegant transformations, such as letting $G=(\sum F_i^2)^{1/2}$, we cannot determine the substantive meaning of the derived scales. It seems at present, we can only theoretically formulate the primitive, generally summated scales with some simplified all-1 and 0-or-1 weighting schemes, such as those represented by the above hypotheses. When the all-1 weighting scheme is applied, however, the validity of a scale based on components instead of individual items may not be improved, since they are "too precise" (in terms of the clarification of dimensionality) on the one hand and too crude (in terms of the uncertainty of the relationships among factors being pooled together) on the other.

The rules-of-thumb represented by the conventional "experts" approach should not be the only way for better weighting, however. Compared with the case of engineering science, we have more expedient statistical means for factoring in psychosocial studies. Therefore, efforts ought to be invested in future studies to work out feasible strategies with more solid theoretical and empirical grounds. There are many ways of constructing a scale that can be explored, indeed. For example, we may try to take the absolute values of the components before summing them up. Space forbids, however, and I will only apply the articulated hypotheses to the scaling of the major theoretical constructs involved in the present study. Later, I shall consider some empirical means as an alternative to the theoretical approach.

Stress

The first general hypothesis (Equation 1) takes root in the maximum stress theory in science. Note the hypothesis and the corresponding scaling method do not limit themselves to the 16 factors extracted from the specific data by the default settings of the statistical (SPSS-X) programs. In other words, it is not dependent on particular manners of factor extraction. We can actually specify different numbers of factors to be extracted. To expand the range of comparison, two larger numbers, namely, 22 and 44, are also used as the criteria respectively. The latter is the maximum number of items and factors. The former is chosen somewhat arbitrary (half the maximum), though also based on an inspection of the distribution of the eigenvalues (nearly 70% of the total variance explained by the 22 factors in contrast to only 57.1% for the first 16 factors). Note, however, if different numbers are specified as different criteria for factor extraction, factor loadings as well as values of the maximum components may vary. Suppose the score on a global life stress scale based on the first hypothesis is symbolized as LSSH1, and abs($LSPCOB_i$) is used to mark the absolute value of the ith component obtained by oblique rotation. The particular equations for scaling life stress based on the first hypothesis, which can be termed the maximum stress theory in this case, can be written as

LSSH1=max(abs(LSPCOB1),...,abs(LSPCOB16)), or
LSSH1=max(abs(LSPCOB1),...,abs(LSPCOB22)), or
LSSH1=max(abs(LSPCOB1),...,abs(LSPCOB44)),

using SPSS-X language. The last equation is somewhat similar to extracting the maximum from all the 44 original items, but the principal components are standardized and optimally ranked and therefore suitable for comparative purposes. It is worth noticing that this scaling strategy is in line with the DSM-III-R suggestions, which state that "When more than one stressor is present, the severity rating will generally be that of the most severe stressor" (American Psychiatric Association, 1987:19).

The second general hypothesis (see Equation 2) can be translated into the following specific form when scaling life stress:

LSSH2=LSPCOB1

where LSSH2 denotes the score on a global life stress scale based on the second hypothesis and LSPCOB1 the first component obtained by oblique rotation. This is probably the simplest way for scaling multi-factorial constructs. Similarly, the first factor (component) can be a result of different methods or criteria used in extraction. Instead of expanding to larger numbers of components, here I intend to examine the difference by comparing the result obtained by the default settings of SPSS-X with that by specifying only 1 factor (the minimum number of components) as the criterion for extraction. Such a solution free from concerns of rotation presumably would have the highest discriminating power as a measurement scale. Note that if I have specified only 1 factor in applying Hypothesis 1, it would have lost its case-specific "maximum" meaning and turned into Hypothesis 2.

As for the third hypothesis, from the usual practice of simple summation we immediately get an equation for the present study:

LSSH3=sum(LSPCOB1 to LSPCOB44).

The only difference is that we are using standardized components instead of original items. Recognizing the utility of factor analysis in data reduction, this hypothesis may narrow down its scope by taking the following forms:

LSSH3=sum(LSPCOB1 to LSPCOB22),

or more conventionally by default setting,

169

LSSH3=sum(LSPCOB1 to LSPCOB16).

Social support

In scaling social support, the first general hypothesis (Equation 1) can be called the maximum support theory. For the present study, I use SSSH1 to symbolize the score on a global social support scale based on this hypothesis, and abs($SSPCOB_i$) to mark the absolute value of the *ith* component obtained by oblique rotation (see factor analysis results presented earlier). Accordingly, I have the following working programs for the scaling of social support based on the maximum support theory:

SSSH1=max(abs(SSPCOB1),...,abs(SSPCOB9)), or
SSSH1=max(abs(SSPCOB1),...,abs(SSPCOB14)), or
SSSH1=max(abs(SSPCOB1),...,abs(SSPCOB29)).

From the second general hypothesis (see Equation 2), similarly, I can derive another type of global social support scales by the simplest method,

SSSH2=SSPCOB1,

in which the first component can be taken from different components pools extracted by different criteria.

For the third general hypothesis (see Equation 3), the following specific programs can be formulated for scaling social support in this study:

SSSH3=sum(SSPCOB1 to SSPCOB29), or
SSSH3=sum(SSPCOB1 to SSPCOB14), or
SSSH3=sum(SSPCOB1 to SSPCOB9).

Depression

Suppose DSH1 is the score on a global depression scale based on the first general hypothesis (Equation 1), and abs($DSPCOB_i$) the absolute value of the *ith* component obtained by oblique rotation (cf. factor analysis results presented earlier). The working programs for scaling depression under the "maximum depression" theory can be shown as follows, using SPSS-X language:

170

DSH1=max(abs(DSPCOB1),...,abs(DSPCOB6)), or
DSH1=max(abs(DSPCOB1),...,abs(DSPCOB12)), or
DSH1=max(abs(DSPCOB1),...,abs(DSPCOB25)).

For the second hypothesis, the "first component" theory (see Equation 2),

DSH2=DSPCOB1.

For the third, simple summation hypothesis (see Equation 3),

DSH3=sum(DSPCOB1 to DSPCOB25), or
DSH3=sum(DSPCOB1 to DSPCOB12), or
DSH3=sum(DSPCOB1 to DSPCOB6).

Personal coping

Suppose HBBH1, ATSSH1 and ATEH1 are the scores on the three personal co-ping proxy scales based on the first general hypothesis (see Equation 1), respectively, and abs($HBPCOB_i$), abs($ASPCOB_i$) and abs($AEPCOB_i$) the absolute values of their ith components obtained by oblique rotation. The working programs for scaling these personal coping proxies based on the "maximum personal coping" theory can be derived accordingly. For the Health Behaviors and Beliefs (HBB) measure,

HBBH1=max(abs(HBPCOB1),...,abs(HBPCOB4)), or
HBBH1=max(abs(HBPCOB1),...,abs(HBPCOB11)).

For the Attitudes Toward Social Support (ATSS) measure,

ATSSH1=max(abs(ASPCOB1),...,abs(ASPCOB3)), or
ATSSH1=max(abs(ASPCOB1),...,abs(ASPCOB9)).

For the Attitudes Toward Elderly (ATE) measure,

ATEH1=max(abs(AEPCOB1),abs(AEPCOB2)), or
ATEH1=max(abs(AEPCOB1),...,abs(AEPCOB4)).

171

Similarly, from the second general hypothesis (see Equation 2) the following specific scaling programs can be formulated for the three personal coping proxies:

HBBH2=HBPCOB1,
ATSSH2=ASPCOB1, and
ATEH2=AEPCOB1.

The third general hypothesis (see Equation 3) provides another rationale for establishing these proxy measures. For the Health Behaviors and Beliefs (HBB) measure,

HBBH3=sum(HBPCOB1 to HBPCOB4), or
HBBH1=sum(HBPCOB1 to HBPCOB11).

For the Attitudes Toward Social Support (ATSS) measure,

ATSSH1=sum(ASPCOB1 to ASPCOB3), or
ATSSH1=sum(ASPCOB1 to ASPCOB9).

For the Attitudes Toward Elderly (ATE) measure,

ATEH1=sum(AEPCOB1,AEPCOB2), or
ATEH1=sum(AEPCOB1 to AEPCOB4).

Practice-oriented unidimensionalization

It should be pointed out that in the summated treatment of the factors (components), a procedure of component scaling could be performed to meet the requirement for additivity. This is similar to the item scaling procedure in unidimensional summated scale development (Donald & Ware, 1984), which is also applicable to the simple summation choice to obtain subscales in place of factor scores in multidimensional scaling. In the above, I did not touch the topic because I wanted to recap the usual practice, which has yet rarely gone beyond a simple summation. As a step forward, however, I need to show how the underlying assumptions could be addressed, and endowed with full meaning in an optimal approach to unidimensionalized scaling.

The additive hypothesis entails linearizing the relationships between the scaling items and some criterion variables. Such criterion variables are useful not just in preparing individual items for unidimensional summation, however. In general, the use of the criterion variables is an important strategy in statistical analysis, and in scale development in particular (e.g., criterion-related validity). By relating to the criterion measures based on our theoretical beliefs in their associations with the constructs to be scaled, we attain an important passageway to unidimensionalization. As discussed in the methodology chapter, multiple regression will yield optimal weights by using such criterion variables. And the statistical procedure has with it serviceable means for searching for violations of assumptions such as linearity and normality. Once serious violations are detected, remedy measures can be taken to transform the data to meet the requirements for such analysis. Nonlinear regression analysis may also be considered. These techniques, therefore, seem to outclass the conventional item scaling procedures.

The above strategy has a practical orientation since it targets specific criterion variables, which are usually of particular research or practice interest. To try out such an approach on the empirical basis, careful consideration of the criterion variables needs be taken for each of the key constructs to be scaled. For an intended Depression Scale (DS) in the present study, the 17-item CES-D employed in the original survey may serve as a criterion. In the absence of a well-established scale in measuring both life events and daily strains, the DS can be utilized as a criterion for scaling life stress based on the hypothetical stress-depression linkage. Similarly, the regression of the personal coping proxy scales may aim at its mediating effect on stress. Finally, based on the supposed extensive effects of social support, various measures of depression, life stress and personal coping may all serve as some criteria for its scaling.

All the criterion variables form certain causal links and flows ending at various measures of depression. The underlying assumptions and hypotheses, if taken as a whole, constitute exactly the causal model I have proposed for substantive inquiry, which has also rendered the context for construct validity. Now the model serves as the basis for further considering criterion-related validity, which again demonstrates the close relationship between scale development and substantive model building and testing.

It should be noted that for the existing 17-item CES-D scale, only some conventional analyses, such as reliability (internal consistency) as well as content validity, will be performed without further pursuit of its dimensionality. The major reason is that the conclusions about its utility have been drawn with the scale being used as-is, that is, usually only such routine tests were performed in arriving at those results. As they are deemed fairly universal, I should be able to use the scale as a criterion measure in developing a new depression scale as well as other needed measures. A reliability analysis using the available data renders Cronbach's $\alpha=.77$ (standardized item $\alpha=.82$) for the 17-item CES-D.[1] And an inspection of the frequency (histograms with normal curves imposed on) shows that the scale does not deviate substantially from normal distribution. To enhance the ultimate criterion while stay with the focus on new scales development, however, one more variable could be selected as an alternative to the 17-item CES-D. After a careful consideration of all the domains examined earlier, self ratings of general health (a single-item indicator) appears to be the other suitable and convenient yardstick for most constructs to be scaled.

Only linear multiple regression analysis is tried for scaling purposes. To avoid the interaction effects among the components, factor solutions from orthogonal rotation are used for regression analysis. This is indeed the advantage of the factor models over regression analysis using individual items. The analysis of residuals is also performed to ensure that no assumptions are seriously violated. The following will briefly report on the results of the multiple regression analyses using factor scores. The Depression Scale (DS) unidimensionalized by using its component scores in regression almost perfectly predicts the 17-item CES-D (R Square=.96). When targeted at self-rated health, foreseeably, R Square falls back to .19 (Multiple R=.44). The results of regression of life stress factors aimed at predicting the scores on the two Depression Scales (using the 17-item CES-D and self-rated health as criteria, respectively) are considerable. For the former, R Square=.26; for the latter, R Square=.45. Since personal coping may impact on both life stress and its disease consequence (depression), the factor scores of each of the proxy measures are regressed on the two corresponding sets of scales (each set contains two scales targeted at either the 17-item CES-D or self-rated health), respectively. However, none of the R Squares obtained exceeds .05, with the exception of the Attitudes Toward Elderly (ATE) scale in predicting life stress (the R Squares still fall below .09). This, on the one hand, indicates no remarkable bearing of the aspects measured on either depression or life stress. On the other, it suggests the proxy scales would hardly perform well in confirming the alleged relationship between the two constructs and personal coping. Since I have a stronger interest here in the

174

role of social support in influencing depression, stress and personal coping, three corresponding sets of results are especially shown in the following tables (see Tables 9.1a to 9.1e). For simplicity, only one scale is selected for each criterion construct in the regression of the social support components. In contrast to the personal coping proxy scales, the results for the Social Support Scale (SSS) are noteworthy. The R Squares are .32 in predicting the regressed depression measure (criterion: the 17-item CES-D), .24 in relation to the regressed life stress scale (criterion: the aforementioned regressed depression measure), and .11 in association with the regressed Health Behaviors and Beliefs measure (criterion: the aforementioned regressed depression measure). The other two personal coping proxy measures are less well predicted by the social support components, and therefore they will less likely be adopted in subsequent substantial model testing. Before I make such a conclusion, however, a more comprehensive examination of the scaling results is necessary, which will be given in the next section. For the purpose of testing the scaling models and methods expounded in the above (named the Chen Approaches to Unidimensionalized Scaling, or CAUS, for easy citation), all the standardized predicted values are saved as the scores of some new scales of depression, stress, social support, and personal coping.

Table 9.1a Regression of the SSS with the DS (RDSCESD)

DEPENDENT VARIABLE..   RDSCESD

	MEAN	STD DEV	LABEL
	-.022	.964	STANDARDIZED PREDICTED VALUE

VARIABLE(S) ENTERED ON STEP NUMBER

		MEAN	STD DEV	LABEL	
1..	SSPCOR9	.172	.971	REGR FACTOR SCORE	9
2..	SSPCOR7	.017	.890	REGR FACTOR SCORE	7
3..	SSPCOR5	.067	.847	REGR FACTOR SCORE	5
4..	SSPCOR2	-.066	1.003	REGR FACTOR SCORE	2
5..	SSPCOR3	.060	.999	REGR FACTOR SCORE	3
6..	SSPCOR8	-.002	.953	REGR FACTOR SCORE	8
7..	SSPCOR4	-.114	.918	REGR FACTOR SCORE	4
8..	SSPCOR6	.166	.696	REGR FACTOR SCORE	6
9..	SSPCOR1	.086	.994	REGR FACTOR SCORE	1

---------- VARIABLES IN THE EQUATION ----------

VARIABLE	B	SE B	BETA	T	SIG T
SSPCOR9	-.024593	.036813	-.024769	-.668	.5044
SSPCOR7	.019773	.041608	.018257	.475	.6348
SSPCOR5	-.618060	.041927	-.543085	-14.741	.0000
SSPCOR2	-.010593	.035474	-.011023	-.299	.7654
SSPCOR3	-.190851	.035282	-.197799	-5.409	.0000
SSPCOR8	.063108	.037404	.062396	1.687	.0922
SSPCOR4	.049093	.039058	.046742	1.257	.2094
SSPCOR6	-.162185	.052884	-.117095	-3.067	.0023
SSPCOR1	-.074795	.037316	-.077095	-2.004	.0456
(CONSTANT)	.073408	.037999		1.932	.0539

MULTIPLE R	.56943
R SQUARE	.32425
ADJUSTED R SQUARE	.31246
STANDARD ERROR	.79925

ANALYSIS OF VARIANCE

	DF	SUM OF SQUARES	MEAN SQUARE
REGRESSION	9	158.16415	17.57379
RESIDUAL	516	329.61994	.63880

F = 27.51071   SIGNIF F = .0000   N OF CASES = 526

176

Table 9.1b Regression of the SSS with the LSS (RLSRDSC)

		MEAN	STD DEV	LABEL	
DEPENDENT VARIABLE..	RLSRDSC	-.031	.947		

VARIABLE(S) ENTERED ON STEP NUMBER		MEAN	STD DEV	LABEL	STANDARDIZED PREDICTED VALUE
1..	SSPCOR9	.155	.928	REGR FACTOR SCORE	9
2..	SSPCOR3	.058	1.004	REGR FACTOR SCORE	3
3..	SSPCOR7	.112	.874	REGR FACTOR SCORE	7
4..	SSPCOR2	-.066	1.023	REGR FACTOR SCORE	2
5..	SSPCOR5	.012	.974	REGR FACTOR SCORE	5
6..	SSPCOR4	-.088	.920	REGR FACTOR SCORE	4
7..	SSPCOR8	.048	1.005	REGR FACTOR SCORE	8
8..	SSPCOR6	.177	.684	REGR FACTOR SCORE	6
9..	SSPCOR1	.101	.996	REGR FACTOR SCORE	1

------------- VARIABLES IN THE EQUATION -------------

VARIABLE	B	SE B	BETA	T	SIG T
SSPCOR9	-.076138	.057329	-.074567	-1.328	.1853
SSPCOR3	-.343535	.051940	-.364107	-6.614	.0000
SSPCOR7	-.098755	.064848	-.091081	-1.523	.1290
SSPCOR2	-.114883	.051887	-.124074	-2.214	.0277
SSPCOR5	-.231259	.054992	-.237842	-4.205	.0000
SSPCOR4	-.007042	.057153	-.006836	-.123	.9020
SSPCOR8	-.248745	.053803	-.263909	4.623	.0000
SSPCOR6	-.130477	.080941	-.094263	-1.612	.1082
SSPCOR1	-.290338	.056612	-.305131	-5.129	.0000
(CONSTANT)	.047085	.056787		.829	.4078

		ANALYSIS OF VARIANCE			
MULTIPLE R	.49195		DF	SUM OF SQUARES	MEAN SQUARE
R SQUARE	.24202	REGRESSION	9	58.43863	6.49318
ADJUSTED R SQUARE	.21578	RESIDUAL	260	183.02392	.70394
STANDARD ERROR	.83901				

F = 9.22408   SIGNIF F = .0000   N OF CASES = 270

Table 9.1c Regression of the SSS with the HBB (RHBRDSC)

	MEAN	STD DEV	LABEL
DEPENDENT VARIABLE..	RHBRDSC	-.157	1.039	STANDARDIZED PREDICTED VALUE

VARIABLE(S) ENTERED ON STEP NUMBER

Step		MEAN	STD DEV	LABEL	STANDARDIZED PREDICTED VALUE
1..	SSPCOR9	.167	.972	REGR FACTOR SCORE	9
2..	SSPCOR7	.009	.880	REGR FACTOR SCORE	7
3..	SSPCOR2	-.062	1.001	REGR FACTOR SCORE	2
4..	SSPCOR3	.030	1.003	REGR FACTOR SCORE	3
5..	SSPCOR5	.055	.873	REGR FACTOR SCORE	5
6..	SSPCOR8	-.007	.975	REGR FACTOR SCORE	8
7..	SSPCOR4	-.125	.911	REGR FACTOR SCORE	4
8..	SSPCOR1	.101	.989	REGR FACTOR SCORE	1
9..	SSPCOR6	.158	.702	REGR FACTOR SCORE	6

------------ VARIABLES IN THE EQUATION ------------

VARIABLE	B	SE B	BETA	T	SIG T
SSPCOR9	-.063415	.045263	-.059308	-1.401	.1618
SSPCOR7	-.204311	.052229	-.173076	-3.912	.0001
SSPCOR2	-.167596	.044052	-.161409	-3.805	.0002
SSPCOR3	-.109796	.043468	-.106020	-2.526	.0118
SSPCOR5	-.111762	.050643	-.093886	-2.207	.0278
SSPCOR8	.083630	.045131	.078428	1.853	.0644
SSPCOR4	.158135	.048910	.138705	3.233	.0013
SSPCOR1	-.050401	.046203	-.047957	-1.091	.2758
SSPCOR6	-.037252	.065135	.025155	.572	.5676
(CONSTANT)	-.126552	.046833		-2.702	.0071

		ANALYSIS OF VARIANCE		
MULTIPLE R	.33034		DF	SUM OF SQUARES	MEAN SQUARE
R SQUARE	.10913	REGRESSION	9	61.98255	6.88695
ADJUSTED R SQUARE	.09362	RESIDUAL	517	506.00344	.97873
STANDARD ERROR	.98931				

F = 7.03662   SIGNIF F = .0000   N OF CASES = 527

178

Table 9.1d Regression of the SSS with the ATSS (RASRDSC)

DEPENDENT VARIABLE..

	MEAN	STD DEV	LABEL
RASRDSC	-.061	.995	

VARIABLE(S) ENTERED ON STEP NUMBER

			STANDARDIZED PREDICTED VALUE
1..	SSPCOR9	.178	.972	REGR FACTOR SCORE	9
2..	SSPCOR7	.018	.880	REGR FACTOR SCORE	7
3..	SSPCOR2	-.067	.998	REGR FACTOR SCORE	2
4..	SSPCOR3	.057	1.002	REGR FACTOR SCORE	3
5..	SSPCOR5	.066	.854	REGR FACTOR SCORE	5
6..	SSPCOR8	-.007	.968	REGR FACTOR SCORE	8
7..	SSPCOR4	-.108	.915	REGR FACTOR SCORE	4
8..	SSPCOR6	.161	.694	REGR FACTOR SCORE	6
9..	SSPCOR1	.076	.982	REGR FACTOR SCORE	1

-------------- VARIABLES IN THE EQUATION --------------

VARIABLE	B	SE B	BETA	T	SIG T
SSPCOR9	-.004701	.042858	-.004594	-.110	.9127
SSPCOR7	-.106999	.049270	-.094599	-2.172	.0303
SSPCOR2	.016000	.041793	.016044	.383	.7020
SSPCOR3	-.041150	.041238	-.041431	-.998	.3188
SSPCOR5	-.062168	.048920	-.053381	-1.271	.2043
SSPCOR8	.186092	.042952	.181068	4.333	.0000
SSPCOR4	.215064	.045976	.197736	4.678	.0000
SSPCOR6	-.104475	.062242	-.072823	-1.679	.0938
SSPCOR1	-.147834	.044021	-.145896	-3.358	.0008
(CONSTANT)	.001373	.044376		.031	.9753

ANALYSIS OF VARIANCE

	DF	SUM OF SQUARES	MEAN SQUARE
REGRESSION	9	46.51235	5.16804
RESIDUAL	543	500.10191	.92100

MULTIPLE R	.29170
R SQUARE	.08509
ADJUSTED R SQUARE	.06993
STANDARD ERROR	.95969

F = 5.61135   SIGNIF F = .0000   N OF CASES = 553

179

Table 9.1e Regression of the SSS with the ATE (RAERDSC)

DEPENDENT VARIABLE..

	MEAN	STD DEV	LABEL
RAERDSC	-.003	.966	

VARIABLE(S) ENTERED ON STEP NUMBER

		MEAN	STD DEV	LABEL	STANDARDIZED PREDICTED VALUE
1..	SSPCOR9	.169	.974	REGR FACTOR SCORE	9
2..	SSPCOR8	.008	.961	REGR FACTOR SCORE	8
3..	SSPCOR5	.064	.856	REGR FACTOR SCORE	5
4..	SSPCOR4	-.096	.912	REGR FACTOR SCORE	4
5..	SSPCOR3	.065	1.002	REGR FACTOR SCORE	3
6..	SSPCOR2	-.067	1.001	REGR FACTOR SCORE	2
7..	SSPCOR7	.020	.882	REGR FACTOR SCORE	7
8..	SSPCOR1	.072	.990	REGR FACTOR SCORE	1
9..	SSPCOR6	.169	.693	REGR FACTOR SCORE	6

---------- VARIABLES IN THE EQUATION ----------

VARIABLE	B	SE B	BETA	T	SIG T
SSPCOR9	.016074	.042468	.016213	.378	.7052
SSPCOR8	.072400	.042987	.072021	1.684	.0927
SSPCOR5	-.079610	.048482	-.070578	-1.642	.1012
SSPCOR4	-.048026	.045804	-.045374	-1.049	.2949
SSPCOR3	-.107585	.040934	-.111615	-2.628	.0088
SSPCOR2	-.016314	.041387	-.016904	-.394	.6936
SSPCOR7	.011158	.048706	.010192	.229	.8189
SSPCOR1	-.091065	.043287	-.093326	-2.104	.0359
SSPCOR6	-.196945	.061810	-.141406	-3.186	.0015
(CONSTANT)	.041812	.044061		.949	.3431

MULTIPLE R   .22106
R SQUARE   .04887
ADJUSTED R SQUARE .03299
STANDARD ERROR   .94960

ANALYSIS OF VARIANCE

	DF	SUM OF SQUARES	MEAN SQUARE
REGRESSION	9	24.97215	2.77468
RESIDUAL	539	486.03748	.90174

F = 3.07704   SIGNIF F = .0013   N OF CASES = 549

180

Examination of scaling hypotheses by comparing derived scales: Criterion-related validity

Tables 9.2a through 9.2f list the scales developed for the key constructs. For each construct or proxy of a construct, a table contains the scales obtained via the theoretical approach, its optimally weighted scales resulted from the multiple regression approach, as well as some simply summated scales consisting of all the individual items or only those items mainly loading on the first factor. To be relatively exhaustive, results from different hypotheses as well as different techniques are encompassed. Also, for depression, the abbreviated forms of CES-D (17-item and 14-item) are included, and for social support, the original LSNS. Some descriptive statistics are displayed, including internal consistency coefficients (Cronbach's α) where applicable, which are conventionally employed as indicators of the reliability of the scales.

These, however, are not enough. As mentioned earlier, comparing scales by α values in the case of multifactorial scaling is misleading. In the absence of data for calculating test-retest reliability (stability) coefficients as well as data for so-called generalizability study, directly considering measurement validity is probably the only yet ultimate means by which different scales can be evaluated. Note, however, it is sometimes hard to distinguish between different kinds of validity, partly because there are various confusions in definition. For the purpose to distinguish between different scaling models and methods by their utility in substantiating the research hypotheses and the causal model, this book is interested in comparing their capacity of manifesting the relationships among the theoretical constructs. Their correlations with the criterion measures, therefore, are taken as a most important and direct test of the scaling hypotheses. But bear in mind that we are only going to test the scaling procedures, since the various items pools have been established with careful consideration of the content and construct validity as exemplified by the logical requirements.

Table 9.2a List of the Depression Scales (DS) and basic statistics

SCALE	ALPHA	STANDARDIZED ITEM ALPHA	MEAN	STD DEV	MINIMUM	MAXIMUM	VALID N	SCALING NOTES
DSH1A	N/A	N/A	1.72	.92	.44	8.06	1486	Hypothesis 1 (oblimin rotation)
DSH1B	N/A	N/A	1.66	.87	.48	7.37	1486	Hypothesis 1 (varimax rotation)
DSH1A12	N/A	N/A	2.16	1.02	.45	9.29	1486	Hypothesis 1 (oblimin, 12 factors)
DSH1A25	N/A	N/A	3.17	1.73	.43	10.65	1486	Hypothesis 1 (oblimin, 25 factors)
DSH2	(same as DSS)*		-.04	.95	-.81	6.13	1486	Hypothesis 1 or 2 (1 factor)
DSH2A7	(same as DSS1BC)*		-.03	1.02	-2.72	8.06	1486	Hypothesis 2 (oblimin rotation)
DSH2B7	(same as DSS1BC)*		-.04	.93	-1.34	7.37	1486	Hypothesis 2 (varimax rotation)
DSH3A	.0720	.0690**	-.05	2.80	-10.52	14.54	1486	Hypothesis 3 (oblimin rotation)
DSH3B	.0109	.0108**	-.12	2.61	-5.13	13.50	1486	Hypothesis 3 (varimax rotation)
DSH3A12	.1638	.1547**	-.04	3.95	-16.37	18.06	1486	Hypothesis 3 (oblimin, 12 factors)
DSH3A25	.1333	.1118**	-.16	6.54	-27.51	34.83	1486	Hypothesis 3 (oblimin, 25 factors)
DSS1A	.8041	.8627	4.12	5.94	.00	42.00	1566	Summated items on 1st component (before rotation)
DSS1BC	.8640	.8660	1.97	4.01	.00	30.00	1567	Summated items on 1st component (after rotation)
DSSD1A	.8619	.8627	-.19	8.32	-5.28	55.05	1566	Summated items (standardized) on 1st component (before rotation)
DSSD1BC	.8666	.8660	-.15	6.63	-3.35	46.94	1567	Summated items (standardized) on 1st component (after rotation)
DSSD	.8395	.8417	-.25	11.36	-13.70	70.89	1567	All summated items (standardized)
DSS	.7837	.8417	14.08	10.54	.00	77.00	1567	All summated items of the DS
CESDTl17	.8079	.8616	6.67	6.20	0	46	1563	CES-D total score (17 items)
CESDTl14	.7816	.8434	6.21	5.50	0	39	1538	CES-D total score (14 items)
RDSCESD	(same as DSH3B)**		.00	1.00	-1.25944	6.04356	1486	Standardized predicted value of depression (regression score targeted at CES-D)
RDSHLTH	(same as DSH3B)**		.00	1.00	-5.01618	1.43698	1486	Standardized predicted value of health (regression score targeted at HEALTH)

Note: *   Based on items that mainly load on the component
        ** Based on the components

Table 9.2b List of the Life Stress Scales (LSS) and basic statistics

SCALE	ALPHA	STANDARDIZED ITEM ALPHA	MEAN	STD DEV	MINIMUM	MAXIMUM	VALID N	SCALING NOTES
LSSH1A	N/A	N/A	2.34	1.16	.76	13.21	485	Hypothesis 1 (oblimin rotation)
LSSH1B	N/A	N/A	2.28	1.14	.73	12.87	485	Hypothesis 1 (varimax rotation)
LSSH1A22	N/A	N/A	2.83	1.67	.82	17.64	485	Hypothesis 1 (oblimin, 22 factors)
LSSH1A44	N/A	N/A	3.76	1.84	1.30	20.78	485	Hypothesis 1 (oblimin, 44 factors)
LSSH2	(same as LSSS)˙		.02	.96	-1.81	3.58	485	Hypothesis 1 or 2 (1 factor)
LSSH2A16	(same as LSSS1BC)˙		.03	1.13	-3.05	4.11	485	Hypothesis 2 (oblimin rotation)
LSSH2B16	(same as LSSS1BC)˙		.09	1.03	-1.23	5.37	485	Hypothesis 2 (varimax rotation)
LSSH3A	.0608	.0775˙˙	.30	4.18	-15.83	18.62	485	Hypothesis 3 (oblimin rotation)
LSSH3B	-.1612	-.1592˙˙	1.13	3.69	-7.88	19.68	485	Hypothesis 3 (varimax rotation)
LSSH3A22	-.0035	.0139˙˙	.85	4.87	-14.90	17.58	485	Hypothesis 3 (oblimin, 22 factors)
LSSH3A44	-.1375	-.1243˙˙	.76	7.20	-21.79	26.70	485	Hypothesis 3 (oblimin, 44 factors)
LSSS1A	.6750	.7611	13.97	10.25	-2.00	62.00	1227	Summated items on 1st component (before rotation)
LSSS1B	.0942	.7104	26.08	66.02	.00	399.00	1650	Summated items on 1st component (after varimax rotation)
LSSS1C	.5718	.5750	3.49	3.14	.00	20.00	1239	Summated items on 1st component (after oblimin rotation)
LSSSD1A	.7587	.7611	1.14	7.25	-13.25	35.84	1227	Summated items (standardized) on 1st component (before rotation)
LSSSD1B	.7073	.7104	.03	3.74	-4.88	19.52	1650	Summated items (standardized) on 1st component (after varimax rotation)
LSSSD1C	.5741	.5750	.23	2.37	-2.40	12.71	1239	Summated items (standardized) on 1st component (after oblimin rotation)
LSSSD	.6324	.6225	.13	10.58	-21.67	60.41	1592	All summated items (standardized)
LSSS	.1613	.6225	47.26	70.14	3.00	445.25	1592	All summated items of the LSS
RLSRDSC	(same as LSSH3B)˙˙		.00	1.00	-2.13783	3.78241	485	Standardized predicted value of depression (regression score targeted at RDSCESD)
RLSRDSH	(same as LSSH3B)˙˙		.00	.99	-3.49624	2.00383	485	Standardized predicted value of health

Note: ˙ Based on items that mainly load on the component ˙˙ Based on the components

183

Table 9.2c List of the Social Support Scales (SSS) and basic statistics

SCALE	ALPHA	STANDARDIZED ITEM ALPHA	MEAN	STD DEV	MINIMUM	MAXIMUM	VALID N	SCALING NOTES
SSSH1A	N/A	N/A	1.77	.70	.41	9.20	556	Hypothesis 1 (oblimin rotation)
SSSH1B	N/A	N/A	1.70	.67	.42	8.81	556	Hypothesis 1 (varimax rotation)
SSSH1A14	N/A	N/A	2.06	.86	.78	8.55	556	Hypothesis 1 (oblimin, 14 factors)
SSSH1A29	N/A	N/A	3.19	1.44	1.35	10.03	556	Hypothesis 1 (oblimin, 29 factors)
SSSH2	(same as SSSS)'		.12	.87	-2.61	2.50	556	Hypothesis 1 or 2 (1 factor)
SSSH2A9	(same as SSSS1C)'		.05	1.10	-2.58	2.60	556	Hypothesis 2 (oblimin rotation)
SSSH2B9	(same as SSSS1B)'		.07	.99	-2.39	2.24	556	Hypothesis 2 (varimax rotation)
SSSH3A	.3058	.2928''	-.36	3.38	-16.48	8.92	556	Hypothesis 3 (oblimin rotation)
SSSH3B	-.2009	-.2236''	.37	2.55	-7.44	8.70	556	Hypothesis 3 (varimax rotation)
SSSH3A14	-.2003	-.1867''	.03	4.07	-16.98	11.03	556	Hypothesis 3 (oblimin, 14 factors)
SSSH3A29	.3864	.3305''	.11	8.34	-27.42	30.35	556	Hypothesis 3 (oblimin, 29 factors)
SSSS1A	.6118	.7341	24.51	7.67	2.00	53.00	1678	Summated items on 1st component (before rotation)
SSSS1B	.6872	.6949	14.53	5.40	-1.00	26.00	1615	Summated items on 1st component (after varimax rotation)
SSSS1C	.7022	.7177	13.10	4.86	-1.00	22.00	1656	Summated items on 1st component (after oblimin rotation)
SSSSD1A	.7352	.7341	.09	5.28	-19.01	10.12	1678	Summated items (standardized) on 1st component (before rotation)
SSSSD1B	.6948	.6949	.13	3.89	-11.67	8.51	1615	Summated items (standardized) on 1st component (after varimax rotation)
SSSSD1C	.7159	.7177	.09	3.43	-10.57	6.36	1656	Summated items (standardized) on 1st component (after oblimin rotation)
SSSSD	.7188	.7101	-.10	10.30	-51.86	27.09	1636	All summated items (standardized)
SSSS	.6531	.7101	67.12	19.24	9.00	133.00	1636	All summated items of the SSS
LSNS	.6935	.6547	32.17	8.85	2	.50	1705	LSNS total score
RSSRDSC	(same as SSSH3B)''		.00	.99	-.98602	8.77085	556	Standardized predicted value of depression (regression score targeted at RDSCESD)
RSSLSDSC	(same as SSSH3B)''		-.02	1.06	-2.30764	4.58884	556	Standardized predicted value of stress (regression score targeted at RLSRDSC)
RSSHBDSC	(same as SSSH3B)''		.00	.99	-2.83850	2.42807	556	Standardized predicted value of HBB (regression score targeted at RHBRDSC)
RSSASDSC	(same as SSSH3B)''		.00	1.00	-2.28193	4.50118	556	Standardized predicted value of ATS (regression score targeted at RASRDSC)
RSSAEDSC	(same as SSSH3B)''		.01	1.00	-2.21806	3.94751	556	Standardized predicted value of ATE (regression score targeted at RAERDSC)

Note: ' Based on items that mainly load on the component
       '' Based on the components

184

Table 9.2d List of the Health Behaviors and Beliefs (HBB) measures and basic statistics

SCALE	ALPHA	STANDARDIZED ITEM ALPHA	MEAN	STD DEV	MINIMUM	MAXIMUM	VALID N	SCALING NOTES
HBH1A	N/A	N/A	1.47	.54	.35	4.57	1520	Hypothesis 1 (oblimin rotation)
HBH1B	N/A	N/A	1.45	.53	.34	4.52	1520	Hypothesis 1 (varimax rotation)
HBH1A11	N/A	N/A	2.08	.90	.99	9.40	1520	Hypothesis 1 (oblimin, 11 factors)
HBH2	(same as HBS)*		.01	1.01	-2.07	3.94	1520	Hypothesis 1 or 2 (1 factor)
HBH2A4	(same as HBS1BC)*		.01	1.03	-2.10	3.32	1520	Hypothesis 2 (oblimin rotation)
HBH2B4	(same as HBS1BC)*		.02	1.01	-1.79	3.30	1520	Hypothesis 2 (varimax rotation)
HBH3A	-.4376	-.4370**	.02	1.76	-5.02	6.48	1520	Hypothesis 3 (oblimin rotation)
HBH3B	-.0116	-.0019**	.02	2.00	-5.64	7.44	1520	Hypothesis 3 (varimax rotation)
HBH3A11	.0018	-.0148**	-.05	3.78	-11.87	16.15	1520	Hypothesis 3 (oblimin, 11 factors)
HBS1A	.3530	.6396	14.61	10.20	4.00	77.00	1632	Summated items on 1st component (before rotation)
HBS1BC	.6999	.6990	4.69	1.44	3.00	9.00	1651	Summated items on 1st component (after rotation)
HBSD1A	.6407	.6396	.04	3.58	-8.10	14.63	1632	Summated items (standardized) on 1st component (before rotation)
HBSD1BC	.6992	.6990	.00	2.36	-2.80	7.25	1651	Summated items (standardized) on 1st component (after rotation)
HBSD	.5675	.5662	.02	4.75	-14.53	18.78	1656	All summated items (standardized)
HBS	.3518	.5662	19.67	10.68	2.00	86.00	1656	All summated items of the HBB
RHBRDSC	(same as HBH3B)**		-.02	1.00	-3.93183	2.79105	1520	Standardized predicted value of depression (regression score targeted at RDSCESD)
RHBRDSH	(same as HBH3B)**		.03	1.00	-3.15270	4.03820	1520	Standardized predicted value of depression (regression score targeted at RDSHLTH)
RHBLSDSC	(same as HBH3B)**		.30	.94	-3.42493	1.98615	1520	Standardized predicted value of stress (regression score targeted at RLSRDSC)
RHBLSDSH	(same as HBH3B)**		-.27	.95	-2.00755	3.29483	1520	Standardized predicted value of stress (regression score targeted at RLSRDSH)

Note: * Based on items that mainly load on the component
:: Based on the components

185

Table 9.2e List of the Attitudes Toward Social Support (ATSS) measures and basic statistics

SCALE	ALPHA	STANDARDIZED ITEM ALPHA	MEAN	STD DEV	MINIMUM	MAXIMUM	VALID N	SCALING NOTES
ASH1A	N/A	N/A	1.29	.30	.18	1.91	1658	Hypothesis 1 (oblimin rotation)
ASH1B	N/A	N/A	1.21	.36	.03	2.50	1661	Hypothesis 1 (varimax rotation)
ASH1A9	N/A	N/A	2.24	1.17	.50	7.51	1658	Hypothesis 1 (oblimin, 9 factors)
ASH2	(same as ASS)*		-.01	1.00	-1.82	1.84	1658	Hypothesis 1 or 2 (1 factor)
ASH2A3	(same as ASS1ABC)*		-.01	1.01	-1.91	1.88	1658	Hypothesis 2 (oblimin rotation)
ASH2B3	(same as ASS1ABC)*		-.01	1.00	-1.73	1.71	1658	Hypothesis 2 (varimax rotation)
ASH3A	-.1201	-.1182**	-.03	1.69	-4.04	3.57	1658	Hypothesis 3 (oblimin rotation)
ASH3B	-.0132	-.0131**	-.03	1.72	-4.11	3.66	1658	Hypothesis 3 (varimax rotation)
ASH3A9	.2785	.2582**	.01	4.42	-19.40	18.48	1658	Hypothesis 3 (oblimin, 9 factors)
ASS1ABC	.8306	.8349	10.05	6.33	.00	20.00	1701	Summated items on 1st component
ASSD1ABC	.8349	.8349	.01	3.88	-6.18	6.13	1701	Summated items (standardized) on 1st component
ASSD	.6991	.6996	.00	4.88	-11.24	10.34	1704	All summated items (standardized)
ASS	.7267	.6996	15.84	7.51	.00	31.00	1704	All summated items of the ATSS
RASRDSC	(same as ASH3B)**		-.01	1.00	-1.57313	1.90332	1658	Standardized predicted value of depression (regression score targeted at RDSCESD)
RASRDSH	(same as ASH3B)**		.02	1.00	-2.12241	1.87864	1658	Standardized predicted value of depression (regression score targeted at RDSHLTH)
RASLSDSC	(same as ASH3B)**		.18	1.05	-1.81076	2.43406	1658	Standardized predicted value of stress (regression score targeted at RLSRDSC)
RASLSDSH	(same as ASH3B)**		-.18	1.05	-2.49634	1.88741	1658	Standardized predicted value of stress (regression score targeted at RLSRDSH)

Note: * Based on items that mainly load on the component
      ** Based on the components

186

Table 9.2f List of the Attitudes Toward Elderly (ATE) measures and basic statistics

SCALE	ALPHA	STANDARDIZED ITEM ALPHA	MEAN	STD DEV	MINIMUM	MAXIMUM	VALID N	SCALING NOTES
AEH1A	N/A	N/A	1.10	.67	.03	4.12	1690	Hypothesis 1 (oblimin rotation)
AEH1B	N/A	N/A	1.08	.64	.03	3.85	1690	Hypothesis 1 (varimax rotation)
AEH1A4	N/A	N/A	1.57	1.04	.23	5.41	1690	Hypothesis 1 (oblimin, 4 factors)
AEH2	(same as AES)*		.00	1.00	-3.98	1.27	1690	Hypothesis 1 or 2 (1 factor)
AEH2A2	(same as AES1BC)*	AES1BC)*	.00	1.03	-3.25	1.94	1690	Hypothesis 2 (oblimin rotation)
AEH2B2	(same as AES1BC)*	AES1BC)*	.00	1.00	-3.04	1.47	1690	Hypothesis 2 (varimax rotation)
AEH3A	-.6454	-.6454**	.00	1.27	-5.16	1.63	1690	Hypothesis 3 (oblimin rotation)
AEH3B	-.0022	-.0022**	.00	1.41	-5.75	1.82	1690	Hypothesis 3 (varimax rotation)
AEH3A4	-.0106	.0513**	.01	2.42	-11.91	10.12	1690	Hypothesis 3 (oblimin, 4 factors)
AES1A	.6543	.6471	3.12	2.59	-6.00	6.00	1690	Summated items on 1st component (before rotation)
AES1BC	.7494	.7511	1.95	2.12	-4.00	4.00	1696	Summated items on 1st component (after rotation)
AESD1A	.6470	.6471	.00	2.30	-8.23	2.58	1690	Summated items (standardized) on 1st component (before rotation)
AESD1BC	.7511	.7511	.00	1.79	-5.05	1.74	1696	Summated items (standardized) on 1st component (after rotation)
AESD	.6456	.6456	.00	2.78	-11.31	3.60	1698	All summated items (standardized)
AES	.6464	.6456	4.11	3.03	-8.00	8.00	1698	All summated items of the ATE
RAERDSC	(same as AEH3B)**		.02	.98	-1.13104	3.54507	1690	Standardized predicted value of depression (regression score targeted at RDSCESD)
RAERDSH	(same as AEH3B)**		-.02	.98	-3.74520	1.17808	1690	Standardized predicted value of depression (regression score targeted at RDSHLTH)
RAELSDSC	(same as AEH3B)**		.06	1.06	-1.25379	4.17344	1690	Standardized predicted value of stress (regression score targeted at RLSRDSC)
RAELSDSH	(same as AEH3B)**		-.06	1.06	-4.19819	1.25947	1690	Standardized predicted value of stress (regression score targeted at RLSRDSH)

Note: * Based on items that mainly load on the component
      ** Based on the components

187

The correlation coefficients of the new scales with the two criterion variables, namely, the 17-item CES-D and self-rated health, are shown in Table 9.3. CESDTL14 is a scale constituted by the 14 CES-D items that were included in the new Depression Scale (see the foregoing discussion). Several conclusions can be drawn from an examination of the effect sizes and significance levels of the relationships demonstrated by the correlation coefficients. First, look at the correlations with the 17-item CES-D. It seems that the 24-item new depression scale performed pretty well when simply summed up as usual (the summated scale is named DSS, $\gamma = .8251$, $p < .01$). Nevertheless, the standardization of the individual items before summation considerably improved measurement validity (i.e., DSSD, $\gamma = .9097$, $p < .01$). And it is noticeable that summing up all the 24 items is no better than summing up only the items mainly loading on the first factor (compare DSS with DSS1A - items before rotation, DSS1BC - items after either varimax or oblimin rotation, as well as DSSD1A and DSSD1BC - standardized items). The most striking is the optimally weighted scale (named RDSCESD) secured by the regression approach, which resulted in almost perfect correlation with the CES-D ($\gamma = .9809$, $p < .01$). Of all the depression scales derived by the theoretical approach, however, only the scales based on Hypothesis 2 (especially the 1 factor solution, named DSH2) had better criterion validity than the simply summated scale (DSS) in relation to the CES-D. Hypothesis 3 (summated components theory), in contrast, resulted in the poorest validity except for DSH3B where varimax rather than oblimin rotation is applied to the 7-factor solution. Simply summing up all possible 25 factors (i.e., the scale DSH3A25) particularly demonstrates how violation of the dimensionality requirement would bring about unexpected result.

Second, consider the correlations of the various depression scales with self-rated health.[2] On the one hand, there are similar or even more outstanding points that could be highlighted on scales DSS (simple summation of individual items), RDSHLTH (optimally weighted scale by the regression approach), and DSH3B (summation of components obtained from varimax rather than oblique rotation). On the other, DSH2 (scale based on Hypothesis 2, 1 factor solution) and DSSD (scale summated from standardized items) did not perform so well as in the case of correlations with the 17-item CES-D. This seemed to discredit the role of standardization and factorization in improving

Table 9.3 Correlation coefficients of the Depression Scales (DS) with criterion variables

	CESDTL17	HEALTH
DSH1A	.5706**	-.2606**
DSH1B	.5850**	-.2614**
DSH1A12	.5475**	-.2726**
DSH1A25	.4433**	-.2362**
DSH2	.8998**	-.3355**
DSH2A7	.6426**	-.0275
DSH2B7	.8009**	-.1335**
DSH3A	.3237**	-.0789**
DSH3B	.7224**	-.4058**
DSH3A12	.0783**	-.0258
DSH3A25	.0001	.0368
DSSD	.9097**	-.3831**
DSS	.8251**	-.4263**
CESDTL17	1.0000	-.2773**
CESDTL14	.9893**	-.2780**
DSS1A	.8609**	-.3158**
DSSD1A	.8977**	-.2912**
DSS1BC	.8862**	-.2433**
DSSD1BC	.8853**	-.2410**
RDSCESD	.9809**	-.2880**
RDSHLTH	-.6412**	.4405**

Note: * p<.05   ** p<.01   (2-TAILED)

the specific criterion-related validity of the summated scale DSS (also compare it with the scales DSS1A through DSSD1BC). Simply summing up all the factors (i.e., the scales DSH3A, DSH3A12 and DSH3A25) were again proven undesirable, though the scale DSH3B using a different rotation seemed to outclass even the scales based on Hypothesis 2 (DSH2 through DSH2B7). As for scales based on the maximum component theory (i.e., DSH1A through DSH1A25), they did not perform so well, nor too bad.

Since there is a fairly established instrument (i.e., the CES-D) available in the area of scaling concern, the practical (regression) approach seemed most suited to develop a new scale using the existing instrument as a criterion. Of all the proposed theoretical treatments of the factor scores, in contrast, only Hypothesis 2 based on 1 factor solution as well as Hypothesis 3 based on varimax rotation of the extracted factors have relatively promised their utility in depression scale development. Summated scales based on individual items have performed well in this case probably due to the unique quality of the items pool, yet whether or not standardization or factorization process will improve criterion-related

189

validity is still in question. With regard to the relationship between depression and self-rated health, the analysis has arrived at considerable association between the two in terms of either a direct correlation or the validity of the depression scales when self-rated health was used as the criterion. As for the 17-item CES-D, a further exclusion of the three "social" items for the sake of avoiding confounding with social support and life stress scales (see preceding sections) seemed having little impact on its validity ($\gamma=.9893$ and $p<.01$ between CESDTL17 and CESDTL14, total scores on the two scales). In fact, this has even slightly improved its validity in relation to self-rated health ($\gamma=.2780$ for CESDTL14 vs. $\gamma=.2773$ for CESDTL17).

Life stress scales

The correlation coefficients between the various life stress scales and selected criterion variables are shown in Table 9.4. For the depression scales, they are chosen based on above results). A conspicuous feature of the correlation coefficients is that their distributions are fairly consistent across the criterion variables. First, the two optimally weighted life stress scales secured by the regression approach (named RLSRDSC and RLSRDSH) resulted in the highest capability of predicting depression, no matter it was measured by which specific scale. Second, standardization and factorization treatments reconfirmed their utility in improving criterion-related validity of summated scales on individual items (compare LSSSD and LSSSD1A with LSSS). Thirdly, similar to the conclusion drawn from Table 9.3, Hypothesis 2 based on 1 factor solution (i.e., LSSH2) also held true for scaling life stress; and it seemed to be the sole employable one of all the scales derived from the theoretical approach. Fourth, summing up items loading mainly on the first factor (e.g., LSSS1A and LSSSD1A) worked almost as well as the most indicative factor score (i.e., LSSH2). Finally, it is noticeable that when self-rated health is used as either a direct or an indirect (through depression) criterion, the results seemed remarkable. This reflects a close relationship between self-rated health and life stress, partly because the latter contained some indicators of ill-health situations. Although the fact indicates no unconscious conceptual confounding, it suggests how specific arrangements of the measurement items or indicators would impact on substantive findings. If my study underscores the relationship between self-rated health and *non-illness* life stress, I may need to eliminate those illness indicators from the life stress scale, and that would probably cause the correlation

190

coefficients fall bellow the current levels. In the present research, however, this is not necessary nor appropriate since my focus is put on affective functioning, and I am interested in how life stress, including the part of ill physical health or even poor general health situations, would effect depression.

Table 9.4 Correlation coefficients of the Life Stress Scales (LSS) with criterion variables

	DSH2	DSH3B	DSSD	DSS	CESDTL17	DSS1A	DSSD1A	DSS1BC	RDSCESD	RDSHLTH	HEALTH
LSSH1A	.1520**	.1643**	.1873**	.1891**	.1747**	.1310**	.1328**	.1319**	.1667**	-.1631**	-.1383**
LSSH1B	.1546**	.1674**	.1912**	.1930**	.1765**	.1369**	.1374**	.1353**	.1715**	-.1642**	-.1339**
LSSH1A22	.1088*	.1090*	.1439**	.1385**	.1249**	.1000*	.1056*	.1047*	.1107*	-.1131*	-.1170*
LSSH1A44	.1266**	.1174*	.1525**	.1496**	.1405**	.1154*	.1188**	.1155*	.1285**	-.1204**	-.1079*
LSSH2	.5346**	.5770**	.5826**	.6208**	.4132**	.5236**	.4790**	.3999**	.4415**	-.6348**	-.5722**
LSSH2A16	.2047**	.2043**	.2138**	.2336**	.1367**	.1716**	.1620**	.1263**	.1554**	-.2401**	-.2518**
LSSH2B16	.3189**	.2904**	.3304**	.3281**	.2357**	.3018**	.2918**	.2524**	.2480**	-.3387**	-.3385**
LSSH3A	-.0480	.0211	-.0233	-.0180	-.0069	-.0498	-.0575	-.0623	-.0083	.0339	.0704
LSSH3B	.3888**	.4385**	.4524**	.4787**	.3369**	.3865**	.3464**	.2912**	.3601**	-.4548**	-.3841**
LSSH3A22	.0042	.0528	.0257	.0198	.0505	.0041	.0026	-.0017	.0316	-.0173	.0569
LSSH3A44	-.0846	-.0801	-.0726	-.0810	-.0479	-.0742	-.0708	-.0609	-.0497	.0957*	-.0346
LSSSD	.5285**	.5789**	.5878**	.6236**	.4528**	.5111**	.4756**	.4069**	.4712**	-.6194**	-.5081**
LSSS	.3772**	.3328**	.4009**	.4052**	.3175**	.3562**	.3515**	.3209**	.3206**	-.3810**	-.3447**
LSSS1A	.5023**	.5290**	.5567**	.5944**	.4280**	.4917**	.4604**	.3945**	.4348**	-.5934**	-.5143**
LSSSD1A	.5187**	.5582**	.5715**	.6165**	.4315**	.5109**	.4712**	.3986**	.4491**	-.6185**	-.5551**
LSSS1B	.3266**	.2716**	.3434**	.3415**	.2777**	.3056**	.3063**	.2843**	.2776**	-.3150**	-.2880**
LSSSD1B	.4758**	.4502**	.5198**	.5278**	.4216**	.4491**	.4386**	.3978**	.4267**	-.5067**	-.4590**
LSSS1C	.3572**	.3713**	.3877**	.4299**	.2605**	.3273**	.3049**	.2535**	.2826**	-.4409**	-.4208**
LSSSD1C	.3572**	.3715**	.3874**	.4299**	.2596**	.3276**	.3048**	.2531**	.2822**	-.4413**	-.4209**
RLSRDSC	.5787**	.5902**	.6303**	.6511**	.4819**	.5556**	.5204**	.4499**	.5055**	-.6403**	-.5016**
RLSRDSH	-.5749**	-.6142**	-.6251**	-.6623**	-.4552**	-.5520**	-.5098**	-.4321**	-.4817**	.6720**	.5498**

Note: * p<.05   ** p<.01   (2-TAILED)

192

Tables 9.5a through 9.5c exhibit the correlations of the personal coping proxy scales with selected life stress and depression scales as well as the general indicator of self-rated health. Since these proxy measures did not have as good theoretical and empirical grounds as those for the other two constructs, the results did not seem quite consistent. Nevertheless, the outstanding performance of the regression scales, the relative merit of the theoretical Hypothesis 2 (1 factor solution), as well as the role of standardization and/or factorization tended to be reconfirmed by the empirical data. It should be pointed out that the properties of the data play an important part in these conclusions. For example, if the data are more heterogenous across scaling items, standardization may prove more beneficial to summated scaling. Note that the variety of scaling procedures did not make very much difference to the Attitudes Toward Elderly (ATE) measure, probably because the scale contained too few (only 4) items. For that possible reason, another exploration is made to pool together the items for all the three proxy measures to form a unified Personal Coping Proxy Scale (PCPS). In that case, the conclusions about the optimally weighted scales acquired by the regression approach still held true, although the scales derived by the theoretical approach performed less consistently. All in all, the results basically rendered support to the original conceptual and scaling scheme of "personal coping" in relation to stress, depression, and general health. However, the interpretation of the correlation coefficients between the Attitudes Toward Social Support (ATSS) measures and the criterion variables demands special attention. The ATSS measures seem largely irrelevant to the scaling of depression. On the other hand, it seems that informal social support oriented elderly persons tended to suffer from higher degree of life stress (see Table 9.5b), though the result was not so consistent across the various ATSS measures. This may have significant implications to social support study, and therefore deserve further research endeavor in the future.

Table 9.5a Correlation coefficients of the Health Behaviors and Beliefs (HBB) measure with criterion variables

	DSH2	DSH3B	DSSD	DSS	CESDTL17	DSS1A	DSSD1A	RDSCESD	RDSHLTH	HEALTH
HBH1A	-.0122	-.0476	-.0271	-.0292	-.0333	-.0152	-.0157	-.0327	.0287	.0883**
HBH1B	-.0154	-.0501	-.0304	-.0331	-.0360	-.0173	-.0173	-.0362	.0331	.0897**
HBH1A11	-.0476	-.0749**	-.0601*	-.0709**	-.0639*	-.0432	-.0402	-.0632*	.0629*	.1183**
HBH2	-.1065**	-.1090**	-.1304**	-.1152**	-.1362**	-.0998**	-.1111**	-.1215**	.0978**	.1095**
HBH2A4	-.0557*	-.0734**	-.0821**	-.0739**	-.0975**	-.0540*	-.0599*	-.0883**	.0608*	.0758**
HBH2B4	-.0620*	-.0787**	-.0891**	-.0793**	-.1046**	-.0598*	-.0669*	-.0940**	.0650*	.0825**
HBH3A	-.0485	-.0489	-.0650	-.0426	-.0803**	-.0482	-.0617*	-.0611*	.0246	.0526*
HBH3B	-.0529*	-.0528*	-.0695*	-.0475	-.0838**	-.0521*	-.0655*	-.0648*	.0295	.0558*
HBH3A11	-.0474	-.0632*	-.0470	-.0613*	-.0419	-.0457	-.0356	-.0367	.0821*	.0199
HBSD	-.0605*	-.0670**	-.0813**	-.0630*	-.0876**	-.0599*	-.0703**	-.0695*	.0478	.0704**
HBS	-.1137**	-.1102**	-.1321**	-.1263**	-.1211**	-.1020**	-.1118**	-.1084**	.1133**	.1353**
HBS1A	-.1278**	-.1313**	-.1456**	-.1448**	-.1323**	-.1126**	-.1204**	-.1238**	.1376**	.1595**
HBSD1A	-.1143**	-.1319**	-.1394**	-.1293**	-.1362**	-.1100**	-.1167**	-.1257**	.1196**	.1384**
HBS1BC	-.0700**	-.0935**	-.0994**	-.0911**	-.1066**	-.0727**	-.0752**	-.0952**	.0836**	.0754**
HBSD1BC	-.0674**	-.0905**	-.0968**	-.0885**	-.1039**	-.0705**	-.0732**	-.0919**	.0799**	.0741**
RHBRDSC	.2048**	.1860**	.2172**	.2239**	.1799**	.1839**	.1850**	.1829**	-.2204**	-.1528**
RHBLSDSC	.1368**	.1333**	.1589**	.1475**	.1542**	.1264**	.1361**	.1426**	-.1323**	-.1245**
RHBRDSH	.2125**	.1834**	.2168**	.2306**	.1651**	.1907**	.1869**	.1736**	-.2323**	-.1307**
RHBLSDSH	.1568**	.1505**	.1781**	.1708**	.1661**	.1439**	.1516**	.1577**	-.1577**	-.1345**

	LSSH2	LSSH3B	LSSSD	LSSS	LSSS1A	LSSSD1A	RLSRDSC	RLSRDSH
HBH1A	-.1114*	-.0180	-.0775*	-.0482	-.0682*	-.0636*	-.0437	.0742
HBH1B	-.1123*	-.0192	-.0803**	-.0455	-.0711*	-.0671*	-.0436	.0739
HBH1A11	-.1017*	-.0030	-.0543*	-.0254	-.0874**	-.0864**	-.0491	.0782
HBH2	-.2349**	-.0427	-.1400**	-.0727**	-.2078**	-.1709**	-.2089**	.2011**
HBH2A4	-.1949**	-.0290	-.1154**	-.0525*	-.1832**	-.1594**	-.1506**	.1516**
HBH2B4	-.2057**	-.0310	-.1199**	-.0550*	-.1902**	-.1637**	-.1632**	.1627**
HBH3A	-.1684**	-.0255	-.0563*	-.0053	-.1044**	-.0749*	-.1801**	.1619**
HBH3B	-.1717**	-.0268	-.0611*	-.0093	-.1097**	-.0796**	-.1820**	.1642**
HBH3A11	-.0348	-.0148	-.0449	-.0009	-.0264	-.0363	-.0548	.0554
HBSD	-.1930**	-.0334	-.0872*	-.0191	-.1340**	-.1076**	-.1919**	.1769**
HBS	-.1735**	-.0359	-.1219**	-.0793**	-.1497**	-.1230**	-.1462**	.1465**
HBS1A	-.1813**	-.0425	-.1410**	-.1064**	-.1753**	-.1433**	-.1407**	.1456**
HBSD1A	-.2480**	-.0583	-.1567**	-.0963**	-.2169**	-.1782**	-.2094**	.2038**
HBS1BC	-.2255**	-.0452	-.1456**	-.0684**	-.2258**	-.1905**	-.1829**	.1836**
HBSD1BC	-.2254**	-.0498	-.1419**	-.0678**	-.2230**	-.1874**	-.1802**	.1829**
RHBRDSC	.2352**	.0673	.2320**	.1745**	.2854**	.2542**	.1711**	-.1835**
RHBLSDSC	.2452**	.0506	.1688**	.0996**	.2352**	.1976**	.2115**	-.2073**
RHBRDSH	.1919**	.0692	.2284**	.1798**	.2598**	.2385**	.1288**	-.1465**
RHBLSDSH	.2529**	.0561	.1919**	.1208**	.2585**	.2214**	.2094**	.2093**

Note: * p<.05 ** p<.01 (2-TAILED)

194

Table 9.5b Correlation coefficients of the Attitudes Toward Social Support (ATSS) measure with criterion variables

	DSH2	DSH1R	DSSD	DEE	CRSHLTH	LSS1A	DSSD1A	RDSCED	RDSHLTH	HEALTH
ASH1A	-.0262	-.0079	-.0021	.0114	.0019	-.0209	-.0200	-.0216	-.0023	-.0595*
ASH1B	-.0234	-.0092	-.0032	.0070	.0054	-.0224	-.0213	-.0024	.0121	-.0435
ASH1A9	.0054	-.0065	.0028	-.0044	.0077	.0321	.0283	-.0064	.0043	-.0050
ASH2	.0265	.0749**	.0549*	.0759**	.0413	.0567*	.0404	.0229	-.0776**	-.0362
ASH2A3	.0192	.0606*	.0505*	.0643*	.0331	.0464	.0352	.0136	-.0657*	-.0038
ASH2B3	.0210	.0645*	.0519*	.0677**	.0353	.0495	.0368	.0158	-.0691**	-.0116
ASH3A	-.0087	-.0048	-.0050	.0054	-.0085	.0130	.0060	-.0158	.0002	.0024
ASH3B	-.0065	-.0001	-.0021	.0095	-.0057	.0158	.0079	-.0134	-.0042	-.0022
ASH3A9	.0413	.0275	.0424	.0281	.0610*	.0578*	.0590*	-.0610*	-.0053	-.0007
ASSD	.0066	.0307	.0225	.0375	.0137	.0337	.0225	.0006	-.0348	-.0092
ASS	.0183	.0526*	.0385	.0570*	.0290	.0481	.0336	.0144	-.0551*	-.0256
ASS1ABC	.0253	.0698**	.0557*	.0724**	.0406	.0551*	.0412	.0216	-.0729**	-.0210
ASSD1ABC	.0233	.0682**	.0537*	.0706**	.0382	.0524*	.0387	.0190	-.0719**	-.0203
RASRDSC	.0452	.0984**	.0653**	.0845**	.0608**	.0558**	.0405	.0519*	-.0928**	-.0823**
RASLSDSC	.0429	.1034**	.0736**	.0955**	.0616**	.0655**	.0480	.0449	-.1018**	-.0639**
RASRDSH	-.0442	-.1045**	-.0738**	-.0954**	-.0628**	-.0649**	-.0476	.0471	.1023**	.0679**
RASLSDSH	-.0424	-.1026**	-.0718**	-.0951**	-.0607**	-.0663**	-.0479	.0443	.1009**	.0682**

	LSSH2	LSSH3B	LSSSD	LSSS	LSSS1A	LSSSD1A	RLSRDSC	RLSRDSH
ASH1A	.0253	-.0096	-.0070	.0221	.0208	.0285	.0168	-.0131
ASH1B	-.0906*	-.0674	-.0665**	-.0273	-.0330	.0355	-.0822	.0848
ASH1A9	-.0009	-.0813	.0118	.0115	.0221	.0053	-.0609	.0458
ASH2	.1999**	.0469	.0768**	.0877**	.2053**	.1426**	.1704**	-.1705**
ASH2A3	.1546**	.0449	.0691**	.0733**	.1854**	.1274**	.1455**	-.1376**
ASH2B3	.1688**	.0461	.0713**	.0777**	.1928**	.1327**	.1538**	-.1482**
ASH3A	.0434	.0063	-.0141	.0298	.0859**	.0478	-.0019	-.0178
ASH3B	.0544	.0083	-.0096	.0337	.0933**	.0535	.0077	-.0274
ASH3A9	.0213	.0648	.0131	-.0193	-.0124	-.0018	.0326	-.0210
ASSD	.1162**	.0263	.0243	.0584**	.1454**	.0934**	.0751	-.0872
ASS	.1602**	.0386	.0466	.0731**	.1734**	.1160**	.1196**	-.1283**
ASS1ABC	.1833**	.0497	.0720**	.0801**	.1957**	.1359**	.1646**	-.1599**
ASSD1ABC	.1804**	.0479	.0713**	.0799**	.1948**	.1347**	.1612**	-.1569**
RASRDSC	.1955**	.0399	.1016**	.0746**	.1406**	.1120**	.1902**	-.1795**
RASLSDSC	.2221**	.0509	.1094**	.0936**	.2003**	.1486**	.2114**	-.2008**
RASRDSH	-.2198**	-.0497	-.1104**	-.0919**	-.1932**	-.1448**	-.2107**	.1995**
RASLSDSH	-.2270**	-.0503	-.1064**	-.0955**	-.2034**	-.1499**	-.2098**	.2023**

Note: * p<.05   ** p<.01   (2-TAILED)

Table 9.5c Correlation coefficients of the Attitudes Toward Elderly (ATE) measure with criterion variables

	DSH2	DSH3R	DSSD	DSS	CESITL17	DSS1A	DSSD1A	RDSCESD	RDSHLTH	HEALTH
AEH1A	.1786**	.1467**	.1867**	.1815**	.1726**	.1505**	.1510**	.1854**	.1684**	-.0750**
AEH1B	.1793**	.1454**	.1862**	.1793**	.1734**	.1485**	.1503**	.1878**	.1661**	-.0714**
AEH1A4	.1027**	.1318**	.1212**	.1312**	.1059**	.0980**	.0845**	.1090**	.1516**	-.0510*
AEH2	-.1789**	-.2054**	-.2001**	-.1999**	-.1852**	-.1490**	-.1420**	-.2044**	-.2160**	.0721**
AEH2A2	-.1685**	-.1645**	-.1767**	-.1739**	-.1630**	-.1450**	-.1378**	-.1817**	-.1764**	.0605*
AEH2B2	-.1772**	-.1781**	-.1880**	-.1854**	-.1736**	-.1517**	-.1442**	-.1930**	-.1903**	.0652**
AEH3A	-.1728**	-.2022**	-.1948**	-.1949**	-.1804**	-.1432**	-.1366**	-.1989**	-.2122**	.0703**
AEH3B	-.1728**	-.2022**	-.1948**	-.1949**	-.1804**	-.1433**	-.1366**	-.1989**	-.2122**	.0703**
AEH3A4	-.0857**	-.0108	-.0663**	-.0573**	-.0576**	-.0758**	-.0774**	-.0637**	.0453	.0346
AESD	-.1756**	-.2020**	-.1945**	-.1942**	-.1787**	-.1441**	-.1374**	-.2007**	-.2130**	.0728**
AES	-.1798**	-.2032**	-.1969**	-.1961**	-.1814**	-.1472**	-.1404**	-.2048**	-.2148**	.0735**
AES1A	-.1840**	-.2125**	-.2054**	-.2053**	-.1906**	-.1544**	-.1462**	-.2111**	-.2198**	.0712**
AESD1A	-.1815**	-.2145**	-.2045**	-.2051**	-.1897**	-.1521**	-.1439**	-.2099**	-.2205**	.0708**
AES1BC	-.1853**	-.1848**	-.1934**	-.1905**	-.1768**	-.1558**	-.1486**	-.2008**	-.1996**	.0711**
AESD1BC	-.1849**	-.1850**	-.1935**	-.1908**	-.1767**	-.1558**	-.1485**	-.2004**	-.1997**	.0714**
RAERDSC	.1877**	.2055**	.2060**	.2048**	.1905**	.1580**	.1505**	.2107**	-.2173**	-.0736**
RAERDSH	.1855**	.2069**	.2051**	.2043**	.1898**	.1555**	.1481**	.2097**	-.2183**	-.0735**
RAELSDSC	.1832**	.2068**	.2035**	.2030**	.1883**	.1531**	.1459**	.2080**	-.2179**	-.0731**
RAELSDSH	-.1826**	-.2067**	-.2031**	-.2026**	-.1879**	-.1525**	-.1453**	-.2075**	-.2177**	.0730**

	LSSH2	LSSH3B	LSSSD	LSSS	LSSS1A	LSSSD1A	RLSRDSC	RLSRDSH
AEH1A	.0815	.0966**	.1527**	.0890**	.1455**	.1411**	.0988*	-.0865
AEH1B	.0784	.0935*	.1472**	.0867*	.1439**	.1392**	.0969*	-.0848
AEH1A4	.1048*	.1029**	.1122**	.0616*	.1098**	.1107**	.1028*	-.1033*
AEH2	-.2313**	-.1880**	-.2020**	-.1129**	-.2534**	-.2273**	-.2953**	.2612**
AEH2A2	-.1939**	-.0819	-.1666**	-.0903**	-.2094**	-.1916**	-.2172**	.1890**
AEH2B2	-.2088**	-.1025*	-.1795**	-.0979**	-.2252**	-.2053**	-.2397**	.2093**
AEH3A	-.2244**	-.1930**	-.1980**	-.1110**	-.2480**	-.2220**	-.2906**	.2576**
AEH3B	-.2244**	-.1930**	-.1980**	-.1110**	-.2480**	-.2220**	-.2907**	.2576**
AEH3A4	-.0988*	-.0868	-.0982*	-.0559*	-.1196**	-.1109**	-.0962*	.0827
AESD	-.2292**	-.1968**	-.2008**	-.1122**	-.2505**	-.2247**	-.2935**	.2608**
AES	-.2327**	-.1926**	-.2031**	-.1131**	-.2531**	-.2273**	-.2963**	.2622**
AES1A	-.2284**	-.1527**	-.1976**	-.1093**	-.2478**	-.2233**	-.2844**	.2507**
AESD1A	-.2253**	-.1534**	-.1961**	-.1083**	-.2465**	-.2218**	-.2829**	.2497**
AES1BC	-.2241**	-.1292**	-.1929**	-.1058**	-.2410**	-.2191**	-.2619**	.2291**
AESD1BC	-.2236**	-.1284**	-.1930**	-.1055**	-.2416**	-.2196**	-.2608**	.2282**
RAERDSC	.2373**	.1649**	.2042**	.1131**	.2561**	.2311**	.2917**	-.2569**
RAERDSH	-.2371**	-.1758**	-.2049**	-.1139**	-.2570**	-.2314**	-.2959**	.2611**
RAELSDSC	.2355**	.1816**	.2042**	.1138**	.2562**	.2304**	.2967**	-.2620**
RAELSDSH	-.2349**	-.1828**	-.2040**	-.1137**	-.2559**	-.2300**	-.2966**	.2621**

Note: * p < .05   ** p < .01   (2-TAILED)

196

The correlation coefficients of the social support scales with selected measures of the major criterion variables are shown in Tables 9.6a through 9.6c. Although too many detailed comparisons are involved, a pattern of distribution can be discerned that is similar to the foregoing conclusions on the depression, life stress and personal coping scales. Among all the scales derived via the theoretical approach, only the scale based on Hypothesis 2 (1-factor solution, named SSSH2) had a generally better measurement effect than a simple summation of the 29 individual items (SSSS) in relation to the various criteria. On the other hand, the scaling results of the first hypothesis (SSSH1A to SSSH1A29) tended to suggest that social support had an effect on the criteria that was generally undesirable. For example, it seemed to testify that the higher the social support, the higher the depression among the elderly respondents. Since this cannot be justified on the current knowledge basis, the more seemly interpretation is that this method of measurement seemingly more accurate than Hypothesis 2 turned out to be of poorest criterion validity. In addition, the simply summated (not standardized) scale using the 29 individual items (SSSS) appeared to have only modestly improved criterion validity in relation to depression, as compared with the original LSNS. Generally, the standardized summated scale based on factor scores (SSSH3A to SSSH3C) did not perform well except for SSSH3B (varimax rotation of the factors extracted with default settings) in some cases. Standardization and factorization, however, helped the summative scales using individual items improve validity.

Since the regression of the social support scale can have various targets, it should be highlighted that the strongest association was naturally found for each social support scale with the variable that was used as a criterion to obtain that specific regression scale. Therefore, social support scales aimed at predicting depression were different from those aimed at predicting life stress in terms of their predictability of the different criterion variables. Compared to the various theoretical models, however, the most powerful associations always resulted from the practical, regression approach.

Table 9.6a Correlation coefficients of the Social Support Scales (SSS) with Depression Scales (DS)

	DSH2	DSH3B	DSSD	DSS	CESDTL17	DSS1A	DSSD1A	RDSCESD	RDSHLTH	HEALTH
SSSH1A	.3838**	.1651**	.3167**	.2300**	.3807**	.3537**	.3929**	.3514**	-.1426**	-.1172**
SSSH1B	.3962**	.1710**	.3286**	.2389**	.3944**	.3610**	.4029**	.3633**	-.1498**	-.1050*
SSSH1A14	.3904**	.1981**	.3308**	.2408**	.3969**	.3340**	.3836**	.3722**	-.1657**	-.1252**
SSSH1A29	.1752**	.0906**	.1452**	.1043*	.1672**	.1513**	.1618**	.1649**	-.0782	-.0564
SSSH2	-.1510**	-.2418**	-.1910**	-.1984**	-.1611**	-.1348**	-.1200**	-.1616**	.2198**	.2230**
SSSH2A9	.0674	-.0189	.0197	-.0083	.0368	.0454	.0715	.0385	.0289	.1011*
SSSH2B9	.0368	-.0660	-.0155	-.0442	.0095	.0207	.0477	.0093	.0699	.1382**
SSSH3A	-.0351	.0417	.0164	.0182	-.1034*	-.0515	-.0598	.0668	-.0635	-.0264
SSSH3B	-.2235**	-.2426**	-.2250**	-.2046**	-.2279**	-.1932**	-.1972**	-.2194**	.2036**	.1741**
SSSH3A14	-.1611**	-.0606	-.1524**	-.1170**	-.2052**	-.1621**	-.1782**	-.1674**	.0556	.0027
SSSH3A29	-.0432	-.0045	-.0549	-.0456	-.0720	-.0249	-.0437	-.0504	.0163	-.0206
SSSSD	-.2454**	-.2752**	-.2759**	-.2523**	-.2665**	-.2366**	-.2391**	-.2359**	.2438**	.1919**
SSSS	-.1355**	-.1789**	-.1590**	-.1478**	-.1387**	-.1307**	-.1288**	-.1239**	.1586**	.1766**
LSNS	-.1041**	-.1511**	-.1299**	-.1294**	-.1060**	-.1072**	-.0985**	-.0879**	.1432**	.1860**
SSSS1A	-.1384**	-.1911**	-.1784**	-.1706**	-.1540**	-.1388**	-.1359**	-.1365**	.1727**	.1637**
SSSSD1A	-.1561**	-.2235**	-.2036**	-.1981**	-.1829**	-.1552**	-.1507**	-.1635**	.1971**	.1770**
SSSS1B	-.0687*	-.1479**	-.1244**	-.1305**	-.0956**	-.0924**	-.0790**	-.0671*	.1330**	.1895**
SSSSD1B	-.0728**	-.1532**	-.1284**	-.1345**	-.0997**	-.0944**	-.0815**	-.0713**	.1390**	.1849**
SSSS1C	-.0812**	-.1573**	-.1326**	-.1390**	-.1099**	-.1002**	-.0875**	-.0825**	.1428**	.1890**
SSSSD1C	-.0873**	-.1645**	-.1385**	-.1448**	-.1162**	-.1042**	-.0917**	-.0889**	.1506**	.1844**
RSRDSC	.6018**	.3596**	.5542**	.4541**	.6374**	.5547**	.5943**	.5694**	-.3435**	-.1700**
RSSLSDSC	.3683**	.3347**	.3951**	.3748**	.3618**	.3374**	.3370**	.3441**	-.3520**	-.2627**
RSSHBDSC	.2306**	.2190**	.2373**	.2372**	.1940**	.1997**	.2057**	.1804**	-.2255**	-.1820**
RSSHBLSD	.2109**	.2410**	.2346**	.2370**	.2001**	.1865**	.1826**	.1849**	-.2361**	-.2358**
RSSASDSC	.1678**	.1502**	.1927**	.2010**	.1389**	.1535**	.1451**	.1340**	-.1975**	-.1408**
RSSASLSD	.1459**	.1380**	.1651**	.1779**	.1072*	.1279**	.1222**	.1050*	-.1778**	-.1302**
RSSAEDSC	.2897**	.2250**	.2992**	.2612**	.3004**	.2661**	.2692**	.2913**	-.2384**	-.1327**
RSSAELSD	.2663**	.2137**	.2795**	.2458**	.2787**	.2456**	.2459**	.2724**	-.2275**	-.1238**

Note: * p<.05   ** p<.01   (2-TAILED)

198

Table 9.6b Correlation coefficients of the Social Support Scales (SSS) with Life Stress Scales (LSS)

	LSSH2	LSSH3B	LSSSD	LSSS	LSSS1A	LSSSD1A	RLSRDSC	RLSRDSH
SSSH1A	.0408	-.0234	.0694	.0835	.0862	.0570	.0740	-.0664
SSSH1B	.0433	-.0193	.0647	.0871*	.0889	.0556	.0774	-.0732
SSSH1A14	.0501	-.0135	.0810	.0576	.1083*	.0691	.0941	-.0778
SSSH1A29	.0490	.0273	.0581	.0048	.0396	.0328	.1350*	-.0942
SSSH2	-.2397**	-.2177**	-.2645**	-.0888*	-.2118**	-.1992**	-.3008**	.2582**
SSSH2A9	-.0952	-.0742	-.0445	-.0029	-.0898	-.0669	-.1073	.0921
SSSH2B9	-.1326*	-.1055	-.0953*	-.0174	-.1235*	-.1011*	-.1545*	.1328*
SSSH3A	.1210*	.0154	.1306**	.1255**	.1503**	.1402**	.0764	-.1015
SSSH3B	-.1379*	-.1679**	-.2041**	-.0340	-.0799	-.0995*	-.1861**	.1503*
SSSH3A14	.0627	.0238	.0271	.0120	.1027*	.0971*	.0595	-.0532
SSSH3A29	-.0299	.0190	.0111	.0294	.0213	.0014	.0563	.0371
SSSSD	-.2107**	-.1876**	-.2974**	-.0865**	-.2115**	-.2142**	.2756**	.2357**
SSSS	-.1526**	-.1238**	-.2188**	-.0569*	-.1401**	-.1461**	.1858**	.1567**
LSNS	-.1650**	-.1169**	-.2004**	-.0951**	-.1981**	-.1676**	.1897**	.1612**
SSSS1A	-.2132**	-.1338**	-.2453**	-.0748**	-.1997**	-.1973**	.2378**	.2125**
SSSSD1A	-.2227**	-.1676**	-.2777**	-.0764**	-.2270**	-.2227**	.2630**	.2370**
SSSS1B	-.2093**	-.1307**	-.2302**	-.1029**	-.2401**	-.2174**	.2226**	.2048**
SSSSD1B	-.2121**	-.1315**	-.2349**	-.0976**	-.2412**	-.2220**	.2238**	.2072**
SSSS1C	-.2107**	-.1392**	-.2311**	-.1047**	-.2426**	-.2180**	.2096**	.1971**
SSSSD1C	-.2135**	-.1408**	-.2366**	-.0989**	-.2441**	-.2231**	.2084**	.1982**
RSSRDSC	.2365**	.1915**	.3125**	.2255**	.2586**	.2312**	.2752**	.2579**
RSSLSDSC	.4473**	.2951**	.4350**	.3117**	.4719**	.4118**	.4920**	.4720**
RSSHBDSC	.2957**	.1025	.2723**	.1818**	.2782**	.2664**	.2144**	.2470**
RSSHBLSD	.2954**	.1432*	.2748**	.1263**	.2735**	.2584**	.2647**	.2663**
RSSASDSC	.3126**	.0952	.2367**	.2214**	.3658**	.3114**	.2508**	.2812**
RSSASLSD	.2938**	.0585	.2180**	.1916**	.3330**	.2921**	.2083**	.2500**
RSSAEDSC	.2493**	.2034**	.2700**	.1964**	.3329**	.2724**	.3564**	.3131**
RSSAELSD	.2398**	.2021**	.2600**	.1931**	.3248**	.2633**	.3487**	.3044**

Note: * p<.05   ** p<.01   (2-TAILED)

Table 9.6c Correlation coefficients of the Social Support Scales (SSS) with personal coping proxies

	HBH2	HBSD	HBSD1A	RHBRDSC	RHBRDSH	RHBLSDSC	RHBLSDSH
SSSH1A	-.0082	-.0084	.0193	-.0177	.0250	.0014	.0001
SSSH1B	-.0068	-.0094	.0249	-.0186	.0236	.0006	.0015
SSSH1A14	-.0765	.0770	-.0464	.0322	-.0138	.0708	-.0655
SSSH1A29	-.0234	-.0469	.0039	-.0287	.0316	.0144	-.0064
SSSH2	.2877**	.3234**	.2727**	-.0907*	.0050	-.2591**	.2300**
SSSH2A9	.1620**	.2071**	.1495**	.0691	-.1655**	-.1145**	.0758
SSSH2B9	.2134**	.2615**	.2000**	.0343	-.1385**	-.1657**	.1252**
SSSH3A	.0034	.0759	-.0313	.1936**	-.2468**	.0413	-.0830
SSSH3B	.2314**	.2607**	.2200**	-.1097	.0603	-.2197**	.2010**
SSSH3A14	.0083	.0202	-.0330	.0700	-.0867*	.0075	-.0254
SSSH3A29	-.0276	-.0105	-.0540	.0335	-.0095	.0267	-.0291
SSSSD	.2453**	.2846**	.2351**	-.0605*	.0134	-.2197**	.1910**
SSSS	.2239**	.2542**	.2173**	-.0561*	.0156	-.2003**	.1732**
LSNS	.2492**	.2702**	.2397**	-.0573*	-.0298	-.2203**	.1909**
SSSS1A	.2479**	.2739**	.2302**	-.0736**	.0001	-.2249**	.1979*
SSSSD1A	.2583**	.2920**	.2417**	-.0623*	.0172	-.2308**	.2006**
SSSS1B	.2739**	.2987**	.2600**	-.0640*	-.0300	-.2426**	.2113**
SSSSD1B	.2814**	.3059**	.2663**	-.0721**	-.0210	-.2510**	.2201**
SSSS1C	.2642**	.2915**	.2557**	-.0538*	-.0399	-.2321**	.2000**
SSSSD1C	.2725**	.2996**	.2633**	-.0620*	-.0310	-.2411**	.2093**
RSSRDSC	-.1107*	-.0945*	-.0857*	.1047*	-.0913*	.1158**	-.1193**
RSSLSDSC	-.2222**	-.2079**	-.2085**	.1594**	-.1130**	.2192**	-.2172**
RSSHBDSC	-.2359**	-.1656**	-.2756**	.3303**	-.3169**	.2701**	-.2974**
RSSHBLSD	-.3551**	-.3438**	-.3688**	.2537**	-.1768**	.3517**	-.3432**
RSSASDSC	-.1560**	-.1063*	-.1748**	.1821**	-.1527**	.1662**	-.1822**
RSSASLSD	-.1709**	-.1112**	-.2005**	.2358**	-.2175**	.1918**	-.2150**
RSSAEDSC	-.0744	-.1114**	-.0240	-.0444	.0724	.0518	-.0345
RSSAELSD	-.0578	-.0927*	-.0076	-.0595	.0869*	.0340	-.0170

Table 9.6c Correlation coefficients of the Social Support Scales (SSS) with personal coping proxies (continued)

	ASH2	ASS1ABC	RASRDSC	RASRDSH	RASLSDSC	RASLSDSH	LSNS
SSSH1A	-.0190	-.0185	.0352	-.0222	.0181	-.0118	.0222
SSSH1B	-.0378	-.0382	.0328	-.0116	.0060	.0005	.0200
SSSH1A14	-.0252	-.0163	-.0162	.0176	-.0181	.0224	-.1266**
SSSH1A29	-.0543	-.0633	.0146	.0169	-.0232	.0229	-.0499
SSSH2	.0363	.0102	-.0287	.0198	-.0156	.0009	.7826**
SSSH2A9	.0021	.0192	-.0937*	.0530	-.0443	.0509	.4381**
SSSH2B9	.0037	.0114	-.0900*	.0555	-.0475	.0495	.5667**
SSSH3A	.1573**	.1706**	.0840*	-.1393**	.1476**	-.1415**	-.0233
SSSH3B	.0779	.0427	.0574	-.0534	.0541	-.0719	.5924**
SSSH3A14	.1140**	.1271**	.0178	-.0665	.0756	-.0759	-.0925*
SSSH3A29	.0789	.0758	.0089	-.0312	.0367	-.0470	.0421
SSSSD	.0867**	.0720**	-.0663**	.0236	-.0115	-.0069	.7839**
SSSS	.1003**	.0931**	-.0490*	-.0017	.0141	-.0271	.8823**
LSNS	.0280	.0243	-.0989**	.0648**	-.0547*	.0445	1.0000
SSSS1A	.0358	.0343	-.1238**	.0839**	-.0715**	.0560*	.7370**
SSSSD1A	.0312	.0285	-.1308**	.0905**	-.0779**	.0628*	.6584**
SSSS1B	-.0038	.0056	-.1647**	.1256**	-.1130**	.1020**	.7196**
SSSSD1B	-.0125	-.0026	-.1730**	.1365**	-.1241**	.1123**	.6959**
SSSS1C	.0030	.0114	-.1526**	.1121**	-.0997**	.0903**	.7355**
SSSSD1C	-.0045	.0041	-.1594**	.1212**	-.1090**	.0990**	.7153**
RSSRDSC	.0402	.0330	.0649	-.0618	.0601	-.0606	-.1285**
RSSLSDSC	.0867*	.0962*	.1542**	-.1571**	.1534**	-.1432**	-.4704**
RSSHBDSC	.2711**	.2731**	.1616**	-.2368**	.2484**	-.2496**	-.3377**
RSSHBLSD	.1836**	.1936**	.1400**	-.1867**	.1926**	-.1885**	-.6591**
RSSASDSC	.3095**	.2802**	.2917**	-.3278**	.3311**	-.3434**	-.1598**
RSSASLSD	.3489**	.3261**	.2781**	-.3391**	.3473**	-.3586**	-.1066*
RSSAEDSC	-.0494	-.0360	.0749	-.0429	.0334	-.0199	-.2015**
RSSAELSD	-.0553	-.0448	.0763	-.0392	.0289	-.0168	-.2039**

Table 9.6c Correlation coefficients of the Social Support Scales (SSS) with personal coping proxies (continued)

	AEH2	AEH3B	AES	RAERDSC	RAERDSH	RAELSDSC	RAELSDSH
SSSH1A	-.0679	-.0675	-.0699	.0658	-.0672	.0677	-.0678
SSSH1B	-.0655	-.0640	-.0679	.0666	-.0667	.0664	-.0663
SSSH1A14	-.0970*	-.0942*	-.0994*	.1001*	-.0997*	.0988*	-.0986*
SSSH1A29	-.0360	-.0278	-.0402	.0566	-.0486	.0434	-.0422
SSSH2	.1050*	.1008*	.1088*	-.1116**	.1098*	-.1081*	.1076*
SSSH2A9	.0655	.0682	.0617	-.0552	.0599	-.0625	.0630
SSSH2B9	.0788	.0799	.0763	-.0720	.0753	-.0770	.0773
SSSH3A	.0157	.0162	.0124	-.0137	.0146	-.0151	.0152
SSSH3B	.0538	.0467	.0598	-.0704	.0642	-.0599	.0589
SSSH3A14	-.0657	.0641	-.0686	-.0540	-.0669	.0666	-.0665
SSSH3A29	-.0370	.0301	.0378	.0123	.0475	-.0432	.0422
SSSSD	.0570*	.0575*	.0606*	-.0533*	-.0552*	-.0561*	.0563*
SSSS	-.0089	-.0075	-.0038	.0050	-.0110	.0101	-.0099
LSNS	-.0062	-.0066	-.0011	.0116	-.0055	.0058	-.0059
SSSS1A	.0014	-.0024	.0060	-.0425	.0076	-.0050	.0044
SSSSD1A	.0376	.0352	.0400	-.0088	.0408	-.0396	-.0393
SSSS1B	-.0045	-.0093	-.0032	-.0143	.0035	-.0001	-.0007
SSSSD1B	-.0010	-.0067	-.0004	-.0144	.0082	-.0043	.0034
SSSS1C	.0067	.0037	.0081	-.0195	.0114	-.0094	.0090
SSSSD1C	.0101	.0064	.0117		.0158	-.0134	.0128
RSSRDSC	-.0984*	-.0929*	-.1030*	.1088*	-.1054*	.1027*	-.1021*
RSSLSDSC	-.1521**	-.1472**	-.1560**	.1584**	-.1572**	.1555**	-.1550**
RSSHBDSC	.0426	.0478	.0407	-.0265	.0333	-.0373	.0382
RSSHBLSD	-.0170	-.0104	-.0181	.0339	-.0273	.0229	-.0220
RSSASDSC	-.0616	-.0613	-.0585	.0598	-.0610	.0615	-.0615
RSSASLSD	-.0194	-.0174	-.0162	.0238	-.0222	.0210	-.0208
RSSAEDSC	-.2212**	-.2176**	-.2247**	.2211**	-.2229**	.2229**	-.2227**
RSSAELSD	-.2236**	-.2212**	-.2270**	.2199**	-.2232**	.2240**	-.2241**

Conclusion on scaling effectiveness

In terms of measurement validity, the results of the empirical study generally falsified Hypothesis 1. The assumption that the role of a psychosocial construct is determined by its first component (extracted by specifying only 1 factor) was proved to have relatively high validity of all the theoretical models. Among the summated components hypotheses, only the one using varimax rotation seemed to have some utility. Generally speaking, standardization and/or factorization treatments lead to some improvement of the criterion-related validity of the scales. As for the practical approach, the regression scales using specific criteria were most valid in predicting the same variables. Generally speaking, the practical approach is more effective than the theoretical approach. Note that this approach is rather robust in that even with many missing cases in regression (see, for example, Table 9.1b: N of cases=270), the resulting scales are usually still most effective of all the scaling results. The advantage of the theoretical approach is in that it is across-the-board, whereas the practically optimal scaling strategy (regression) is criterion-specific. This fact hints on the application of the latter. In dealing with complicated multivariate relationships among theoretical constructs, one may have to make difficult trade-offs and decide on where the focal-point relationship is which should be heightened or maximized.

Although the above conclusions in terms of measurement validity are encouraging with regard to the CAUS, i.e., both the theoretical and the practical approaches to unidimensionalized scaling, there are some problems with the idea of validity itself. The pursuit of validity seems to imply that the construct to be measured, no matter how rough, incomplete, or even inconceivable, is a set or determined goal for measurement. This is not conducive to theory development indeed. Methodologically, although validity can be marred either by exaggeration or by underrepresentation of what is measured, the idea itself provides no lead to a way out. By articulating the logical requirement (cf. Chapter Three), however, a solid ground can be established for measurement "validity;" and by basing on such a ground we can strive for the best measurement results without fearing the confounding problem. This introduces a simple idea of measurement power or scaling effectiveness, that is, the degree of association(s) with a criterion or a set of criteria that can be attained by a specific measure or scale. The idea is that the associations may be insignificant not because there are no such significant associations but because the measure is not powerful or the scale is not good enough. This justifies the use of multiple scaling methods (the

CAUS) in measuring complex theoretical constructs, including theory-based and practice-oriented approaches, to achieve different research objectives (e.g., general vs. specific).

By aiming at maximum measurement power based on the fulfillment of the logical requirement and by not taking the construct to be scaled as absolute, full possibilities are unveiled for scale as well as theory development. And the rule is simplified: the higher the association with the criterion, the better the measure developed. And even if there is an undesirable outcome, we may ponder on its theoretical meaning without simply abandoning the measure, which could be the case by conventional validity requirement. Taking the poor performance of Hypothesis 1 as an example. If we do not take the construct being measured as a rigid entity simply to be approached, we will detect some new possibilities in measurement. Basically, Hypothesis 1 involves inconsistency of the construction of measurement across different cases. By comparing Hypothesis 1 and Hypothesis 2, we see how substitution of the main factor (the first factor) with other components would affect the quality of social support, stress, and so forth. This may open up a new topic for substantive social support or life stress study, i.e., whether or not consistency is an important quality of social support or life stress. In such a sense, Hypothesis 1, in conjunction with Hypothesis 2, is quite effective in detecting the relationship between social support consistency and depression. All these demonstrate how the expansion of the notion of validity could bring in more elegant thoughts and designs in measurement.

These conclusions and discussions will direct the use of relatively effective measures of the theoretical constructs in ensuing substantive analysis, though the models used are far from perfect and the possibilities in scaling are not exhausted. By these empirically proven approaches to measurement, however, we will have some finer means and more confidence in substantive hypothesis testing. Particularly, the role of social support would be better illuminated via the simultaneous treatment of measurement scales and substantive models.

Notes

1. An earlier study of the Chinese elderly in Hong Kong obtained Cronbach's $\alpha=.80$ and split-half reliability coefficient$=.74$ (p<.001) for the complete 20-item CES-D (Chi & Boey, 1992).

2. The signs of the correlation coefficients of one regressed depression scale (i.e., RDSHLTH) with the 17-item CES-D (CESDTL17) and self-rated health (HEALTH) should be reversed since the regression of the former had been reversed once when targeted at self-rated health.

10 Substantive analysis and model testing

Since the general measures of the key constructs are obtained, substantive analysis ranging from univariate statistics to complex model testing can be made empirically succinct and theoretically relevant. In this chapter, some univariate statistics are first obtained to show the parameters of the distributions of some major variables. Then, some bivariate analyses are performed. Such analyses highlight different portions of the structural model. The full test of the substantive model, however, requires truly multivariate analyses with adequate statistical control. A single-equation multiple regression is conducted to show the results of the common practice, though it is a path analysis or a set of structured regression equations that would give the most accurate findings. Since the statistical program EQS has the merit of simplicity in contrast to the more complex package LISREL, it is utilized in this study and introduced to the reader. On the whole, the findings reconfirm significant associations among affective functioning (depression), life stress and social support with appropriate understanding of the relationship among mental health, social well-being, and quality of life. The role of personal coping in assuaging stress and depression is also betokened. The hypothetical impact of aging, however, gains only minimal support from the empirical data. Gender difference, on the other hand, is relatively noticeable. The implications of these results are discussed. Evidence is also obtained for the difference between Chinese and Chinese-American elderly, though the result does not lend itself to the myth that Chinese culture is tied with extremely low rates or levels of depression.

Chapter six briefly mentioned some demographic characteristics of the elderly sample in describing the data sets. This chapter focuses on the statistics of four key theoretical constructs, namely, depression, life stress, social support, and personal coping. With multiple selected scale sets, the relationships among the key constructs are analyzed. Statistical control is achieved via a single multiple regression method as well as the structural equations modeling approach to clarify the pathways of various effects. The role of stress in effecting depression and the mediating and moderating role of social support is investigated by testing the major research hypotheses, particularly by comparing the partial and the zero-order correlation coefficients as well as distinguishing between the direct and the indirect effects.

Depression among Chinese and Chinese-American elderly

It has been pointed out that "CES-D has not yet been shown to be a useful tool for determination of community prevalence rates of depressive disorder, either as a first-stage screening method or as an independent assessment of illness" (Rabkin & Klein, 1987:78). Nevertheless, there is evidence that á score of 16 (for the complete 20-item scale) is equivalent to 6 symptoms reported as occurring for most of the previous week, or to more than half of the symptoms for fewer days (ibid.). Probably that is why the instrument, which puts emphasis on duration of symptoms, continues to be used in epidemiological studies of depressive symptomatology or prevalence of depression among various populations. Especially, the CES-D scale has been applied to Chinese Americans (Kuo, 1984; Ying, 1988), Chinese population in Hong Kong (Chan, 1991; Chi & Boey, 1992, 1994), and Mainland Chinese (Lin, 1989). It was the only depression scale employed in the original cross-national survey in Beijing, Shanghai, Guangzhou, and Los Angeles. Because of its more or less validated linkage with accepted clinical diagnosis, it can be utilized to preliminarily assess depression among Chinese and Chinese-American elderly and, more importantly, serve as a criterion for defining critical points of the new depression scales developed in last chapter. It is worth mentioning that in studying Mainland Chinese, Lin (1989) has made an effort in adapting the CES-D to the cultural setting. As a result of modification, he recommended the use of a 16-item scale as an abbreviated version. In this study, I will show how a different abbreviation of the CES-D, namely the 17-item scale analyzed in last chapter, works for the Chinese and Chinese-American aging populations.

A descriptive procedure rendered a mean score of 6.67, with a standard deviation of 6.20 and a range of 0 through 46, on the 17-item scale for 1,563 valid cases. In comparison, Lin (ibid.) obtained a mean score of 5.122 for his 16-item scale, which excluded 4 positive items of the original CES-D and was applied to a younger adult population (mean age=43.2 vis-a-vis 69.19 in this study). The maximum score for a 17-item subscale is 51, whereas for a 16-item subscale it is 48. If we want the diagnostic criterion for the 17-item scale to be proportional to that for the original 20-item CES-D, then we will have a cutoff point at 13.60 (=51x16/60). For a 16-item subscale, the cutoff point should be 12.80. Comparing the differences between the mean scores and such diagnostic criteria, the ratio for this study (6.67/13.60=0.490) was higher than Lin's 16-item scale (5.122/12.80=0.400), yet lower than the original 20-item CES-D in his study (10.296/16=0.643). This reflects the mean level of depression with some comparability to previous studies. A more appropriate comparison can be made with Chi and Boey's (1992) study, in which they found a mean score of 12.25 (SD=8.15) for male and 15.77 (SD=9.34) for female respondents who were 70 years of age or older. Their ratios to the cutoff point on the 20-item CES-D employed were 12.25/16=0.766 and 15.77/ 16=0.986, respectively. There are, of course, considerable variations among the findings. The results, however, all challenge the popular point of view that the Chinese tend to score lower on depression scales (cf. Lin, 1989; Nakane et al., 1991). Using the proportionate cutoff point (13.6, rounded to 14) for the 17-item scale in the present study, we have a percentage of 9.9% for the respondents who could be considered as "depressed." This figure is much higher than some previous studies conducted in the Chinese communities (Kleinman, 1982). For example, in their survey conducted in Taiwan, Hwu and colleagues (1989) obtained some extremely low prevalence rates, e.g., 0.6% for major depression and 0.12% for bipolar disorder (1-year prevalence rate) in the urban areas. It is noticeable that if we round the proportionate cutoff point to 13, the percentage of the depressed would be even higher (up to 11.5%) in this study.

Table 10.1 contains some depression scales derived in last chapter and selected based on the conclusions of scale development. By using 9.9% as a relative diagnostic criterion and by examining the distributions of the new scales as well as their relationship with the 17-item CES-D, I suggest some cutoff points for these scales to address practical concerns in mental health (see Table 10.1). However, it should be reminded that these cutoff points depend on the utility of the 17-item CES-D in the research setting, which eventually requires validation with more detailed clinical diagnosis. This is not, however, the focus of the

Table 10.1 Depression measured by multiple selected scales and suggested cutoff points

SCALE	MEAN	STD DEV	MINIMUM	MAXIMUM	CUTOFF POINT	VALID N	SCALING NOTES
CESDTL17	6.67	6.20	0	46	14.0	1563	CES-D total score (17 items)
DSS	14.08	10.54	.00	77.00	28.0	1567	All summated items of the DS
DSSD	-.25	11.36	-13.70	70.89	13.0	1567	All summated items (standardized)
DSS1A	4.12	5.94	.00	42.00	11.0	1566	Summated items on 1st component
DSSD1A	-.19	8.32	-5.28	55.05	9.1	1566	Summated items (standardized) on 1st component
DSH2	-.04	.95	-.81	6.13	1.1	1486	Hypothesis 1 or 2 (1 factor)
DSH3B	-.12	2.61	-5.13	13.50	3.3	1486	Hypothesis 3 (varimax rotation)
RDSCESD	.00	1.00	-1.25944	6.04356	1.1	1486	Standardized predicted value of depression (regression score targeted at CES-D)
RDSHLTH	.00	1.00	-5.01618	1.43698	-1.4*	1486	Standardized predicted value of health (regression score targeted at HEALTH)

Note: * Lower instead of higher values are indicative of depression.

present study, which intends to use these scales as continuous measures to study the relationship of the theoretical constructs with one another and with some other variables.

Social network support

Social network and social support have been commonly measured in terms of a significant area of human functioning. Nevertheless, unlike affective functioning where the state of depression can now be quite professionally determined, efforts made in the social domain to imitate a diagnosis of some clinically significant status seems to be rather premature. Therefore, establishing a criterion for a social support or network scale to indicate the entry point to the "isolated" or "socially impoverished" group often looks somewhat arbitrary. However, it seems that social welfare professionals need to strive for a consensus on practically feasible cutoff points on various scales, on which they can base their decision-making as to when social and professional intervention is required.

In describing this social dimension, the Lubben Social Network Scale (LSNS) may serve a role similar to that of the CES-D in the area of mental functioning delineated in the above. A descriptive procedure rendered a mean score of 32.17, with a standard deviation of 8.85 and a range of 2 through 50, on the 10-item LSNS scale for 1,705 valid cases. Compared to Lubben's original elderly study where the LSNS was established among a sample whose majority were white (Lubben, 1988), this result is much higher than the average score from that study (25.1, standard deviation 9.6). These results seem to suggest that the Chinese elderly were more privileged in terms of informal social networks. However, whether this is mainly due to the Chinese familism or to some other factors demands further investigation.

Lubben (1987) has presented evidence that scores in the lower quartile of the LSNS are associated with significantly increased risks of extended hospital stays. Through a rationale somewhat similar to that of the CES-D, he suggests that scores below 20 (out of a possible 50 points) on the LSNS would qualify as a preliminary cutoff point for screening those elderly who are apt to be at greater risk of extremely limited social networks (Lubben, 1988). However, he points out that more research needs to be done, and as yet few studies have focused on this topic. Utilizing that cutoff point (20 and below) for the scale employed in the present study, we have a percentage of 10.8% for the respondents who could be considered as "isolated."

Table 10.2 compares the descriptive statistics of the LSNS with those of the new social support scales derived in last chapter and selected based on the scale development conclusions. By using 10.8% as a diagnostic reference for the new scales and by examining their distributions as well as their relationship with the LSNS, I suggest some cutoff points for these scales to address practical concerns in social work practice. However, it should be reminded that these cutoff points depend on the utility of the LSNS in the research setting, which eventually requires validation with more detailed clinical diagnosis in social as well as other functional areas, if criterion variables in these areas are used. This is, however, not the focus of the present study, which is intended to use these scales as continuous measures to study the relationship of the key theoretical constructs with one another as well as with some additional variables.

Stress and coping

The selection of the stress scales and the personal coping proxy measures is similar to the assortment of depression and social support scaling results. The means and ranges of the scores on the stress and coping instruments to be used are included in Table 9.2b and Tables 9.2d through 9.2f, respectively. Here no cutoff point will be given to any selected measure, however. First, the overall scaling of life stress as well as personal coping has a meaning more theoretical than practical (or clinical). Few, if any, have expected as yet a helping profession to act on such kind of measures based on some critical points. Second, no scaling efforts in these aspects have indeed succeeded in establishing such meaningful and reliable cutoff points. Third, no existing scales were employed in the original survey, which lends no ground for such manipulations in the present study. I will not, therefore, further pursue this dimension. Since the current study is going to examine the utility of the global scales in substan-

Table 10.2 Social support measured by multiple selected scales and suggested cutoff points

SCALE	MEAN	STD DEV	MINIMUM	MAXIMUM	CUTOFF POINT	VALID N	SCALING NOTES
LSNS	32.17	8.85	2	50	20.0	1705	LSNS total score
SSSS	67.12	19.24	9.00	133.00	42.0	1636	All summated items of the SSS
SSSSD	-.10	10.30	-51.86	27.09	-14.0	1636	All summated items (standardized)
SSSS1A	24.51	7.67	2.00	53.00	13.5	1678	Summated items on 1st component (before rotation)
SSSSD1A	.09	5.28	-19.01	10.12	-7.1	1678	Summated items (standardized) on 1st component (before rotation)
SSSH2	.12	.87	-2.61	2.50	-1.1	556	Hypothesis 1 or 2 (1 factor)
SSSH3B	.37	2.55	-7.44	8.70	-3.0	556	Hypothesis 3 (varimax rotation)
RSSRDSC	.00	.99	-.98602	8.77085	0.8*	556	Standardized predicted value of depression (regression score targeted at RDSCESD)
RSSLSDSC	-.02	1.06	-2.30764	4.58884	1.4*	556	Standardized predicted value of stress (regression score targeted at RLSRDSC)

Note: * Higher instead of lower values are indicative of isolation.

212

tive analysis, I will not go into the detailing of their individual items either. Rather, I shall concentrate on the interrelationships among the theoretical constructs by scrutinizing into their correlation coefficients. This is the task for the following two sections

In concluding this whole section, it should be noted and underscored that a subject can be categorized into different groups if different depression scales are employed. This is also true to the assessment of social support, life stress, or personal coping. Although in generating some general population rates like community prevalence we are able to concert the results by assigning proper cutoff points to different scales, we could be disturbed by the distinct differences of different scales as individual screening tools. The point is, however, a thorough comparison of all the scales is wanting, and no scale could claim itself as the best one of all the possible measurement tools. It is, therefore, imprudent or even dangerous to decide the whole thing based on any single available scale. The advantage of the multiple measurement approach is in that it reveals all kinds of possibilities in scaling and assessment. The necessity of a more comprehensive approach to screening and diagnosis, therefore, is made evident.

The fact that the signs of the items of a scale could be reversed by rearranging their codings indicates that the traditional negative perspective of mental health can hardly be maintained in the operationalization process. The purposive reversal of the signs as a methodological doctrine actually also breaks up the boundaries between social support and social stress (in the "informal" sense) as well as between life stress and life satisfaction or well-being. Indeed, when we start to inspect the relationships among mental and social functioning and overall quality of life, we do not want to confine ourselves to only half of each domain below or above some threshold point. In the following, all such constructs will be treated as continuous, cross-border variables. For example, I will be talking about a broader conception of affective functioning even though I use the subheading of "depression."

Correlates of depression

Quality of life and affective functioning

Table 10.3 shows the zero-order correlation coefficients of the scores on the multiple selected depression scales with those on the multiple selected life stress scales. The highest correlation is between RDSHLTH (regressed depression scale using self-rated health as the criterion) and RLSRDSH (regressed life stress scale using the above regressed depression scale as the criterion) ($\gamma=0.672$, $p<0.01$). As a whole, the correlation matrix displayed remarkable positive relationship between affective functioning and quality of life, or in other words, between depression and life stress. This conclusion sounds eloquent since it gained support from the results of not just a single pair of scales, especially those of probably questionable utility, but a whole bunch of measurement tools developed by diverse theoretical and practical means. With the potential confounding problem being taken care of beforehand, however, whether the highest correlation coefficient ($\gamma=0.672$) has set the limit for scaling manipulation is still open to inquiry.

Social support and affective functioning

Table 10.4 shows the zero-order correlation coefficients of the scores on the multiple selected depression scales with those on the multiple social support scales. Generally, social support is negatively associated with depression, though the relationship is not so close as between life stress and depression. The performance of the social support scale obtained by regression using a regressed depression scale as the criterion, again, is outstanding. The highest correlation coefficient is found between that social support scale (named RSSRDSC) and CESDTL17 (the 17-item CES-D) ($\gamma=0.637$, $p<0.01$). Note that the correlation coefficient here has a positive value while actually indicates a negative relationship between the two constructs, since the regression of the social support scale using a depression scale as a criterion has reversed its sign once. On the whole, an ameliorative effect of social support on depression is reconfirmed at the zero-order correlation level, though the relationship is gener-

214

Table 10.3 Correlations between depression and life stress using multiple scales

	LSSS	LSSSD	LSSS1A	LSSSD1A	LSSH3B	LSSH2	RLSRDSC	RLSRDSH
CESDTL17	.3175**	.4528**	.4280**	.4315**	.3369**	.4132**	.4819**	-.4552**
DSS	.4052**	.6236**	.5944**	.6165**	.4787**	.6208**	.6511**	-.6623**
DSSD	.4009**	.5878**	.5567**	.5715**	.4524**	.5826**	.6303**	-.6251**
DSS1A	.3562**	.5111**	.4917**	.5109**	.3865**	.5236**	.5556**	-.5520**
DSSD1A	.3515**	.4756**	.4604**	.4712**	.3464**	.4790**	.5204**	-.5098**
DSH3B	.3328**	.5789**	.5290**	.5582**	.4385**	.5770**	.5902**	-.6142**
DSH2	.3772**	.5285**	.5023**	.5187**	.3888**	.5346**	.5787**	-.5749**
RDSCESD	.3206**	.4712**	.4348**	.4491**	.3601**	.4415**	.5055**	-.4817**
RDSHLTH	-.3810**	-.6194**	-.5934**	-.6185**	-.4548**	-.6348**	-.6403**	.6720**

Note: * p<.05   ** p<.01   (2-tailed)

Table 10.4 Correlations between depression and social support using multiple scales

	LSNS	SSSS	SSSSD	SSSS1A	SSSSD1A	SSSH3B	SSSH2	RSSRDSC	RSSLSDSC
CESDTL17	-.1060**	-.1387**	-.2665**	-.1540**	-.1829**	-.2279**	-.1611**	.6374**	.3618**
DSS	-.1294**	-.1478**	-.2523**	-.1706**	-.1981**	-.2046**	-.1984**	.4541**	.3748**
DSSD	-.1299**	-.1590**	-.2759**	-.1784**	-.2036**	-.2250**	-.1910**	.5542**	.3951**
DSS1A	-.1072**	-.1307**	-.2366**	-.1388**	-.1552**	-.1932**	-.1348**	.5547**	.3374**
DSSD1A	-.0985**	-.1288**	-.2391**	-.1359**	-.1507**	-.1972**	-.1200**	.5943**	.3370**
DSH3B	-.1511**	-.1789**	-.2752**	-.1911**	-.2235**	-.2426**	-.2418**	.3596**	.3347**
DSH2	-.1041**	-.1355**	-.2454**	-.1384**	-.1561**	-.2235**	-.1510**	.6018**	.3683**
RDSCESD	-.0879**	-.1239**	-.2359**	-.1365**	-.1635**	-.2194**	-.1616**	.5694**	.3441**
RDSHLTH	.1432**	.1586**	.2438**	.1727**	.1971**	.2036**	.2198**	-.3435**	-.3520**

Note: * p<.05   ** p<.01   (2-tailed)

ally not so striking as that between depression and life stress (compare Table 10.4 with Table 10.3). It is worth mentioning that as compared with the Lubben Social Network Scale (LSNS), the simply summated SSS (labeled SSSS in Table 10.4) only marginally improved measurement power (in terms of the capability of detecting the relationship between social support and depression). The treatment of standardization, however, more than doubled the measurement power, or scaling effectiveness. And the extraordinary performance of the regressed social support scale RSSRDSC seems to have made ample room for scaling improvement, with some correlation coefficients being increased by more than five times.

Personal coping and affective functioning

Tables 10.5a through 10.5c give the zero-order correlation coefficients of the scores on the multiple selected depression scales with those on the multiple selected personal coping proxies. On the whole, the correlations are much weaker than those shown in the two preceding tables, which may partially reflect the fact that we do not have a comprehensive personal coping scale. Especially, the measure of Attitudes Toward Social Support (ATSS) seems largely irrelevant to the scaling of affective functioning. If the results suggest anything, it is the more informal-social-support-oriented elderly that seem more depressed. In comparison, the measures of Attitudes Toward Elderly (ATE) as well as Health Behaviors and Beliefs (HBB) are more closely correlated with depression, though the highest values of the correlation coefficients are still only slightly higher than 0.2.

Table 10.5a Correlations between depression and health behaviors and beliefs using multiple scales

	HBS	HBSD	HBS1A	HBSD1A	HBH3B	HBH2	RHBRDSC	RHBLSDSC
CESDTL17	-.1211**	-.0876**	-.1323**	-.1362**	-.0838**	-.1362**	.1799**	.1542**
DSS	-.1263**	-.0630*	-.1448***	-.1293***	-.0475	-.1152**	.2239***	.1475**
DSSD	-.1321***	-.0813**	-.1456***	-.1394***	-.0695**	-.1304***	.2172***	.1589**
DSS1A	-.1020**	-.0599*	-.1126**	-.1100**	-.0521*	-.0998**	.1839**	.1264**
DSSD1A	-.1118**	-.0703**	-.1204***	-.1167***	-.0655*	-.1111**	.1850**	.1361**
DSH3B	-.1102**	-.0670**	-.1313***	-.1319***	-.0528*	-.1090**	.1860**	.1333**
DSH2	-.1137**	-.0605*	-.1278***	-.1143***	-.0529*	-.1065**	.2048***	.1368**
RDSCESD	-.1084**	-.0695**	-.1238***	-.1257***	-.0648*	-.1215**	.1829**	.1426**
RDSHLTH	.1133**	.0478	.1376**	.1196**	.0295	.0978**	-.2204**	-.1323**

Note: * p<.05   ** p<.01   (2-tailed)

Table 10.5b Correlations between depression and attitudes toward social support using multiple scales

	ASS	ASSD	ASS1ABC	ASSD1ABC	ASH3B	ASH2	RASRDSC	RASLSDSC
CESDTL17	.0290	.0137	.0406	.0382	-.0057	.0413	.0608*	.0616*
DSS	.0570*	.0375	.0724***	.0706***	-.0095	.0759***	.0845**	.0955**
DSSD	.0385	.0225	.0557*	.0537*	-.0021	.0549*	.0653**	.0736**
DSS1A	.0481	.0337	.0551*	.0524*	.0158	.0567*	.0558*	.0655**
DSSD1A	.0336	.0225	.0412	.0387	.0079	.0404	.0405	.0480
DSH3B	-.0526*	-.0307	.0698**	.0682**	-.0001	.0749**	.0984**	.1034**
DSH2	.0183	.0066	.0253	.0233	-.0065	.0265	.0452	.0429
RDSCESD	.0144	.0006	.0216	.0190	-.0134	.0229	.0519*	.0449
RDSHLTH	-.0551*	-.0348	-.0729**	-.0719**	-.0042	-.0776**	-.0928**	-.1018**

Note: * p<.05   ** p<.01   (2-tailed)

Table 10.5c Correlations between depression and attitudes toward elderly using multiple scales

	AES	AESD	AES1A	AESD1A	AEH3B	AEH2	RAERDSC	RAELSDSC
CESDTL17	-.1814**	-.1787**	-.1906**	-.1897**	-.1804**	-.1852**	.1905**	.1883**
DSS	-.1961**	-.1942**	-.2053**	-.2051**	-.1949**	-.1999**	.2048**	.2030**
DSSD	-.1969**	-.1945**	-.2054**	-.2045**	-.1948**	-.2001**	.2060**	.2035**
DSS1A	-.1472**	-.1441**	-.1544**	-.1521**	-.1433**	-.1490**	.1580**	.1531**
DSSD1A	-.1404**	-.1374**	-.1462**	-.1439**	-.1366**	-.1420**	.1505**	.1459**
DSH3B	-.2032**	-.2020**	-.2125**	-.2145**	-.2022**	-.2054**	.2055**	.2068**
DSH2	-.1798**	-.1756**	-.1840**	-.1815**	-.1728**	-.1789**	.1877**	.1832**
RDSCESD	-.2048**	-.2007**	-.2111**	-.2099**	-.1989**	-.2044**	.2107**	.2080**
RDSHLTH	.2148**	.2130**	.2198**	.2205**	.2122**	.2160**	-.2173**	-.2179**

Note: * p<.05   ** p<.01   (2-tailed)

Table 10.6 Aging and affective functioning: Correlations

	AGE
CESDTL17	.0757**
DSS	.0823**
DSSD	.0802**
DSS1A	.0631*
DSSD1A	.0626*
DSH3B	.0650*
DSH2	.0533*
RDSCESD	.0412
RDSHLTH	-.0795**

Note: * p<.05   ** p<.01   (2-tailed)

The multiple selected depression scales all indicate a positive relationship with age (see Table 10.6 on the last page). Note, a negative sign is needed for the correlation between AGE and RDSHLTH because the value of the latter was reversed once in its regression using self-rated health as a criterion. All in all, the results suggest that the older old would probably not be better off in terms of the status of affective functioning, as opposed to some suggestion from the literature. On the other hand, they do not show that aging is associated with the decline of affective functioning to any considerable degree either, since the effect size is generally too small. Such conclusions, nevertheless, apply only to the aging group and cannot do justice to the comparison between the elderly and the non-elderly populations.

Gender difference in depression

A significant gender difference in depression is found no matter which scale is used (see Table 10.7). Female elderly respondents tend to score higher than their male counterparts. This result is in accord with most previous findings reported in literature. Nevertheless, this does not automatically lead to the conclusion that elderly Chinese and Chinese-American women are more depressed than elderly men. There might be some other factors functioning in it. For example, the mental health reporting behavior may not tend to be the same between the two genders. However, these need be pursued with great care, and any difference should in no way be taken as presuming some superior property of men over women.

Table 10.7 Gender difference in affective functioning: T-Tests

VARIABLE	# OF CASES	MEAN	STD. DEV.	STD. ERROR	F VALUE	2-TAIL PROB.	POOLED VARIANCE ESTIMATE T VALUE	DEGREES OF FREEDOM	2-TAIL PROB.	SEPARATE VARIANCE ESTIMATE T VALUE	DEGREES OF FREEDOM	2-TAIL PROB.
CESDTL17												
GROUP 1	734	5.9319	5.322	.196	1.65	.000	-4.50	1560	.000	-4.57	1535.34	.000
GROUP 2	828	7.3394	6.828	.237								
DSS												
GROUP 1	737	11.9742	9.159	.337	1.52	.000	-7.63	1564	.000	-7.72	1550.98	.000
GROUP 2	829	15.9723	11.302	.393								
DSSD												
GROUP 1	737	-2.2165	9.729	.358	1.62	.000	-6.57	1564	.000	-6.66	1541.23	.000
GROUP 2	829	1.5127	12.380	.430								
DSS1A												
GROUP 1	736	3.1658	4.979	.184	1.74	.000	-6.09	1563	.000	-6.19	1526.56	.000
GROUP 2	829	4.9783	6.565	.228								
DSSD1A												
GROUP 1	736	-1.4134	6.895	.254	1.81	.000	-5.53	1563	.000	-5.63	1517.14	.000
GROUP 2	829	.8974	9.278	.322								
DSH3B												
GROUP 1	703	-.6057	2.386	.090	1.31	.000	-6.92	1483	.000	-6.97	1481.87	.000
GROUP 2	782	.3193	2.729	.098								
DSH2												
GROUP 1	703	-.1898	.818	.011	1.59	.000	-5.90	1483	.000	-5.97	1460.20	.000
GROUP 2	782	.0975	1.032	.037								
RDSCESD												
GROUP 1	703	-.1113	.891	.034	1.47	.000	-4.12	1483	.000	-4.16	1472.50	.000
GROUP 2	782	.1014	1.079	.039								
RDSHLTH												
GROUP 1	703	.2147	.870	.033	1.50	.000	8.03	1483	.000	8.11	1469.41	.000
GROUP 2	782	-.1935	1.067	.038								

Note: GROUP 1 - Male   GROUP 2 - Female   (independent samples)

Because of the widespread geographical distribution of the research sites ranging from Northern, Eastern, and Southern China to North America, it is quite plausible to assume a research dimension of cultural differentiation. Because of the "assimilation" or "acculturation" process, the sample here in Los Angeles would have experienced some kind of cultural change. Even within the People's Republic of China, different regions have been influenced by Western culture to different degrees in recent years. For example, the city of Guangzhou as a show widow for foreign trade may have had a larger and longer exposure to outer commercial world than Beijing. These cities are historically considered as important cultural centers of the Chinese society. Therefore, if depression has a great deal to do with cultures, then we should be able to see some difference among these different research sites.

Empirical data do render some support to such a hypothesis. The results, however, are not consistent. Tables 10.8a and 10.8b show that if depression is measured by either the 17-item CES-D (CESDTL17) or the new summated Depression Scale (DSS), there is no significant difference that can be found among the four sites (Beijing, Shanghai, Guangzhou, and Los Angeles). This also holds true if the two optimally weighted depression scales (RDSCESD and RD-SHLTH) are used. Considerable significance levels, nevertheless, are attained when other depression scales are used (see Tables 10.8c through 10.8f). The variation of the mean scores, however, does not coincide with some readily presumed direction. The Los Angeles sample tends to resemble the Beijing sample more than the samples from Shanghai and Guangzhou. This is interesting indeed, while the reason for this may demand a much more exhaustive and detailed exploration.

Table 10.8a Cultural differentiation in affective functioning (measured by 17-Item CES-D): One-Way ANOVA

SOURCE	D.F.	SUM OF SQUARES	MEAN SQUARES	F RATIO	F PROB.
BETWEEN GROUPS	3	110.0682	36.6894	.9530	.4142
WITHIN GROUPS	1559	60019.5210	38.4987		
TOTAL	1562	60129.5893			

GROUP	COUNT	MEAN	STANDARD DEVIATION	STANDARD ERROR	MINIMUM	MAXIMUM	95 PCT CONF INT FOR MEAN
GRP 1	500	6.8880	6.6907	.2992	.0000	46.0000	6.3001 TO 7.4759
GRP 2	366	6.2213	5.1708	.2703	.0000	41.0000	5.6898 TO 6.7528
GRP 3	493	6.6917	5.9904	.2698	.0000	45.0000	6.1616 TO 7.2218
GRP 5	204	6.9167	7.1119	.4979	.0000	45.0000	5.9349 TO 7.8985
TOTAL	1563	6.6737	6.2045	.1569	.0000	46.0000	6.3659 TO 6.9815

Note: Group 1=Beijing   Group 2=Shanghai   Group 3=Guangzhou   Group 5=Los Angeles

Table 10.8b Cultural differentiation in affective functioning (measured by DSS): One-Way ANOVA

SOURCE	D.F.	SUM OF SQUARES	MEAN SQUARES	F RATIO	F PROB.
BETWEEN GROUPS	3	524.1093	174.7031	1.5751	.1935
WITHIN GROUPS	1563	173357.1058	110.9131		
TOTAL	1566	173881.2151			

GROUP	COUNT	MEAN	STANDARD DEVIATION	STANDARD ERROR	MINIMUM	MAXIMUM	95 PCT CONF INT FOR MEAN
GRP 1	500	14.7100	10.7760	.4819	.0000	70.0000	13.7632 TO 15.6568
GRP 2	363	13.1488	8.9958	.4695	1.0000	56.0000	12.2254 TO 14.0721
GRP 3	500	14.0440	10.2761	.4596	.0000	68.0000	13.1411 TO 14.9469
GRP 5	204	14.3039	12.8939	.9028	.0000	77.0000	12.5239 TO 16.0839
TOTAL	1567	14.0830	10.5373	.2662	.0000	77.0000	13.5608 TO 14.6051

Note: Group 1=Beijing   Group 2=Shanghai   Group 3=Guangzhou   Group 5=Los Angeles

Table 10.8c Cultural differentiation in affective functioning (measured by DSSD): One-Way ANOVA

SOURCE	D.F.	SUM OF SQUARES	MEAN SQUARES	F RATIO	F PROB.
BETWEEN GROUPS	3	1041.8314	347.2771	2.6996	.0444
WITHIN GROUPS	1563	201067.4044	128.6420		
TOTAL	1566	202109.2358			

GROUP	COUNT	MEAN	STANDARD DEVIATION	STANDARD ERROR	MINIMUM	MAXIMUM	95 PCT CONF INT FOR MEAN	
GRP 1	500	.6082	11.6984	.5232	-13.7021	64.8340	-.4197 TO	1.6360
GRP 2	363	-1.4789	9.5940	.5036	-12.3478	55.4196	-2.4692 TO	-.4887
GRP 3	500	-.4942	11.0936	.4961	-13.7021	64.4196	-1.4689 TO	.4806
GRP 5	204	-.4345	13.6902	.9585	-13.7021	70.8915	-1.4554 TO	2.3244
TOTAL	1567	-.2497	11.3605	.2870	-13.7021	70.8915	-.8126 TO	.3113

Note: Group 1=Beijing Group 2=Shanghai Group 3=Guangzhou Group 5=Los Angeles

Table 10.8d Cultural differentiation in affective functioning (measured by DSS1A): One-Way ANOVA

SOURCE	D.F.	SUM OF SQUARES	MEAN SQUARES	F RATIO	F PROB.
BETWEEN GROUPS	3	611.1909	203.7303	5.8290	.0006
WITHIN GROUPS	1562	54594.0230	34.9514		
TOTAL	1565	55205.2139			

GROUP	COUNT	MEAN	STANDARD DEVIATION	STANDARD ERROR	MINIMUM	MAXIMUM	95 PCT CONF INT FOR MEAN	
GRP 1	500	4.7620	6.0540	.2707	.0000	42.0000	4.2301 TO	5.2939
GRP 2	366	3.1175	5.0019	.2615	.0000	37.0000	2.6003 TO	3.6316
GRP 3	496	4.0524	5.8449	.2624	.0000	40.0000	3.5368 TO	4.5681
GRP 5	204	4.5343	7.1102	.4978	.0000	42.0000	3.5528 TO	5.5159
TOTAL	1566	4.1232	5.9393	.1501	.0000	42.0000	3.8289 TO	4.4176

Note: Group 1=Beijing Group 2=Shanghai Group 3=Guangzhou Group 5=Los Angeles

Table 10.8e Cultural differentiation in affective functioning (measured by DSSD1A): One-Way ANOVA

SOURCE	D.F.	SUM OF SQUARES	MEAN SQUARES	F RATIO	F PROB.
BETWEEN GROUPS	3	1205.0973	401.6991	5.8575	.0006
WITHIN GROUPS	1562	107120.5833	68.5791		
TOTAL	1565	108325.6807			

GROUP	COUNT	MEAN	STANDARD DEVIATION	STANDARD ERROR	MINIMUM	MAXIMUM	95 PCT CONF INT FOR MEAN
GRP 1	500	.7719	8.5701	.3833	-5.2837	55.0530	.0189 TO 1.5249
GRP 2	366	-1.5067	7.0608	.3691	-5.2837	50.8368	-2.2325 TO -.7809
GRP 3	496	-.4462	8.2143	.3688	-5.2837	52.4237	-1.1708 TO .2785
GRP 5	204	.4179	9.6422	.6751	-5.2837	53.0742	-.9132 TO 1.7490
TOTAL	1566	-.1926	8.3197	.2102	-5.2837	55.0530	-.6049 TO .2198

Note: Group 1=Beijing Group 2=Shanghai Group 3=Guangzhou Group 5=Los Angeles

Table 10.8f Cultural differentiation in affective functioning (measured by DSH2): One-Way ANOVA

SOURCE	D.F.	SUM OF SQUARES	MEAN SQUARES	F RATIO	F PROB.
BETWEEN GROUPS	3	22.7055	7.5685	8.5628	.0000
WITHIN GROUPS	1482	1309.9201	.8839		
TOTAL	1485	1332.6257			

GROUP	COUNT	MEAN	STANDARD DEVIATION	STANDARD ERROR	MINIMUM	MAXIMUM	95 PCT CONF INT FOR MEAN
GRP 1	499	.0945	1.0084	.0451	-.8115	5.7223	.0058 TO .1832
GRP 2	327	-.2219	.7006	.0387	-.7774	4.3174	-.2982 TO -.1457
GRP 3	457	-.0927	.9139	.0427	-.8115	5.7327	-.1767 TO -.0087
GRP 5	203	.0484	1.1403	.0800	-.8115	6.1287	-.1094 TO .2062
TOTAL	1486	-.0390	.9473	.0246	-.8115	6.1287	-.0872 TO .0092

Note: Group 1=Beijing Group 2=Shanghai Group 3=Guangzhou Group 5=Los Angeles

Social support, life stress, and personal coping

Table 10.9 contains the zero-order correlation coefficients of the scores on the multiple selected life stress scales with those on the multiple selected social support scales. The results generally support the hypothesis that more social support is associated with less life stress. Especially, scales using the optimal weighting approach provide considerable correlation coefficients (the highest correlation coefficient almost reaches 0.5).

Tables 10.10a through 10.10c give the zero-order correlation coefficients of the scores on the multiple selected life stress scales with those on the multiple selected personal coping proxy measures. In contrast to the other two personal coping proxies, the measures of Attitudes Toward Social Support (ATSS) have gone against our expectation. They seem to suggest that the more an elderly person is attitudinally informal social support oriented, the more likely s/he will experience higher life stress. It is noticeable that the ATSS has a similar, though generally weaker, association with depression as described earlier. From the standpoint of scale development, we may conclude that the ATSS is a poor proxy measure of personal coping if we take the latter as some fixed or rigid construct to be approached (the conventional conception of measurement validity). Guided by the appropriate theoretical framework and scaling approaches, however, it is rather effective in revealing some significant substantial meaning. The findings show that even though informal social support does have notable positive impact on affective functioning and quality of life of the Chinese and Chinese-American elderly, their preference for it may not necessarily have the same effect, and in fact may even bring to them some adverse consequence.

Table 10.9 Correlations between life stress and social support using multiple scales

	LSNS	SSSS	SSSSD	SSSS1A	SSSSD1A	SSSH3B	SSSH2	RSSRDSC	RSSLSDSC
LSSS	-.0951**	-.0569**	-.0865**	-.0748**	-.0764**	-.0340	-.0888**	.2255**	.3117**
LSSSD	-.2004**	-.2188**	-.2974**	-.2453**	-.2777**	-.2041**	-.2645**	.3125**	.4350**
LSSS1A	-.1981**	-.1401**	-.2115**	-.1997**	-.2270**	-.0799	-.2118**	.2586**	.4719**
LSSSD1A	-.1676**	-.1461**	-.2142**	-.1973**	-.2227**	-.0995*	-.1992**	.2312**	.4118**
LSSH3B	-.1169**	-.1238**	-.1876**	-.1338**	-.1676**	-.1679**	-.2177**	.1915**	.2951**
LSSH2	-.1650**	-.1526**	-.2107**	-.2132**	-.2227**	-.1379*	-.2397**	.2365**	.4473**
RLSRDSC	-.1897**	-.1858**	-.2756**	-.2378**	-.2630**	-.1861**	-.3008**	.2752**	.4920**
RLSRDSH	.1612**	.1567**	.2357**	.2125**	.2370**	.1503*	.2582**	-.2579**	-.4720**

Note: * p<.05   ** p<.01   (2-tailed)

Table 10.10a Correlations between life stress and health behaviors and beliefs using multiple scales

	HBS	HBSD	HBS1A	HBSD1A	HBH3B	HBH2	RHBRDSC	RHBLSDSC
LSSS	-.0793**	-.0191	-.1064**	-.0963**	-.0093	-.0727**	.1745**	.0996**
LSSSD	-.1219**	-.0872**	-.1410**	-.1567**	-.0611*	-.1400**	.2320**	.1688**
LSSS1A	-.1497**	-.1340**	-.1753**	-.2169**	-.1097**	-.2078**	.2854**	.2352**
LSSSD1A	-.1230**	-.1076**	-.1433**	-.1782**	-.0796**	-.1709**	.2542**	.1976**
LSSH3B	-.0359	-.0334	-.0425	-.0583	-.0268	-.0427	.0673	.0506
LSSH2	-.1735**	-.1930**	-.1813**	-.2480**	-.1717**	-.2349**	.2352**	.2452**
RLSRDSC	-.1462**	-.1919**	-.1407**	-.2094**	-.1820**	-.2089**	.1711**	.2115**
RLSRDSH	.1465**	.1769**	.1456**	.2038**	.1642**	.2011**	-.1835**	-.2073**

Note: * p<.05   ** p<.01   (2-tailed)

226

Table 10.10b Correlations between life stress and attitudes toward social support using multiple scales

	ASS	ASSD	ASS1ABC	ASSD1ABC	ASH3B	ASH2	RASRDSC	RASLSDSC
LSSS	.0731**	.0584*	.0801**	.0799**	.0337	.0877**	.0746**	.0936**
LSSSD	.0466	.0243	.0720**	.0713**	-.0096	.0768**	.1016**	.1094**
LSSS1A	.1734**	.1454**	.1957**	.1948**	.0933**	.2053**	.1406**	.2003**
LSSSD1A	.1160**	.0934**	.1359**	.1347**	.0535	.1426**	.1120**	.1486**
LSSH3B	.0386	.0263	.0497	.0479	.0083	.0469	.0399	.0509
LSSH2	.1602**	.1162*	.1833**	.1804**	.0544	.1999**	.1955**	.2221**
RLSRDSC	.1196**	.0751	.1646**	.1612**	.0077	.1704**	.1902**	.2114**
RLSRDSH	-.1283**	-.0872	-.1599**	-.1569**	-.0274	-.1705**	-.1795**	-.2008**

Note: * p<.05   ** p<.01   (2-tailed)

Table 10.10c Correlations between life stress and attitudes toward elderly using multiple scales

	AES	AESD	AES1A	AESD1A	AEII3B	AEH2	RAERDSC	RAELSDSC
LSSS	-.1131**	-.1122**	-.1093**	-.1083**	-.1110**	-.1129**	.1131**	.1138**
LSSSD	-.2031**	-.2008**	-.1976**	-.1961**	-.1980**	-.2020**	.2042**	.2042**
LSSS1A	-.2531**	-.2505**	-.2478**	-.2465**	-.2480**	-.2534**	.2561**	.2562**
LSSSD1A	-.2273**	-.2247**	-.2233**	-.2218**	-.2220**	-.2273**	.2311**	.2304**
LSSH3B	-.1926**	-.1968**	-.1527**	-.1534**	-.1930**	-.1880**	.1649**	.1816**
LSSH2	-.2327**	-.2292**	-.2284**	-.2253**	-.2244**	-.2313**	.2373**	.2355**
RLSRDSC	-.2963**	-.2935**	-.2844**	-.2829**	-.2907**	-.2953**	.2917**	.2967**
RLSRDSH	.2622**	.2608**	.2507**	.2497**	.2576**	.2612**	-.2569**	-.2620**

Note: * p<.05   ** p<.01   (2-tailed)

227

Tables 10.11a through 10.11c give the zero-order correlation coefficients of the scores on the selected social support scales with those on the selected personal coping proxy measures. To this point, the measures of Health Behaviors and Beliefs seem to have fulfilled the expectation that higher scores would reflect more desirable (or positive) categories of personal coping in relation to affective functioning, quality of life, and social support. As for the Attitudes toward Social Support (ATSS) measures, it is interesting that they have consistent positive correlations with social support as well as with life stress scores. It seems to suggest that an informal social support attitudinal orientation would be conducive to both life stress and social support. The Attitudes toward the Elderly measures, in contrast, performed somewhat inconsistent in this case. However, a positive relationship between the ATE and the SSS seems to be bolstered by the stronger evidence derived from the practical approach with optimal weights secured by the regression method (note the negative signs of the correlation coefficients are due to the negative relationship between ATE and DS or LSS).

Table 10.11a Correlations between social support and health behaviors and beliefs using multiple scales

	LSNS	SSSS	SSSSD	SSSS1A	SSSSD1A	SSSH3B	SSSH2	RSSHBDSC	RSSHBLSD
HBS	.1832**	.1827**	.1870**	.1873**	.1883**	.1934**	.2150**	-.1908**	-.2803**
HBSD	.2702**	.2542**	.2846**	.2739**	.2920**	.2607**	.3234**	-.1656**	-.3438**
HBS1A	.1502**	.1493**	.1470**	.1476**	.1465**	.1601**	.1744**	-.2117**	-.2623**
HBSD1A	.2397**	.2173**	.2351**	.2302**	.2417**	.2200**	.2727**	-.2756**	-.3688**
HBH3B	.2584**	.2432**	.2675**	.2651**	.2795**	.2497**	.3016**	-.1243**	-.3052**
HBH2	.2492**	.2239**	.2453**	.2479**	.2583**	.2314**	.2877**	-.2359**	-.3551**
RHBRDSC	-.0573*	-.0561*	-.0605*	-.0736**	-.0623*	-.1097**	-.0907*	.3303**	.2537**
RHBLSDSC	-.2203**	-.2003**	-.2197**	-.2249**	-.2308**	-.2197**	-.2591**	.2701**	.3517**

Note: * p<.05   ** p<.01   (2-tailed)

Table 10.11b Correlations between social support and attitude toward social support using multiple scales

	LSNS	SSSS	SSSSD	SSSS1A	SSSSD1A	SSSH3B	SSSH2	RSSASDSC	RSSASLSD
ASS	.0660**	.1325**	.1350**	.0944**	.0890**	.1048*	.0702	.2715**	.3078**
ASSD	.0940**	.1499**	.1564**	.1312**	.1258**	.0953**	.0810*	.2116**	.2532**
ASS1ABC	.0243	.0931**	.0720**	.0343	.0285	.0427	.0102	.2802**	.3261**
ASSD1ABC	.0285	.0949**	.0740**	.0364	.0305	.0418	.0134	.2760**	.3236**
ASH3B	.1173**	.1574**	.1801**	.1589**	.1576**	.1083*	.1092*	.1312**	.1636**
ASH2	.0280	.1003**	.0867**	.0358	.0312	.0779	.0363	.3095**	.3489**
RASRDSC	-.0989**	-.0490*	-.0663**	-.1238**	-.1108**	.0574	-.0287	.2917**	.2781**
RASLSDSC	-.0547*	.0141	-.0115	-.0715**	-.0779**	.0541	-.0156	.3311**	.3473**

Note: * p<.05   ** p<.01   (2-tailed)

Table 10.11c Correlations between social support and attitude toward elderly using multiple scales

	LSNS	SSSS	SSSSD	SSSS1A	SSSSD1A	SSSH3B	SSSH2	RSSAEDSC	RSSAELSD
AES	-.0011	-.0038	.0606*	.0060	.0400	.0598	.1088**	-.2247**	-.2270**
AESD	-.0021	-.0043	.0597*	.0021	.0374	.0497	.1023*	-.2201**	-.2236**
AES1A	-.0069	-.0118	.0514*	-.0094	.0416	.0575	.1042**	-.2093**	-.2081**
AESD1A	-.0080	-.0117	.0513*	-.0067	.0402	.0511	.1008*	-.2066**	-.2061**
AEH3B	-.0066	-.0075	.0575*	-.0024	.0352	.0467	.1008*	-.2176**	-.2212**
AEH2	-.0062	-.0089	.0570*	-.0014	.0376	.0538	.1050*	-.2212**	-.2236**
RAERDSC	.0050	.0123	-.0533*	-.0116	-.0425	-.0704	-.1116**	-.2211**	-.2199**
RAELSDSC	.0058	.0101	-.0561*	-.0050	-.0396	-.0599	-.1081*	-.2229**	-.2240**

Note: * p<.05   ** p<.01   (2-tailed)

Statistical control via multiple regression

Regression is one of the most versatile procedures for data analysis. As a computerized statistical program, it can supply us with more precise as well as more comprehensive information like partial correlation, multiple correlation, as well as a variety of statistics associated with the regression modeling.

In the foregoing section, I examined the relationships among the key constructs by calculating their correlation coefficients. Such coefficients were calculated with neither experimental nor statistical control. In other words, the relationships exhibited could be spurious. A coefficient might be significant without any true connection between the two constructs it was supposed to represent, because such a coefficient could be made significant potentially by some other variables. For such a concern, the utility of the multiple regression procedure is in that it contains the statistics called partial correlation coefficients, which are the measures of the degree of dependence between variables after adjusting for the linear effect of one or more of the other variables. On the other hand, all the detailed statistics can be pooled together to provide a general indicator of the degree of dependence of a variable on its various determining factors, such as the overall impact of stress, social support, and personal coping upon affective functioning (depression). The multiple regression procedure can calculate the multiple correlation coefficient to summarize data as well as to quantify relationships among the variables.

It should be noted, however, that the regression model is different from the correlation model. The application of multiple regression is aimed at predicting values of new observations based on a previously derived model, which always distinguishes between a dependent variable and one or more independent variables. The correlation model, on the other hand, focuses on the degree of relation, or association, between variables. Since such an association or relationship is the basis for predictability, the study of correlation can be regarded as more fundamental than regression. Whereas the relative importance of various factors in influencing the dependent variable is of most research interest, this study is intended to solicit both kinds of information.

Since I am working from a theoretical model and the variables have been chosen and arranged to fit that model (cf. chapter four), I can enter all of them into the regression equation at once. To focus on the psychosocial mechanism of affective functioning, my dependent variable here is depression. The question is, however, which scale should be used for each construct, since I have developed multiple measures for the dependent and independent variables? Quite naturally, one may think about the ones representing the highest correlations of the independent variables with affective functioning or depression. This is indeed the ideal choice for featuring the psychosocial mechanism of affective functioning. Nevertheless, a single multiple regression model cannot handle the relationships among the independent variables very well. And, unlike the regression approach adopted for scale development, missing values will directly impact on substantive results. Therefore, three criteria seem in order for the selection of a measure for each construct in the substantive analysis: a) the power of detecting the relationship between the independent and the dependent variables, b) the independence of the independent variable from other independent variables, and c) the number of valid cases the measure covers. After a careful inspection of all the scaling results (cf. Tables 10.3 through 10.5c and 10.9 through 10.11c), the following measures are chosen: DSS for depression, LSSSD for life stress, SSSSD for social support, and RHBRDSC for Health Behaviors and Beliefs as a personal coping proxy.

Table 10.12 contains the result of the multiple regression. SHANGHAI, CANTON and LACHN are dummy variables created from the categorical variable SITEID, representing respectively the survey sites Shanghai, Guangzhou (Canton) and Los Angeles. Here Beijing is taken as the reference site for the purpose of comparison. For the gender variable, female is taken as the reference. Of all the independent variables (predictors), life stress as measured by the standardized summative scale LSSSD, plays an extraordinary role in determining the degree of depression, as indicated by the standardized regression coefficient (BETA), partial correlation coefficient (PARTIAL), as well as the significance level (SIG T). And by comparing its zero-order correlation coefficient with depression with its partial correlation coefficient with depression, we can see the effect of statistical control in reducing the spurious portion of the relationship (the magnitude is reduced from .62 to .56). The most dramatic change, however, is found in the relationship of both social support (as measured by SSSD) and personal coping (as represented by the Health

231

Behaviors and Beliefs measure RHBRDSC) with depression (as measured by DSS). The magnitude of the correlation of SSSD with DSS is slashed from -.25 to less than -.10; and that of RHBRDSC with DSS, from .22 to less than .09 (the negative sign is offset since the regression targeting depression has already assigned a negative sign for the Health Behaviors and Beliefs measure). Recall the two leading hypotheses in the psychosocial studies of depression as reviewed in Chapter 2. The partial correlation coefficients can be regarded as the direct effects of social support as well as the proxy of personal coping. The considerable "spurious" portions in their zero-order correlation coefficients, on the other hand, may be attributed to the "buffering" effects of the two variables. Note, however, this buffering not only takes effect on stress but also moderates the influence of the two variables on each other, the impact of aging, gender difference, and especially, site variation (indicating some sort of cultural differentiation). It is noticeable that the role of Chinese-American identity as represented by the Los Angeles site ID (LACHN) is escalated after all the statistical control is applied (compare its zero-order correlation coefficient with depression with the partial correlation coefficient in Table 10.12). The differences within the total group of the Chinese elderly are almost negligible as compared with the Los Angeles sample. This further confirms the existence of such a dimension as well as clarifies the direction of cultural differentiation (cf. foregoing ANOVA results), though the findings here are not statistically significant.

On the whole, the independent variables largely account for the affective functioning of the Chinese and Chinese-American elderly (Multiple R=.639), and the role of life stress remains dominant in the multivariate analysis. Other factors play only a small part in influencing depression after controlling for level of stress. Before multiple statistical control, these variables in order of importance (effect size) are social support, personal coping (proxy), gender, age, and site. After statistical control, the rank order becomes gender first, then social support, coping, site, and age. Statistical control enhanced the role of gender while reduced the role of age. It seems that in terms of the net (direct) effect of gender, female elderly still tend to be more depressed, and the effect size is even larger than that of social support. On the other hand, statistical control seems in favor of the "protective aging" hypothesis, since the partial correlation coefficient turned out to be negative. Nevertheless, the correlation coefficient is not significant nor large enough.

Path analysis

The R square (coefficient of determination) contained in Table 10.12 seems to approve the results of the regression equation, though a large standard error indicates some problem in the goodness of fit of the theoretical model used. The partial correlation approach did not accomplish everything, however. Although we were able to distinguish the direct effect of each independent variable, the "buffering" mechanism we are interested in is not made clear. As a matter of fact, it is even overshadowed since with the regression model, we had to dodge any strong relationship among the independent variables in order to reduce the redundancy problem. Our purpose of analysis, however, is not to dismiss the role of social support by singling out only a small portion of the net or direct effect. We should not disregard, for example, the correlation between social support and life stress. To deal with the more complicated mediating mechanism, we need a procedure to further clarify the pathways of its buffering effect. Structural equations modeling, specifically path analysis, seems to be a more powerful tool that can serve this purpose. Since the path model allows for, and indeed aims at, more complicated relationships among independent and dependent variables, the selection of measures can be done under mainly two criteria: a) the power of detecting the relationship between the independent and the dependent variables, and b) the number of valid cases the measure covers. In the following, while the same measures will continue to be employed, we need not worry so much about the correlations among the independent variables (see Table 10.13).

Table 10.12 Psychosocial mechanism of affective functioning: multiple regression

DEPENDENT VARIABLE: DSS   TOTAL CASES = 1708

VARIABLE	B	SE B	BETA	CORREL	PART COR	PARTIAL	T	SIG T
LACHN	1.332716	.758253	.041028	.008115	.035621	.046268	1.758	.0790
SSSSD	-.082146	.022034	-.080301	-.252263	-.075559	-.097777	-3.728	.0002
MALE	-1.788189	.446335	-.084695	-.189460	-.081196	-.104994	-4.006	.0001
AGE	-.007451	.032551	-.004731	.082331	-.004639	-.006032	-.229	.8190
SHANGHAI	-.089832	.571631	-.003880	-.048695	-.003185	-.004141	-.157	.8751
RHBRDSC	.766692	.232340	.072717	.223934	.066877	.086632	3.300	.0010
LSSSD	.568419	.021941	.570594	.623633	.525041	.563836	25.907	.0000
CANTON	-.144807	.565331	.006269	-.002532	.005191	.006750	.256	.7979
(CONSTANT)	15.188558	2.306777					6.584	.0000

MULTIPLE R   .63917
R SQUARE   .40854
ADJUSTED R SQUARE   .40526
STANDARD ERROR   8.12633

ANALYSIS OF VARIANCE

	DF	SUM OF SQUARES	MEAN SQUARE
REGRESSION	8	65685.39747	8210.67468
RESIDUAL	1440	95093.65706	66.03726

F = 124.33397   SIGNIF F = .0000

RESIDUALS STATISTICS:

	MIN	MAX	MEAN	STD DEV	N
*PRED	-.5994	51.5518	14.2035	6.7617	1458
*RESID	-21.7993	40.6289	-.0186	8.1903	1414
*ZPRED	-2.1800	5.5631	.0179	1.0039	1458
*ZRESID	-2.6825	4.9997	-.0023	1.0079	1414

Table 10.13 Correlation matrix input in path analysis

	DSS	LSSSD	SSSSD	RHBRDSC	AGE	MALE	LACHN
DSS	1.0000						
LSSSD	.6236**	1.0000					
SSSSD	-.2523**	-.2974**	1.0000				
RHBRDSC	.2239**	.2320**	-.0605*	1.0000			
AGE	.0823**	.1149**	-.1584**	.0305	1.0000		
MALE	-.1895**	-.1627**	-.0295	-.2436**	-.0395	1.0000	
LACHN	.0081	-.0269	-.0216	-.1659**	.0753**	.0747**	1.0000

Note: * p<.05   ** p<.01   (2-tailed)

A regression equation in the context of a causal model is called a structural equation. Structural equation models are virtually always multiple equation models. Based on the causal modeling efforts made in chapters three and four, several structural equations can be derived that would provide a more accurate description of the interrelationships among the variables. Nevertheless, in the process of model specification for actual data analysis, it is realized that the working model set up earlier (cf. Diagram 6.1 in chapter six) needs some additional modification. Since the above results show that the impact of the personal coping proxy HBB on depression is close to that of social support, a path seems needing to be added to directly connect personal coping and depression. On the other hand, with the multivariate analysis technology available to date, the resolution of a nonrecursive model would go well beyond the scope of this book. Therefore, not even the impact of depression on social support will be considered in the following analysis such that not too many technical complications would be introduced.

The statistical procedure for path analysis is EQS. The subject under investigation suits the application of the tool with a large sample size. EQS is "a simple, consistent, yet technically advanced and accurate approach to structural modeling" (Bentler, 1989). The statistical theory underlying this computer program allows for the estimation of parameters and testing of models using traditional multivariate normal theory, but also enables the use of the more general elliptical and arbitrary distribution theories, based on a unified generalized least squares or minimum chi-square approach (ibid.). Parallel to this advantage of generality is its simplicity. Nevertheless, the program has no

235

data-cleaning features such as procedures for handling missing data, nor is it powerful enough to deal with categorical variables. Due to these concerns, the correlation matrix shown in Table 10.13, instead of the raw data, is used as program input. Since EQS performs better with covariance data, standard deviations are also provided to transform the correlations into covariances. Note, for the dimension of site difference or cultural differentiation, only the dummy variable LACHN (standing for the Los Angeles Chinese American elderly group) is used. This is because the partial correlation results in the above showed the differences among elderly persons at different sites in China are much smaller, and therefore they altogether may serve as the reference for comparison with their American counterpart.

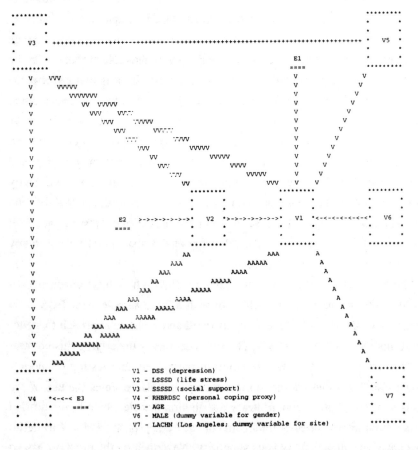

Diagram 10.1 A path diagram plotted by EQS

236

Adding a residual (error) item to each dependent variable (in EQS terminology), the program rendered a diagram representing the path model actually used in the structural equations analysis (see Diagram 10.1). In this diagram, a line of "A"s represents an upwardly moving arrow whereas "V"s indicate a downward direction. The covariation of the two independent variables V3 (social support) and V5 (age), as suggested in Table 10.13 (γ=-.1584, p<0.01), is also taken into consideration by linking them with "+"s.

Parameters of the model are estimated by using three methods that are readily available for analysis with covariance data matrix in EQS. These are Lease Squares (LS), Generalized Least Squares (GLS) and Maximum likelihood (ML) techniques based on multinormal distribution theory. The program messages show that all three types of estimates for all parameters seem to be technically acceptable (no special problems were encountered during optimization). The values of the residual covariance matrices are all small and rather evenly distributed, which is exemplified by the Least Squares (LS) solution contained in Table 10.14. The frequency distribution of the standardized residuals is centered around zero. All these indicate that the model is a pretty good representation of the data. The probability values for the chi-square statistic, however, are very small, which indicate that the residuals are nevertheless different from zero in the population. The Bentler-Bonett Normed and Nonnormed Fit Indices (NFI & NNFI) and the Comparative Fit Index (CFI) are further inspected. For the LS solution, NFI=0.860, NNFI=0.743, and CFI=0.866. The Maximum likelihood (ML) method yields similar measurement levels of fit. Yet for the Generalized Least Squares (GLS) solution, NFI=0.986, NNFI= 0.974, and CFI=0.986, which indicate that it is more desirable than the LS solution. Table 10.15 displays the measurement equations (first row) with standard errors (second row) and test statistics (third row) obtained by all three estimation methods. The test statistics are univariate large-sample normal Z-tests of the null hypothesis that a given parameter is zero in the population. Absolute values exceeding 1.96 (for a 0.05 level test) indicate that the null hypothesis can be rejected, i.e., that the structural coefficient is not zero. Note, in the LS solution there are several standard errors equal to or approaching zero. In this case the test statistic cannot be defined. The other two solutions, on the other hand, suggest that all the parameter estimations are statistically significant. In

237

Table 10.14 Residual covariance matrices (LS solution)

Residual Covariance Matrix (S-Sigma) :

		DSS V1	LSSSD V2	SSSSD V3	RHBRDSC V4	AGE V5	MALE V6	LACHN V7
DSS	V1	0.000						
LSSSD	V2	0.000	0.000					
SSSSD	V3	0.000	0.501	0.312				
RHBRDSC	V4	0.000	0.000	0.015	0.000			
AGE	V5	0.000	4.319	1.344	0.130	0.000		
MALE	V6	0.000	-0.861	-0.152	-0.122	-0.132	0.000	
LACHN	V7	0.000	-0.091	-0.071	-0.053	0.161	0.012	0.000

Average absolute covariance residuals   = 0.2955
Average off-diagonal absolute covariance residuals = 0.3792

Standardized Residual Matrix:

		DSS V1	LSSSD V2	SSSSD V3	RHBRDSC V4	AGE V5	MALE V6	LACHN V7
DSS	V1	0.000						
LSSSD	V2	0.000	0.000					
SSSSD	V3	0.000	0.005	0.003				
RHBRDSC	V4	0.000	0.000	0.001	0.000			
AGE	V5	0.000	0.061	0.020	0.019	0.000		
MALE	V6	0.000	-0.163	-0.029	-0.244	-0.039	0.000	
LACHN	V7	0.000	-0.027	-0.022	-0.166	0.075	0.075	0.000

Average absolute standardized residuals   = 0.0339
Average off-diagonal absolute standardized residuals = 0.0450

Table 10.15 Measurement equations with standard errors and test statistics

LS Solution

DSS =V1= .580*V2 + .889*V4 + -.066*V3 + .061*V5 + -3.995*V6 + .267*V7 + 1.000 E1
        .001   .035   .000   .000   2.336   .877
   746.571   25.451 -1587.539 5149.286 -1.710   .304

LSSSD =V2= 2.265*V4 + -.297*V3 + 1.000 E2
        .084   .001
    27.011 -587.196

RHBRDSC =V4= -.006*V3 + 1.000 E3
        .000
   -252.223

GLS Solution

DSS =V1= .568*V2 + .769*V4 + -.082*V3 + -.007*V5 + -1.781*V6 + 1.333*V7 + 1.000 E1
     .021   .232   .021   .030   .458   .656
  27.272 3.311 -3.997   -.240 -3.889 2.033

LSSSD =V2= 1.617*V4 + -.303*V3 + 1.000 E2
       .267   .023
    6.050 -13.137

RHBRDSC =V4= -.008*V3 + 1.000 E3
        .002
    -3.411

Table 10.15 Measurement equations with standard errors and test statistics (continued)

ML Solution

```
DSS =V1=    .568*V2 +    .769*V4 +   -.082*V3 +   -.007*V5 +  -1.776*V6 +   1.336*V7 +   1.000 E1
            .020         .202         .020         .030         .392         .613
          28.519        3.813       -4.082        -.247       -4.527        2.179

LSSSD =V2=  2.273*V4 +  -.292*V3 +   1.000 E2
            .239         .023
           9.521      -12.607

RHBRDSC =V4= -.006*V3 +  1.000 E3
             .002
           -2.504
```

Table 10.16 Standardized solutions of path analysis

LS
```
DSS     =V1= .582*V2 +  .084*V4 +  -.064*V3 +   .039*V5 +  -.190*V6 +  .008*V7 +  .750 E1
LSSSD   =V2= .214*V4 + -.289*V3 +   .929 E2
RHBRDSC =V4= -.062*V3 +  .998 E3
```

GLS
```
DSS     =V1= .566*V2 +  .069*V4 +  -.082*V3 +  -.005*V5 +  -.080*V6 +  .040*V7 +  .785 E1
LSSSD   =V2= .145*V4 + -.304*V3 +   .938 E2
RHBRDSC =V4= -.086*V3 +  .996 E3
```

ML
```
DSS     =V1= .575*V2 +  .074*V4 +  -.081*V3 +  -.005*V5 +  -.085*V6 +  .041*V7 +  .775 E1
LSSSD   =V2= .215*V4 + -.284*V3 +   .930 E2
RHBRDSC =V4= -.061*V3 +  .998 E3
```

addition, the covariance between the two independent variables SSSSD and AGE (< -10) is also significant.

To further compare the causal effects of different variables, Table 10.16 exhibits the standardized solutions obtained by the three methods. The results consistently indicate that life stress as measured by LSSSD (V2) plays an extraordinary part in effecting depression. Whereas the LS method dramatizes the role of gender (MALE=V6) and age (V5) while downplaying the part of site difference or cultural differentiation (LACHN=V7), the other two solutions suggest that social support (SSSSD=V3) and gender almost have the same size of effect. The role of personal coping as measured by the Health Behaviors and Beliefs proxy (RHBRDSC=V4) is slightly less weighted than that of social support. Although cultural differentiation, as measured by a major site difference (LACHN=V7, i.e., whether or not living in Los Angeles rather than a city in China), is still next in importance, its influence is as large as eight times the impact of chronological aging. In terms of directionality, the results suggest that stress is the main producer of depression, whereas social support and personal coping have some ameliorating effects directly on depression (Note: a negative sign is already implied in RHBRDSC due to its scaling regression aimed at depression). Female elderly tend to be more depressed than male elderly, and elderly persons living in the American metropolis Los Angeles more depressed than their counterparts in the three Chinese cities. In addition, aging has a negative association with depression, though its effect size is close to zero. It is noticeable that both social support and personal coping have much stronger effects in resistance to life stress than in direct relation to depression. The magnitude level of the impact of social support in improving personal coping, however, is nearly the same as its role in improving affective functioning. Diagram 10.2 reproduces the modified path model with the graphical image similar to that in the original modeling. The estimated path coefficients obtained by the GLS method are displayed along with the model. The residual items (E's), however, are omitted to let the image remain simple (cf. Diagram 9). The path coefficients for E1, E2 and E3 are 0.785, 0.938 and 0.996, respectively. The correlation between age and social support as shown in Diagram 9 is also omitted, which amounts to a coefficient of -0.160 in the GLS solution.

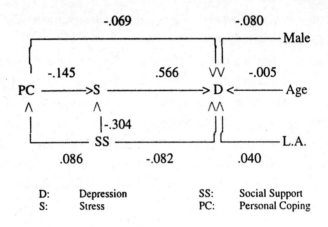

<pre>
        -.069   -.080
  ┌─────────────────────────┐ ┌────────── Male
  │   ││ │
  │ -.145   .566   ││   -.005
  PC ──────>S ──────────────> D <────── Age
  ^   ^   ^^
  │ |-.304   ││
  └───────── SS ────────────┘└────────── L.A.
      .086   -.082   .040
</pre>

D:	Depression	SS:	Social Support
S:	Stress	PC:	Personal Coping

Diagram 10.2 Psychosocial determinants of depression:
A modified and tested model

Table 10.17a shows the total effects with nonstandardized values. Table 10.17b is the nonstandardized indirect effects with standard errors and test statistics. Again, in the LS solution there are several standard errors equal to or approaching zero, and thus the test statistic cannot be defined. The other two solutions, on the other hand, suggest that all the indirect effect estimations are statistically significant. Table 10.18 contains total and direct effects with standardized values, which provides an opportunity to make some meaningful comparisons. The measure of an indirect effect is given by the product of all the coefficients represented by the arrows indirectly liking two variables. There may be many sequences by which a variable can influence another variable, and the total indirect effect is a number indicating the size of the summarized effect. EQS computes only the total indirect effects; total effects are defined as the sum of direct and indirect effects (Bentler, 1989).

The point is, the role of social support and personal coping (as measured by the specific scales) in alleviating depression is realized mainly through their indirect effects (see Table 10.18). Indirect effect on depression constitutes a portion as much as 73.6% ([-0.181]/[-0.246]) of the total effect for social support and a percentage of 59.8% (0.125/0.209) for personal coping in the LS solution. In the GLS solution, the corresponding percentages are 69.3% ([-0.185]/

Table 10.17a Total effects with nonstandardized values

```
DSS    =V1=    .580*V2  +  2.203*V4  +   -.252*V3  +      .061*V5  +   -3.995*V6  +    .267*V7  +
               1.000 E1  +   .580 E2  +   2.203 E3

LSSSD  =V2=   2.265*V4  +   -.311*V3  +   1.000 E2  +   2.265 E3

RHBRDSC =V4=  -.006*V3  +   1.000 E3
```

GLS Solution

```
DSS    =V1=    .568*V2  +  1.688*V4  +   -.268*V3  +   -.007*V5  +  -1.781*V6  +   1.333*V7  +   1.000 E1
               .568 E2  +  1.688 E3

LSSSD  =V2=   1.617*V4  +   -.316*V3  +   1.000 E2  +   1.617 E3

RHBRDSC =V4=  -.008*V3  +   1.000 E3
```

ML Solution

```
DSS    =V1=    .568*V2  +  2.061*V4  +   -.261*V3  +   -.007*V5  +  -1.776*V6  +   1.336*V7  +
               1.000 E1  +   .568 E2  +   2.061 E3

LSSSD  =V2=   2.273*V4  +   -.305*V3  +   1.000 E2  +   2.273 E3

RHBRDSC =V4=  -.006*V3  +   1.000 E3
```

243

Table 10.17b Indirect effects with standard errors and test statistics

LS Solution

```
DSS    =V1=    1.314*V4  +   -.186*V3  +   .580 E2   +  2.203 E3
               .047           .000          .001         .033
               28.015        -568.287      746.571      66.419


LSSSD  =V2=    -.014*V3  +   2.265 E3
               .000          .103
               -27.975       22.015
```

GLS Solution

```
DSS    =V1=    .919*V4   +   -.185*V3  +   .568 E2   +  1.688 E3
               .156           .015          .021         .232
               5.906         -12.101       27.272       7.276


LSSSD  =V2=    -.012*V3  +   1.617 E3
               .006          .298
               -2.200        5.425
```

ML Solution

```
DSS    =V1=    1.292*V4  +   -.178*V3  +   .568 E2   +  2.061 E3
               .143           .015          .020         .197
               9.031         -11.694       28.519       10.485


LSSSD  =V2=    -.013*V3  +   2.273 E3
               .006          .264
               -2.065        8.623
```

[-0.267]) and 54.3% (0.082/0.151). And in the ML solution, the corresponding portions are 68.1% ([-0.175]/[-0.257]) and 62.9% (0.124/ 0.197). In this specific path model using a particular set of measurement scales, the indirect effects of both social support and personal coping are embodied mainly in the mediation of life stress. This conclusion is corroborated by the fact that the total effects of social support and personal coping on life stress are generally stronger than their impacts on depression. Especially, for social support, its influence on personal coping is slim (magnitude < 0.09), and therefore its indirect effect on depression through personal coping is conceivably marginal. This conclusion is also substantiated by the fact that the indirect effect of social support on life stress is merely up to a coefficient of 0.013.

Table 10.18 Total and direct effects with standardized values

Total:

    DSS =V1= .582*V2 + .209*V4 + -.246*V3 + .039*V5 + -.190*V6 + .008*V7
             + .750 E1 + .541 E2 + .209 E3

    LSSSD =V2= .214*V4 + -.302*V3 + .929 E2 + .214 E3

    RHBRDSC=V4= -.062*V3 + .998 E3

Indirect:

    DSS =V1= .125*V4 + -.181*V3 + .541 E2 + .209 E3

    LSSSD =V2= -.013*V3 + .214 E3

GLS Solution

Total:

    DSS =V1= .566*V2 + .151*V4 + -.267*V3 + -.005*V5 + -.080*V6 + .040*V7
             + .785 E1 + .531 E2 + .150 E3

    LSSSD =V2= .145*V4 + -.316*V3 + .938 E2 + .145 E3

    RHBRDSC=V4= -.086*V3 + .996 E3

Indirect:

    DSS =V1= .082*V4 + -.185*V3 + .531 E2 + .150 E3

    LSSSD =V2= -.012*V3 + .145 E3

ML Solution

Total:

    DSS =V1= .575*V2 + .197*V4 + -.257*V3 + -.005*V5 + -.085*V6 + .041*V7
             + .775 E1 + .535 E2 + .197 E3

    LSSSD =V2= .215*V4 + -.297*V3 + .930 E2 + .214 E3

    RHBRDSC=V4= -.061*V3 + .998 E3

Indirect:

    DSS =V1= .124*V4 + -.175*V3 + .535 E2 + .197 E3

    LSSSD =V2= -.013*V3 + .214 E3

11 Conclusion

This book is aimed at advancing the state of the art of psychosocial research by raising some basic theoretical and methodological issues in measurement and analysis. It tries to distinguish between different research purposes, and attempts to clarify some logical requirements specifically for scaling in a relational analysis, which is different from the assessment of individual variables or the test of isolated constructs. In this regard, the issue of confounding among different constructs is related to the limitation of traditional validity concept as an inadequate yardstick in measurement. An awareness of the logical requirements under a more comprehensive conceptual framework is deemed crucial to research workers engaged in a relational analysis. At the heart of the inquiry, the book testifies that theoretical constructs in psychosocial fields tend to be multidimensional (the premise is, they must be gauged with multi-item scales to ensure appropriate measurement coverage); yet a clear guideline for dealing with the results of a dimensional analysis has been long overdue. Acknowledging the merit of an integral approach to measurement and analysis while noticing the potential side-effect of such advanced techniques as FASEM modeling on theory development, the book stresses the desirability of maintaining the integrity of theoretical constructs and the need for global measures in research and practice. As an alternative line of thought to that of confirmatory factor analysis, use of factor-based subscales, and a focus on between-factor relationships, the book holds out a theme of unidimensionalized scaling of the theoretical constructs, which would not only establish their scalability after dimensional analysis (this is especially important for practical purpose), but also prove their usefulness by allowing for theoretical reasoning at more general levels.

The further issue is with the ways in which unidimensionalization can be accomplished systematically and reasonably. People actually "unidimensionalize" scales every day, though they may not be aware that they are performing such a theoretically and methodologically critical task. A clear guide is in pressing need, especially in view of some research workers repeating a procedure that can hardly be claimed as legitimate, or even just plausible. This book attempts to articulate a systematic approach to thinking and exploration in this respect. Summarizing the experience that we already have as well as borrowing from science and engineering, the Chen Approaches to Unidimensionalized Scaling (CAUS) lays the groundwork for theorizing current practice and providing future guidance.

Multiple measurement is a necessary consequence of the unidimensionalized scaling approach. The logical requirement for a meaningful relational analysis, in its extreme the mutual exclusiveness of the constructs involved in the same analysis, serves as a precondition and, in turn, provides a rationale for seeking measurement or scaling effectiveness by every means developed or to be developed under the CAUS. Here the traditional idea of validity is not considered an adequate guide for scaling individual constructs for relational analyses, nor a good indicator of the power of the measures as a whole in detecting the potential relationships.

This concluding chapter summarizes the major accomplishments and some constraints of the study. In addition to some general conclusions, specific results are recapped in light of measurement devices and scaling methods, as well as substantive hypotheses and models. The relevance to practice and policy making as well as suggestions to future research are also discussed.

Psychosocial research and the saving of theory:
Toward unidimensionalized scaling

The rise of dimensional analysis in psychosocial research has irrationalized the blind application of traditional unidimensional scaling techniques. The set of extracted factors or components, however, do not themselves reconcile the difficulty of multidimensionality. The use of factor-based subscales seems to fail a theory, each time when any of its constructs is identified with more than one factor, by declaring that it is not scalable and thus testable at the level of

247

generalization it is intended or supposed to be. The systematic effort of unidimensionalization started in this book is an attempt to "save" scientific theory in psychosocial fields by maintaining the integrity of its constructs and creating opportunity to test it as-is at the general levels. With such systematic effort, the use of global measures will be more grounded, and the test of some "grand" theory or theories built with some "metaconstructs" will no longer be so illusive a task. Of course, the line of thought toward unidimensionalized scaling is complementary rather than contradictory to such fine approaches as FASEM modeling or the conventional use of LISREL techniques in psychosocial research. The currently prevalent methods, however, should not be taken as the only way or simply the major direction for research development. As a matter of fact, since the trend of thought does not emphasize or even allow for general measures or global scales, one cannot use a construct like "social support" unless it is broken down into various "latent" pieces in an advanced analysis. Inasmuch as it downplays other approaches (and only in such a sense), I hold the "advanced" technology responsible for putting a barrier to theory advancement.

Indeed, while confirmatory factor analysis provides details commensurate with the delicacy of the FASEM model, it does not directly address the original theoretical ideas. Such technology often appears to be excessively complicated, and thus is awkward in practical applications. A simple path model, in contrast, clearly lays out the causal relations as embodied in the original theories. On a synthetical basis, its analysis is relatively simple, and the results are easier to interpret and understand. The simple path model is preconditioned on valid and effective general measures of the constructs involved in the analysis, whereas the current analytical approach tends to deny the possibility of such measures. In this regard, the book has exemplified that important psychosocial constructs are scalable at the general levels as the theories have implied. And the methodology proposed under the CAUS, combined with theoretical causal modeling and empirical path analysis, has shown to have some research advantages. Since the CAUS only employs principal components method in dimensional analysis as the first step of scale building (also called "exploratory factor analysis"), it does not resort to confirmatory analysis, which is the core of FASEM involving factor analytic assumptions (Kim & Mueller, 1978). Without the concern that such assumptions might be wrong, the CAUS will always achieve the best scaling results, especially with a multiple measurement approach advocated in this book.

Validity, relation, and unconfounded logic

In this book, relational analysis, which tends to be a core concern in contemporary psychosocial research, is distinguished from traditional psychological tests that have served as the soil for growing many of the fundamental psychometric ideas. In order to understand the significance of some of the major conclusions of the book, we must distinguish between two different research purposes in measurement, that is, individual tests (assessment of isolated constructs) and scaling for relational analyses. For individual tests, the major technical problem or concern could be inadequate coverage of a field, such as reducing life stress to merely some life events. For a relational analysis, the potential danger could not only be insufficient but also excessive coverage that might cause confounding among different constructs. It is indicated that owing to the difference in research purpose, indiscriminately applying the validity requirement could be very problematic. Indeed, blindly looking after "valid" measures of individual constructs may not avoid, or may even cause, the confounding problem in a relation analysis. This is because validity represents a rigid, isolation requirement that does not suit the analysis of the relationship between constructs. The logical requirement articulated in this book focuses on the relative conceptual boundaries among related constructs. Generally speaking, the validity of an individual construct must be considered in conjunction with its potential overlapping with other constructs, which usually has significant bearings on various relational findings. Of course sometimes we need to analyze the relationship among similar yet not identical constructs, in which case the overlapping among the constructs can be significant and unavoidable. The point is, however, the boundaries of the constructs must be clear and the meaning of the conclusion is contingent upon the definition. In other words, the definition and measurement of the constructs involved in the same relational analysis must be consistent with the interpretation of the research findings. This is the logical requirement for a relational analysis in its very general format. The most stringent testing environment in a relational analysis is the requirement for mutual exclusiveness of the measures of all related constructs. This unconfounded analytical logic warrants the authenticity of the relational findings by precluding any artificial boost, which is not uncommon in various research reports. The logic of mutual exclusiveness may incur a cost in the content and construct validity of individual measures. Being aware of all such issues and difficulties, however, will help us understand the

249

nature, including the dilemmas, of psychosocial research.

Supplemental to the general understanding of the confounding issue, a special problem with conceptual boundaries can be noted by relating to the practice of questionnaire design, in which reversing the coding of some items is methodologically desirable. This suggests that a general demarcation line between stress and support (or well-being) is impossible, impractical, or unnecessary. In such case, the logical requirement articulated in this book, other than the idea of validity, is especially relevant to developing appropriate measures for a meaningful relational analysis.

The empirical part of this book employs the mutual exclusiveness principle. Some other criteria are also used in the selection of items for each scale, including: a) good item coverage of the content area, or item sampling adequacy; b) parsimony; and c) relevance and good characteristics of individual items. It should be noted that the "good coverage" requirement often disqualifies single-indicator measures in psychosocial research. Therefore, the issues in multi-item scaling discussed in the theory part are very important to the empirical inquiry.

For the Social Support Scale (SSS), 29 individual indicators are selected from the data used for analysis and demonstration. They fall into three major categories: a) network composition/resources, including living arrangements, sizes of family and friends/neighbors networks, and frequencies of contacts (network interaction); b) support acts, consisting of financial aid, task help, advice/information, and emotional support; and c) support appraisal, comprising satisfaction with living arrangements, feeling of close network members, and perception of the quality and reliability of relationship in terms of financial, task-oriented, and emotional help. This items pool has an emphasis on support acts and behaviors, and integrates more objective facts of network resources with more subjective indicators of support appraisal. It also incorporates support received by the elderly with support provided by the elderly.

The Life Stress Scale (LSS) takes into account both conventionally recognized life events and more enduring situations, in order to incorporate various biopsychosocial factors with the general stress model on affective functioning. From the available data 44 individual items are obtained that fall into 7 major categories, namely, a) physical health conditions and events (including major events, chronic conditions, stressful symptoms, functional status, and subjective ratings), b) physical build (over- and underweight), c) cognitive functioning (memory), d) socioeconomic status (education, unemployment

/retirement, income, and ethnic/regional issue), e) living circumstances (changes and events, home conditions), f) work stress, and g) development (aging) stress. Unfortunately, information regarding some significant sources of stress such as marital discord and friction with children is not available, which may have blunted the power and effectiveness of the scales.

The potential problem of confounding with both stress and social support is especially heeded for the Depression Scale (DS).Under the established criteria, 25 items are garnered from the available data, which can be classified into the following symptom categories: a) mood disturbance, b) loss of interest, c) psychomotor disturbance, d) decreased energy (fatigue), e) sleep disturbance, f) decreased appetite/constipation, g) concentration problem, h) dissatisfaction, and i) hopelessness.

Owing to the limitation of available data, personal coping can only be operationalized into some proxy measures concerning certain health- and illness-related behaviors as well as respondents' attitudes toward a number of social arrangements. The focus on these aspects, nevertheless, may be of special interest since health is usually the primary concern in old age, whereas attitudes have been typically overlooked in previous research. After careful consideration, 11 individual items are selected for a Health Behaviors and Beliefs (HBB) measure, 9 items for an Attitudes Toward Social Support (ATSS) measure, and 4 items for an Attitudes Toward Elderly (ATE) measure.

The codings of some original items are reversed when being pooled together for each scale, which demonstrates the possibility of breaking through the conceptual boundary in each field. For the social support scale, for example, the items are coded in a manner in which possibly neutral situations are assigned the value of 0, whereas potentially stressful cases are given negative valences. This coding scheme helps all the nominal weights to remain positive.

On the whole, an appropriate understanding of social support, stress and depression is established by tracing the roots of confusion and delineating a comprehensive conceptual scheme of social well-being, mental health, and quality of life. The stringent logical requirements for a relational analysis are observed, which may also be taken in a new sense of construct validity (i.e., not just in terms of the test of an individual and isolated construct, but in terms of the analysis of the relationship among different constructs) indispensable for a meaningful analysis in social and behavioral sciences. This approach to conceptualization and operationalization is based on the specific purposes of the study.

Multiple measurement, scaling effectiveness, and standardization of research results

To "standardize" the study of a field like social support, theorists have tried to classify its contents into different categories. The dimensional analysis in this book using empirical data, however, does not seem to exactly or necessarily confirm the initial conceptual scheme that conforms to the typical understanding of the field. Factor analysis applied to the 29 item SSS does not clearly distinguish between network resources, support acts and support appraisal. This makes it difficult to derive specific sets of subscales under such theories as the social isolation hypothesis or the quality of relationship (in terms of appraisal of support) hypothesis. The finding has significant implications to scaling strategies. It is clear that although substantive studies of social support have derived numerous scaling schemes, they have susceptible utility in dealing with the reality.

On the other hand, the incompatibility of research results due to the variation of scale instruments is a concern in generalizing the empirical findings from a field of psychosocial research. It seems that the best we can do is to first standardize our research procedures. In terms of general-level theory testing, the logical requirement for operationalization and scaling should be met and the valid range of individual constructs should be clarified. Dimensional analysis should be performed, then different approaches to unidimensionalization should be tried. Finally, multiple measures derived from different approaches should be compared to achieve higher measurement effectiveness, or greater power of detecting the relationship among different constructs. Such standardized procedure will undoubtedly help standardize substantive research results, although the variety of ways of operationalizing a content area would make a universal scale almost impossible especially in a relational analysis.

The empirical part of the book endeavors to develop some specific sets of social support, life stress and depression scales using empirical data on the Chinese and Chinese-American elderly. The purpose is two-fold. On the one hand, I need to test the scaling models derived from the CAUS. On the other, measurement scales suitable for the Chinese and Chinese Americans, especially for the elderly, are awfully underdeveloped, despite that these populations constitute the largest congregations of people in the world.

Proceeding with the theme of unidimensionalization, multiple measures are developed for the key theoretical constructs. The four sets of scale items are developed by following the logical requirements for content and construct validity. Their dimensionality is clarified by factor analysis. A few primary scaling hypotheses are articulated and used to construct different types of scales, and such hypotheses are validated/falsified by comparing the utility of the corresponding unidimensionalized scales in relation to certain criterion variables. The empirical results generally falsified Hypothesis 1, which states that the effect of a multidimensional measure is determined by its maximum component score (the maximum component theory). Hypothesis 2, the assumption that the role of a psychosocial variable is determined by its first component, is proved to have relatively high validity of all the theoretical models. Note this is especially true when only one component is specified in factor extraction, while in such case the difference between Hypothesis 1 and Hypothesis 2 is eliminated. Among the summated treatments of the components based on Hypothesis 3, only the one using varimax rotation seemed to have some utility. Generally speaking, standardization and/or factorization treatments lead to some improvement of the measurement power of the scales. As for the practical approach, the regression scales using specific criteria were most valid in predicting the same variables. On the whole, the practical approach is more effective than the theoretical approach. The advantage of the theoretical approach is in that it is more general, whereas the practically optimal scaling strategy via regression is criterion-specific. These attributes determine their utility in different research situations.

The concept of measurement power or scaling effectiveness is based on the logical requirements for avoiding confounding, which defies the rigidity of the constructs to be scaled, and intended to achieve the best assessment effects - in this case the maximum degree of association(s) of a specific scale with a criterion or a set of criteria. The idea is that the associations may be insignificant not because there are no such significant associations but because the measure is not powerful or the scale is not effective enough. This justifies the use of multiple scaling methods under the CAUS, including theory-based and practice-oriented approaches, in measuring complex theoretical constructs to achieve different research objectives (e.g., general vs. specific).

The general scaling models flowing from the CAUS may result in various measurement tools that will have extensive applications beyond the scope of this book. The CAUS, with the articulated standard, normal, uniform and universal scaling treatments, renders some solid grounds for comparing all kinds of substantive results obtained with various research designs and data collection instruments.

Social support, stress, and depression in a context of aging and Chinese culture

Stress and social support are two leading approaches to contemporary psychosocial studies of affective functioning and depression. The genuine effects of stress and social support, however, are not made very clear in empirical research because of various confusions among theoretical constructs as well as serious limitations in multidimensional scaling methods. Having addressed some of the fundamental issues in measurement and analysis, the book is in a position to inquire into the psychosocial mechanism of affective functioning among the Chinese and Chinese American elderly.

The four key variables, especially depression and social support, are assessed among the research sample. The cultural meaning of the findings is discussed. With multiple selected sets of scales, the relationships among the key constructs are analyzed. Measures used in analyses include the summative scale for depression (DSS; because of the unique property of the items pool, it worked as well as the more theoretically and methodologically based scales), the standardized summative scales for life stress and social support (LSSSD and SSSSD; mainly to avoid the missing data problem), and the regressed scale for the personal coping proxy Health Behaviors and Beliefs (RHBRDSC).

The role of stress in effecting depression and the moderating and mediating role of social support is investigated by testing the major research hypotheses. Statistical control is achieved via the single multiple regression method as well as the structural equations modeling approach to clarify the pathways of various effects. The preliminary causal modeling is done by incorporating the major perspectives identified in the research literature. It builds on the "stress buffering" as well as the "main effect" hypotheses and takes into account some other key variables. A balance is struck between simplicity and accuracy. The theoretical model is modified to suit the data, which is fully examined for use as an empirical means of test. The data, containing 1,504 elderly Chinese in Beijing, Shanghai and Guangzhou and 204 elderly Chinese-Americans in Los Angeles, were collected in cross-national surveys conducted by an inter-university and interdisciplinary research team during 1990-1992.

The simple regression analysis emphasizes on obtaining partial correlation co-

254

efficients of depression with other theoretical constructs and basic variables. The findings address the major individual hypotheses listed in chapter six, with one additional result regarding the relationship between the personal coping proxy and depression. The conclusions are:

(1) Stress is positively related to depression. Although statistical control had a negative impact on the correlation coefficient, stress remains to be an outstanding predictor of depression (PARTIAL=0.5638, Beta=0.5706).

(2) Social support is negatively related to depression. The size of the net or direct effect of social support (PARTIAL=-0.0978, BETA=-0.0803), however, is less than half of the zero-order correlation (=-0.2523), which suggests the significance of exploring its indirect effect on depression.

(3) Personal coping, as represented by the Health Behaviors and Beliefs proxy, is also negatively related to depression. Similarly, the size of the direct effect of the personal coping proxy (PARTIAL=-0.0866, BETA=-0.0727) is less than half of the zero-order correlation (=-0.2239).

(4) The zero-order correlation (=0.0823) between age and depression is against the hypothesis that the older the age, the less likely the depression. But statistical control reversed this conclusion. The result, however, is not statistically significant, and the effect size is minimal (PARTIAL=-0.0060, BETA=-0.0047), which does not render much support for the hypothesis of "protective aging".

(5) In contrast to the effect of aging, gender seems to make a bigger difference in depression than both social support and personal coping, partly because it is influenced less by statistical control. And the result is statistically significant.

(6) Site difference (cultural differentiation) accounts for the variation in depression to certain degree. Some notable difference is found among sites within China by zero-order correlation as well as by one-way analysis of variance. With statistical control via multiple regression, however, the within-China difference is reduced to the minimum while the China-America difference is intensified.

On the whole, a multiple correlation coefficient in the amount of 0.6392 is obtained, which indicates the goodness of fit of the single regression model (R Square=0.409). To further clarify the mediating role of social support as well as the indirect effects of other variables, nevertheless, a structural equations modeling approach is needed. By using the statistical program EQS, path analysis reconfirmed the correlates of depression by further enhancing the role of stress and slightly reducing the function of other variables. It also further

255

clarified the relationships between stress, social support, and personal coping. The conclusions are (specific path coefficients are obtained through the Generalized Least Squares method):

(1) Social support is negatively associated with stress (path coefficient=-0.304).

(2) Social support is positively associated with desirable coping (path coefficient =0.086).

(3) Positive personal coping is negatively related with stress (path coefficient=-0.145).

Despite the important meaning of the path coefficients, the value of path analysis is in that it clarifies direct as well as indirect effects (total effects are the sum of direct and indirect effects). Results show that the role of social support as well as personal coping (as measured by the specific scales) in alleviating depression is realized mainly through their indirect effects. Indirect effect on depression constitutes a portion as much as 69.3% of the total effect for social support and a percentage of 54.3% for personal coping in the General Least Squares (GLS) solution. For the particular path model used in analysis, the indirect effects of both social support and personal coping are exerted mainly through the mediation of life stress. Therefore, the stress buffering hypothesis is proven to have a stronger position than the direct effect hypothesis, not only for the role of social support but also for the role of personal coping (the role of personal coping is thus perfectly integrated with the depression-life stress-social support model). In concluding on this, however, caution should be taken since EQS only gives the total indirect effects that also include the pathways through all other variables. The most noticeable pathway is the correlation between age and social support, which amounts to a coefficient of -0.160 in the GLS solution (indicating some inescapable decline in support networks associated with aging in later life).

All in all, the findings reconfirm significant associations among affective functioning (depression), life stress and social support under appropriate understanding of the relationships among mental health, social well-being, and quality of life. The role of personal coping in assuaging stress and depression is also betokened. The hypothetical impact of aging, however, gains only minimal support from the empirical data. Gender difference, on the other hand, is relatively noticeable. Evidence is also obtained for the difference between Chinese and Chinese-American elderly. It should be noted that as space forbids, alternative scales are not tried for each construct. Especially, the optimal and most effective regression scales are not used due to the missing data problem. This notwithstanding, the multiple measurement approach is strongly advocated and, if data permit, the optimal scales should be used, with which the substantive results would probably be even more remarkable.

The limitation of research

As is with any single piece of research, not all the theoretical issues involved in the current topic are fully addressed in the book. Other restraints include some obstacles or barriers encountered in carrying out the empirical research design and measurement/analysis tasks.

First of all, some caveats about the CAUS. Different research situations and objectives demand different approaches. The CAUS is inductive in nature, mainly applying to retrospective studies. This study proposed only a few specific models out of a large number of possible solutions. Therefore, more specific scaling models need to be articulated in a understandable and applicable language. Besides, even the conclusions regarding the models tested in the current study are not all conclusive. They need to be tested in more diverse designs with various data. Especially, better data allowing for the regression scales may do a better justice to the role of social support as well as personal coping. An additional point is that the CAUS should in no way be regarded as a denial of the FASEM or LISREL approach. Just as a global scale is needed and simplicity desired, confirmatory factor analysis is also needed and precision desired, at least in some different situations.

It should also be noted that the discussion on measurement and scaling excluded the method factor as well as the influence of mood and etc., which have been the focus of some psychometric elaborations. The alternative way of scaling explicated in this book, however, provides a new basis for further elaborating on these issues.

Lack of relevant data was an empirical barrier to more precise and comprehensive model testing. Especially, information is wanting for the internal factors that contribute to depression. The role of a diathesis, for example, could not be tested simply because the original surveys were not designed to tap into the physiological and genetic aspects. The role of cognitive functioning in depression seems also too detailed for a general community survey study like such to encompass. I am not especially interested in those aspects; yet a

257

thorough investigation of the psychosocial dynamics of affective functioning requires proper control of those variables, especially in view of the endogenous perspective of depression. Indeed, the contribution of social support could be very modest compared to factors such as family history of depression. Yet, it is noticeable that few social studies in the literature included family history of affective disorders, probably because that usually belongs to a different research paradigm.

For those variables present in the data sets, available measures were not as perfect as I would desire since they were not particularly designed for the purposes of this study. Depression could not be measured in a more thorough way since the only scale used in the original survey was not even complete. Especially, no available personal coping scale is included in the original surveys, and I could only come up with some proxy measures to proceed with the needed analysis. All these, however, do not defy the value of the study. The defects of the specific measures and scales are compensated by the comprehensiveness of the data and richness of other relevant information. In fact, I was able to form fairly good, though not ideal, item pools for developing needed social support, life stress and depression scales. For personal coping, it is also not unhelpful to focus on specific aspects like health behaviors and beliefs, as well as the sorts of social attitudes of the elderly that are typically underrepresented in research literature.

It should be noted that the items used do not have a unified metric base, and most of them are variables with limited numbers of categories, including even dichotomies. This will pose a serious problem for such scaling treatment as factor analysis. Yet, as Kim, Nie and Verba (1977) illustrate, if the goal is to search for clustering patterns, the use of factor analysis as a heuristic device even under severe measurement distortions (e.g., on data containing dichotomies or variables with a limited number of categories) may be justified. Since my objective is simply a summary of information contained in the data, I have actually used component scores without recourse to factor analytic assumptions (Kim & Mueller, 1978). The linear combination of observed data by which components analysis standardizes and summarizes the information involves no more than mathematical transformations of the raw variables via orthogonal regression. To meet its requirements, dichotomous variables could be recoded as dummy variables. Of course, if the empirical data have more desirable metric properties, it is certainly advantageous and helpful to demonstrating the utility of the CAUS as well as other major ideas contained in the book.

By design, the empirical part is in the main not a cross-cultural, cross-gender, or cross-generational comparative study. The book is mainly concerned with whether or not the research hypotheses and the causal model derived from the Western and general literature still hold true among the Chinese aging population, using appropriate measures. Although comparing Western view of depression including causation, coping, and norms with the Chinese view is very interesting, it will be further pursued, hopefully, in a separate work. Similar plans are there for the gender and aging aspects. Although the current study does contain all these dimensions, more detailed illustrations of the similarities and differences as well as possible value judgments are not included due to the foci on other issues that are deemed more relevant and important to the major topics here. Accordingly, while cultural influences on all the key variables are noted to ensure appropriate conceptualization and measurement, this dimension is examined only in terms of potential differentiation in depression in empirical data analysis.

Technically, the study had to strike a balance between elegance and simplicity, or between desirability and feasibility. Focusing on some initial work like the CAUS, I was not able nor intending to make the book more complicated by going beyond some generally applied assumptions such as linearity and additivity. In the structural equations modeling, depression is treated only as a dependent variable. That is, its impacts on or reactions to other variables are not considered, although theoretically its negative effect on social support has been made fairly clear. Similarly, the functions of other variables such as aging and cultural differentiation are simplified (e.g., their impacts on support, stress and coping are mostly omitted). Such treatments are to maintain the manageability (recursiveness) of the model so that the project can be completed within the time and space limits. These are done, however, probably at the price of goodness of fit of the model, and should partly account for the error items of which the coefficients are quite notable.

In many ways, the study is confined to the state of the art of the field. As is the case in science, the theories articulated as primitive results of the CAUS were born with their weakness. What should be reminded is, however, that the theories articulated in this book are neither to be accepted nor convicted insightlessly. What is needed is the proper utilization of the theories now available as well as the development of new theoretical paradigms.

Fortunately, we seem always able to resort to the practical approach, and it is not impossible to design and collect data for the purpose of scaling on a better and better empirical basis. The missing information in the data sets used in the current study, however, sets the limit for the application of the optimal, more effective regression scales. And some shortcomings in data formats also had an impact on the findings. In addition, necessary data for certain statistical analyses, including test-retest reliability, were not available.

Finally, in terms of the techniques used in empirical path analysis, methods and statistics more robust than the LS, GLS, and ML approaches available in EQS were not applied. Those methods require the use of raw data. But for the concerns of dealing with missing data as well as treatment of categorical variables, I have chosen to use correlation coefficients rather than the raw data as the input matrix.

The scaling conclusions directed the use of relatively effective measures of the theoretical constructs in substantive analysis, though the models used were far from perfect and the possibilities in scaling manipulation are not exhausted. Conceivably, scales based on the more effective theoretical treatments as well as those optimally regressed scales should be recommended. The application of the regression approach, however, demands quality data with minimum missing information. Since factor scores are virtually also regression scores, they have the same concern in application. In this particular study, all selected scales seem to have worked well in gauging depression and specific aspects of personal coping since there are only few cases missing in these fields. In the domains of life stress and social support, however, there are substantial amounts of information missing due to the effect of listwise deletion on large numbers of individual scaling (regression) items. In such cases, I had to back up to the conventional summative scales, though standardization as well as factorization could be used to improve their performance.

Championing a multiple measurement approach, the substantive results are remarkable in terms of the relationships among the theoretical constructs. The highest zero-order correlation coefficients of depression with stress and social support reached 0.672 and -0.637 (negative sign is added to offset the impact of previous regression), respectively, with a significance level of $P < 0.01$ for both. Excluding those life stress and social support scales that involved regression (for concerns about missing data), the maximum correlation coefficient with depression remained high (0.6236) for life stress while dropped drastically (down to -0.2759) for social support. Similar situation is found in the correlation between stress and social support (maximum coefficient down from -0.4920 to -0.2974). These facts have grave implications to subsequent multivariate analyses, where I had to turn to some summative scales to soothe the data missing problem.

Relevance to practice and policy making

As an exploration from the standpoint of a helping profession, the results of this study are more relevant to practice and policy making than to psychometric or sociological theory building. What psychometricians and sociologists might think all too obvious could be lamentable hurdles to psychosocial "engineering." The purpose of the study is to bridge over the gap between the pure and the applied behavioral and social sciences, as well as the discrepancy between general research paradigms and specific research populations. It tries to concretize and streamline the thoughts and ideas that might be helpful to practical scale developers by articulating the Chen Approaches to Uni-dimensionalized Scaling (CAUS). It also attempts to advance substantive learning by basing research hypotheses on structural equations modeling with the Chinese and Chinese-American elderly population.

On one hand, some scaling models such as the maximum component theory and the summated components theory are generally falsified, whereas some other methods such as the first principal component theory are proven more valid and thus recommended. In particular, the usually most effective optimal regression approach should be considered in scaling practice whenever the objectives are pertinent and the data permit. Depending on the properties of the item pools, sometimes the simple summative scales, or those with additional treatments like standardization and/or factorization, might work and could be particularly useful when other scaling methods are not applicable. These results are especially suggestive to professional practice where appropriate measurement is the basis of any quantitative work.

On the other hand, substantive results suggest that in order to allay affective disfunction among the population, specifically the Chinese and Chinese-American elderly, comprehensive policy measures must be taken to reduce stress or to promote overall quality of life, including health promotion, socioeconomic reform, and improvement of working and living conditions. Social support as well as personal coping have considerable bearing on both life stress and depression, but their role should not be so exaggerated as to overshadow the primary task in improving the quality of life.

It seems reconfirmed that aging, or more exactly continuing aging, is not a cause of affective disfunction. Yet, some decline of social support is evidenced in such a developmental process. Since social support has extensive impacts, including a positive effect on personal coping, an effort of community networking might be especially relevant to effective intervention in later life. This provides a direction for gerontological social work and community organization. As for the gender difference in depression, additional data analysis suggests that female elderly Chinese and Chinese-Americans also suffer from a generally higher degree of life stress. The social meaning of these differences can be understood from different stances, among which the feminist point of view has gained much influence. In terms of the site variations that are assumed to contain a dimension of cultural differentiation, the Chinese-American elderly living in Los Angeles are more depressed than their counterparts in Chinese cities. The difference, nevertheless, is not very significant, and the Chinese elderly do have a generally high score on various depression scales. This finding challenges the notion that traditional Chinese culture is closely tied with extremely low levels of depression, and more active policies are demanded in its treatment and prevention in that particular cultural setting.

Suggestions to future research

Based on the idea of measurement power as well as the logical requirements for precluding confounding, the specific scaling techniques, methods, models and hypotheses can be various to achieve scaling effectiveness. The evaluation of item relevance and sampling adequacy must be based on substantive knowledge and is a skillful process. With regard to the logical requirements, it has been noted that some conceptual boundaries represented by the distinction between positive and negative items are unnecessary or undesirable. This is because the signs as well as the codings could be reversed, and reconciling these codes in a unified scale is considered essential. On the other hand, some borderlines distinguishing different content areas are helpful or probably imperative. It seems that with a support-stress continuum, a scale can run the gamut of all degrees of support (or stress, if signs or codings are simply reversed). Therefore, the measure of social support and life stress are distinguished only in terms of a special "informal, social" area and the rest of life aspects (the latter should further exclude the areas of affective functioning and etc., depending on the topic and purpose of research).

The overall, continuous scaling of depression is based on the assumption of continuity and generality, especially with regard to minor depression which is more frequently seen among the aging population. Clinical diagnosis of depression, in contrast, relies on some cutoff point that might, in a sense, appear arbitrary. An important conclusion of this study is that a patient may be scored on different scales very differently. Since no single scale has so far established its superiority over all other scales, it is essential to employ multiple measures in clinical practice to avoid mistakes. For the purpose of research, the removal of such a cutoff point and the treatment of depression as a continuous variable would allow us to run the gamut of affective functioning and examine its asso-ciation with other variables with a full range of possibilities and opportunities.

In designing the tests of substantive analyses, the meaning of "buffering" should be clarified with regard to specific pathways and indirect effects in a potential causal modeling. The issue of causation, however, should be heeded. Since the current study only employed a relatively simple model, more complete modeling and analytic techniques are needed in the future.

The indirect or mediating effects of social support and personal coping mirror the significance of stress study in the etiology of depression. The unclear relationship between stress and depression in psychosocial research is probably mainly due to poor measurement, e.g., the limitation of the life events approach. In fact, this study has seen an extraordinarily strong linkage between life stress and depression. It is argued that to reduce life stress it is essential to take care of a broad spectrum of human needs and conditions, not just some life events of which many seem unavoidable. The argument supported by this study has profound implications to social service practice. Nevertheless, the concept of life stress or quality of life has its boundaries, depending on its relationship with other constructs involved in the same study, and the parts of other constructs usually need to be excluded or a confounding issue will be aroused sooner or later.

Generally speaking, the practical approach to scale construction as articulated under the CAUS is especially effective when scales are developed without enough theoretical foundation. However, the regression scaling must have a statistical (population) basis before the resulting scales can be applied to the individual level. It should be noted that regression is used here merely to summarize the information contained in the data. It involves no prediction-related issue like the distribution concern.

In order to perform needed scaling test, the researcher needs to select criterion variables with care. In particular, when one conceives of the effect of social support, s/he should make the notion specific, inclusive (all-sided), and relevant. In addition, one should heed the potential impact of any artificially boosted measurement precision (e.g., from the ordinal level to the interval level), which was not included in the discussion of the results in the current study.

To sum up, this study breaks new ground for scientific inquiry and debate. Although separate subscales may be meaningful for some specific purposes, they do not defy the value of generalization in psychosocial research, which is instrumental to both theoretical development and practical work. It is proved that theoretical constructs like social support, life stress and depression are scalable at the general level, where they are defined and intended to use, in a reasonable fashion without resorting to some higher level of abstraction in psychometric thinking. The book reveals some unique opportunities for promoting the leading research hypotheses in a broad range of psychosocial studies. A multiple measurement approach to psychosocial research is advocated, and more refined and befitting methods and models under the CAUS are expected.

Appendix

1a. Lubben Social Network Scale (LSNS) items and scaling methods

[Any answer is more than 10 persons, code=10]

B1. a. Please tell me how many of your ... [*categories 1 to 6*] are still living?

    b. How many of your ... [*Read categories 1 to 6*] live in the Beijing/ Guangzhou/Shanghai/Los Angeles area?

    c. How many of your ... [*Read categories 1 to 6*] do you talk to or write to at least once a month?

	a. How many living?	b. # live in same area	c. # talked to at least once a month?
1) Parents	—	—	—
2) Siblings	—	—	—
3) Children	—	—	—
4) Children In-law	—	—	—
S) Grand-children	—	—	—
6) Other Relatives	—	—	—

COMPUTE B1C=SUM(B1C1 to B1C6)
RECODE B1C (0=0)(1=1)(2=2)(3,4=3)(5 THRU 8=4)(9 THRU HI=5) INTO **LSNS1**

B2. Tell me about the FAMILY MEMBERS/RELATIVE (not include spouse) with whom you have the most contact. How often do you see or hear from that person?

O = < monthly   1 = monthly   2 = 2-3 times a month
3 = weekly   4 = 2-3 times a week   5 =daily (4 times+a week)

COMPUTE LSNS2=B2

B3. How many RELATIVES (include spouse) do you feel CLOSE to? That is, how many of them do you feel at ease with, can talk to about private matters, or can call on for help? *[If 10 or more than 10, code=10]*

Record #: __

RECODE B3 (0=0)(1=1)(2=2)(3,4=3)(5 THRU 8=4)(9 THRU HI=5) INTO LSNS3

B4. Do you have any CLOSE FRIENDS OR NEIGHBORS? That is, do you have any friends or neighbors with whom you feel at ease can talk to about private matters? If so, how many? *[If 10 or more than 10, code=10]*

Record #: __

RECODE B4 (0=0)(1=1)(2=2)(3,4=3)(5 THRU 8=4)(9 THRU HI=5) INTO LSNS4

B5. How many of these FRIENDS OR NEIGHBORS do you see or hear from at least once a month? *[If 10 or more than 10, code=10]*

Record #: __

RECODE B5 (0=0)(1=1)(2=2)(3,4=3)(5 THRU 8=4)(9 THRU HI=5) INTO LSNS5

B6. Tell me about the FRIEND OR NEIGHBOR with whom you have the most contact. How often do you see or hear from that person?

O = < monthly   1 = monthly   2 = 2-3 times a month
3 = weekly   4 = 2-3 times a week   5 =daily (4 times+ a week)

COMPUTE **LSNS6**=B6

B7. When you have an important decision to make, do you have someone you can talk to about it?

Always	Very Often	Often	Sometimes	Seldom	Never
5	4	3	2	1	0

COMPUTE **LSNS7**=B7

B8. When other people you know have an important decision to make, do they talk to you about it?

Always	Very Often	Often	Sometimes	Seldom	Never
5	4	3	2	1	0

COMPUTE **LSNS8**=B8

B9. How often do you help your family, friends or neighbors with tasks like shopping, cooking dinner, home repairs, cleaning house, child care, filling out forms, etc.? Would you say ...

Always	Very Often	Often	Sometimes	Seldom	Never
5	4	3	2	1	0

COMPUTE **LSNS9**=B9

G6. Who do you live with and how many of them? In general, how well do you get along with that/these person?

a. Who?	b.#?	c. How well get along?					
		Very well	Somewhat well	So-so	Not very well	Not well at all	Some well, some not well
1) living alone	NA						
2) Spouse	___	5	4	3	2	1	8
3) Children	___	5	4	3	2	1	8
4) In-laws	___	5	4	3	2	1	8
5) Grandchildren	___	5	4	3	2	1	8
6) Parents	___	5	4	3	2	1	8
7) Siblings	___	5	4	3	2	1	8
8) Other Relatives	___	5	4	3	2	1	8
9) Friends or non-related Persons (e.g. paid helper)	___	5	4	3	2	1	8
10) Other, specify:	___	5	4	3	2	1	8

LSNS10 -
IF (G601A=1) LSNS10=0; IF (G610A=1) LSNS10=1; IF (G602A=1) LSNS10
=5; IF (SUM(G603A,G604A,G605A,G606A,G607A,G608A,G609A) >1)
LSNS10=4.

The overall scale:

COMPUTE **LSNS**=SUM.8(LSNS1 TO LSNS10)

* For the standard format of the LSNS, see Lubben, James E. (1988), "Assessing Social Networks among Elderly Populations," *Family and Community Health,* 11(3):42-52.

Ib. Items used for the Social Support Scale (SSS) development

Network Composition

Living arrangements

COMPUTE **SSS1**=LSNS10 (see Appendix Ia)

Network size

COMPUTE **SSS2**=B1C (see Appendix Ia)

COMPUTE **SSS3**=B5 („)

Frequency of network interaction

COMPUTE **SSS4**=B2=LSNS2 (see Appendix Ia)

COMPUTE **SSS5**=B6=LSNS6 („)

COMPUTE **SSS6**=B7=LSNS7 („)

COMPUTE **SSS7**=B8=LSNS8 („)

Support Acts

Financial

B17. During the <u>PAST 12 MONTHS</u>, how often did these people provide you financial assistance when you needed it?

	Always	Most times	Some- times	Seldom	Never	NA
a. Children, children-in-law, or grand-children	4	3	2	1	0	8
b. Extended family	4	3	2	1	0	8
c. Friends, neighbors	4	3	2	1	0	8

COMPUTE SSS8=B17ABCD=MAX(B17A TO B17C)

I1. At the present, what are the sources of your (and your spouse's) money income?

Sources	Yes	No
2) Son/daughter-in-law in household	1	0
3) Son/daughter-in-law not in household	1	0
4) Daughter/son-in-law in household	1	0
5) Daughter/son-in-law not in household	1	0
9) Other relatives or something else	1	0

I2. What is the most important source of income?

Son/daughter-in-law in household	2
Son/daughter-in-law not in household	3
Daughter/son-in-law in household	4
Daughter/son-in-law not in household	5
Other relatives or something else	9

COMPUTE SSS9=SUM(I12,I13,I14,I15,I19)
IF (I2=2 OR I2=3 OR I2=4 OR I2=5 OR I2=9) SSS9=5

B11. a. How much financial assistance do you (or you & your spouse) provide to your children, children-in-law, and/or grandchildren?

b. your extended family (excluding spouse, children, children-in-laws, and grandchildren)?

c. your friends or neighbors?

	A great deal	Quite a bit	Some	Very little	Not at all	NA
a. Children	4	3	2	1	0	8
b. Extended family	4	3	2	1	0	8
c. Fri./neighbors	4	3	2	1	0	8

COMPUTE **SSS10**=B11ABC=MAX(B11A TO B11C)

Task-oriented

C23. Please <u>recall the last time</u> you were sick enough to think about going to a doctor. a. How much help did you receive from your family and friends? Would you say you received...

All the help you needed	3
Some help but needed more	2
Or, not much help at all	1

COMPUTE **SSS11**=C23a

D1. c. <u>IN THE PAST MONTH</u>, did you get any help in doing that?

	c. Help?		
	Yes	No	NA
1) Shopping for personal items (such as toilet items or medicine)?	1	0	9
2) Managing your money (e.g. keeping track of expenses/ paying bills)?	1	0	9
3) Using the telephone?	1	0	9
4) Washing yourself?	1	0	9
5) Climbing 2-3 flights of stairs?	1	0	9
6) Walking about 200-300 meters?	1	0	9
7) Doing heavy work in or around the house (such as washing floor, moving furniture)?	1	0	9
8) Taking a bus or train by yourself?	1	0	9
9) Lifting or carrying something as heavy as 25 pounds (such as 11-12 kg of rice)?	1	0	9

COMPUTE SSS12=HELP9=SUM(D1C1 TO D1C9)

COMPUTE SSS13=B9=LSNS9 (see Appendix Ia)

Advice/Information

H1. c. Did your family plan with you for your retirement? Would you say that they planned with you...

Very seriously	5
Seriously	4
Somewhat seriously	3
Not very seriously	2
Not seriously at all	1

RECODE H1c (1=0)(2=1)(3=2)(4=3)(5=4) INTO **SSS14**

272

C22. When you are sick, what do your family and friends usually encourage you to do?

	Yes	No
a. Do they encourage you to see a doctor right away?	1	0
b. Do they encourage you to wait a while before deciding whether or not to go to the doctor?	1	0
c. Do they encourage you to avoid going to the doctor for as long as possible?	1	0

IF (C22c=1) C22=0
IF (C22b=1) C22=1
IF (C22a=1) C22=2
COMPUTE SSS15=C22

J2. Are you consulted in the decisions made by your family? Would you say you are consulted ...

Most of the times	Sometimes	Not very often	Never
4	3	2	1

A. [UNDER WHAT CONDITION, WHEN ASKED]

a. R is alone	1
b. Children or family present	2
c. Other	3

IF (J2A=3) J2=J2-0.5
IF (J2A=2) J2=J2-1
COMPUTE SSS16=J2-1

Emotional

B12. a. How much is your (husband/wife) willing to listen when you need to talk about your worries or problems? Would you say <u>a great deal</u>, <u>quite a bit</u>, some, <u>very little</u>, or <u>not at all</u>?

b. How much are your children, children-in-laws and grandchildren willing to listen when you need to talk about your worries or problems?

c. How much are members of your extended family (excluding spouse, children and children-in-laws) willing to listen when you need to talk about your worries or problems?

d. How much are your friends or neighbors willing to listen when you need to talk about your worries or problems?

	A great deal	Quite a bit	Some	Very little	Not at all	NA
a. Spouse	5	4	3	2	1	8
b. Children, children-in-law, grandchildren	5	4	3	2	1	8
c. Extended family	5	4	3	2	1	8
d. Friends/neighbors	5	4	3	2	1	8

COMPUTE SSS17=B12ABCDE=MAX(B12A TO B12E)-1

B18. Do you feel that people around you are critical of what you do?

a. How much is your spouse critical of you or what you do?

b. How much are your children, children-in-law, or grandchildren critical of you or what you do?

c. How about members of your extended family (other relatives excluding spouse, children, children-in-laws)?

d. How about your friends, or neighbors?

	A great deal	Quite a bit	Some	Very little	Not at all	NA
a. Spouse	4	3	2	1	0	8
b. Children, children-in-law, grandchildren	4	3	2	1	0	8
c. Extended family	4	3	2	1	0	8
d. Friends/neighbors	4	3	2	1	0	8

COMPUTE SSS18=1-B18ABCDE=1-MIN(B18A TO B18E)

B10. a. How often do you comfort and/or encourage members of your immediate family (spouse, children. children-in-law, and/or grandchildren) when they feel down?

b. How about extended family members (all other relatives except immediate family)?

c. How about friends or neighbors?

	Always	Most times	Some- times	Seldom	Never	NA
a. Immediate family	4	3	2	1	0	8
b. Extended family	4	3	2	1	0	8
c. Friends, neighbors	4	3	2	1	0	8

COMPUTE SSS19=B10ABC=MAX(B10A TO B10C)

Support Appraisal

Living arrangements

G7. How satisfied are you with your current living arrangement?

Very satisfied	Somewhat satisfied	Indifferent	Somewhat dissatisfied	Very dissatisfied
5	4	3	2	1

COMPUTE SSS20=G7-3

Network size

COMPUTE SSS21=B3 (see Appendix Ia)

COMPUTE SSS22=B4 (,,   )

COMPUTE SSS23=MAX(G602C TO G610C)-3 (see Appendix Ia)

Financial assistance

B16. a. If needed, how much can you count on your children, children-in-law, or grandchildren to help you meet your expenses?

b. How much can you count on members of your extended family (other relatives excluding spouse, children, children-in-laws) to help you meet your expenses?

c. How much can you count on friends, or neighbors to help you meet your expenses?

	A great deal	Quite a bit	Some	Very little	Not at all	NA
a. Children, children-in-law, grandchildren	4	3	2	1	0	8
b. Extended family	4	3	2	1	0	8
c. Friends/neighbors	4	3	2	1	0	8
d. Others	4	3	2	1	0	8

COMPUTE **SSS24**=B16ABCD=MAX(B16A TO B16D)

Task-oriented help

B14. How much can you count on ...

a. your spouse to care for you when you are ill?
b. your children, children-in-law, or grand-children to care for you when you are ill?
c. members of your extended family (other relatives excluding spouse, children, children-in-laws) when you are ill?
d. your friends, neighbors to care for you when you are ill?

	A great deal	Quite a bit	Some	Very little	Not at all	NA
a. Spouse	4	3	2	1	0	8
b. Children, children-in-law, grandchildren	4	3	2	1	0	8
c. Extended family	4	3	2	1	0	8
d. Friends/neighbors	4	3	2	1	0	8

COMPUTE **SSS25**=B14ABCDE=MAX(B14A TO B14E)

Emotional support

J1. In your family, do you think you receive the respect you deserve from your family members? Would you say you receive...

Very much respect	Some respect	Not too much respect	Very little respect
4	3	2	1

    A. [UNDER WHAT CONDITION, WHEN ASKED]
        a. R is alone   1
        b. Children or family present   2
        c. Other   3

IF (J1A=3) J1=J1-0.5
IF (J1A=2) J1=J1-1
COMPUTE **SSS26**=J1-1

F1. During the past week,

	Rarely or none (<1 day)	Some or a little (1-2 days)	Occasionally (3-4 days)	Most/all the time (5-7 days)
12) you felt lonely	0	1	2	3
16) you felt that people dislike you	0	1	2	3
13) people were unfriendly	0	1	2	3

RECODE F112 (0=0)(1=-1)(2=-2)(3=-3) INTO **SSS27**
RECODE F116 (0=0)(1=-1)(2=-2)(3=-3) INTO **SSS28**
RECODE F113 (0=0)(1=-1)(2=-2)(3=-3) INTO **SSS29**

2. Items used for the Life Stress Scale (LSS) development

Physical Health Conditions and Events

Major events

E2. Did you have any serious but not life-threatening illness or accidental injury that occurred or got worse <u>in the past 3 years</u>?

       Yes   1   No   0

COMPUTE **LSS1**=E2

C5. <u>IN THE PAST YEAR</u>, how many separate injuries or illnessés including flare-ups of chronic conditions, have you experienced?

Record number: ___

COMPUTE **LSS2**=C5

Chronic conditions

C2. Do you have any chronic or recurring health conditions, that is, health conditions that you experience most of the time or that occur over and over?

       Yes   1   No   0

       a. How many chronic health conditions do you have?

       Record number: ___

IF (C2=0) C2a=0
COMPUTE **LSS3**=C2a

279

C4. a. <u>IN THE PAST YEAR</u>, have you had any of the following symptoms continually?

b. [For every YES, ask] How often did you have these conditions?
(daily=DL=4, several times a week=SW=3, several times a month=SM=2, once a month=OM=1, less than monthly=LM=0)

	a. Have? Yes No	b. How often? DL SW SM OM LM
3) Pain in the heart. Tightness or heaviness in the chest	1 0	4 3 2 1 0
4) Trouble breathing or shortness of breath	1 0	4 3 2 1 0
5) Repeated pain in the stomach	1 0	4 3 2 1 0
6) Frequent headaches	1 0	4 3 2 1 0
7) Spells of dizziness/poor balance	1 0	4 3 2 1 0

RECODE C4b3 C4b4 C4b5 C4b6 C4b7 C4b13 (4=5)(3=4)(2=3)(1=2) (0=1)
IF (C4a3=0) C4b3=0, ...
COMPUTE **LSS4**=C4b3
COMPUTE **LSS5**=C4b4
COMPUTE **LSS6**=C4b5
COMPUTE **LSS7**=C4b6
COMPUTE **LSS8**=C4b7

Functional status

D1. Now I will ask you about some activities of daily living. Please tell me about doing them yourself.

a. Because of a health or physical problem, do you have any difficulty doing ... [READ EACH QUESTION] by yourself?

b. By yourself, how much difficulty do you have? [A little=LT, A lot=AT, Unable to do=UD]

	a. Have?		b. How much?		
	Yes	No	LT	AT	UD
1) Shopping for personal items (such as toilet items or medicine)?	1	0	1	2	3
2) Managing your money (e.g. keeping track of expenses/paying bills)?	1	0	1	2	3
3) Using the telephone?	1	0	1	2	3
4) Washing yourself?	1	0	1	2	3
5) Climbing 2-3 flights of stairs?	1	0	1	2	3
6) Walking about 200-300 meters?	1	0	1	2	3
7) Doing heavy work in or around the house (such as washing floor, moving furniture)?	1	0	1	2	3
8) Taking a bus or train by yourself?	1	0	1	2	3
9) Lifting or carrying something as heavy as 25 pounds (such as 11-12 kg of rice)?	1	0	1	2	3

IF (D1a1=0) D1B1=0, ...
COMPUTE LSS9=SUM(D1B1 TO D1B9)

C14. Do you have trouble biting or chewing any kinds of foods, such as firm meat or apples?

Yes   1   No   0

COMPUTE LSS10=C14

C6. DURING THE PAST YEAR, how much do health troubles stand in the way of your doing the things you want to do, e.g., keep you from working at a job, doing work around the house, or doing something for your self?

Not at all 1 [skip a.]   Somewhat a little bit 2   A great deal 3

a. DURING THE PAST YEAR, how many days did you cut down on your usual activities because of a health problem?   Number of days: ___

RECODE C6 (1=0)(2=1)(3=2) INTO LSS11
IF (C6=1) C6a=0
COMPUTE LSS12=C6a

C2b. Now, please think of the most serious of your chronic health conditions. How would you rate its severity? Would you say it is ...

Very severe	Somewhat severe	Not too severe	Not severe at all
4	3	2	1

COMPUTE LSS13=C2b

C12. How is your eyesight (with glasses or contacts, if needed)?

Excellent	good	Fair	Poor	Nearly/completely blind
5	4	3	2	1

COMPUTE LSS14=4-C12

C13. How is your hearing (with hearing aid, if needed)?

Excellent	good	Fair	Poor	Nearly/completely blind
5	4	3	2	1

COMPUTE LSS15=4-C13

Physical Build

C11. a. What is your current weight?   Record weight (lb): ___
     b. What is your current height?   Record height (in): ___

COMPUTE BADWEIGHT (based on the Metropolitan Life Tables):
Appropriate   0
Over/under weight   1

COMPUTE LSS16=BADWEIGHT

C11. c. About your weight, do you think that you are...

Overweight		Just right	Underweight	
Very much	Somewhat	Just right	Somewhat	Very much
5	4	3	2	1

RECODE C11c (5,1=2)(4,2=1)(3=0) INTO **LSS17**

Cognitive Functioning

K1. Could you please tell me how well do you remember things now?

Very well	Moderately well	Can get by	Poorly	Very poorly
5	4	3	2	1

COMPUTE **LSS18**=4-K1

K2. Compared to other people your age, would you say that your memory is...

Excellent	Better	Good	Poor	Much worse
5	4	3	2	1

COMPUTE **LSS19**=3-K2

Socioeconomic Status

Education

A4. a. Have you received any formal education?   Yes 1   No 0

b. How many years of formal education have you completed? [e.g., No formal education=0, elementary school=1-6, middle school=7-9, high school=10-12, college or beyond=13-25]   Total number of years: ___

c. Are you able to read?
Yes   3
Can read a little   2
Can not read at all 1

IF (A4a=0) A4b=0
RECODE A4b (0=4)(1 THRU 6=3)(7 THRU 9=2)(10 THRU 12=1)(13 THRU HI=0) INTO **LSS20**
RECODE A4c (3=0)(2=1)(1=2) INTO **LSS21**

Unemployment/Retirement

E4. In the past 3 years, have you involuntarily lost a job for reasons other than retirement?

Yes   1   No   0

COMPUTE LSS22=E4

H1. At this time, do you consider yourself... [CHOOSE ONLY ONE RE-SPONSE CATEGORY]
Completely retired   1
Partially retired (still work some)   2
Employed full-time (not retired)   3
Unemployed   4
Never employed   5

RECODE H1 (4=4)(1=3)(2=2)(5=1)(3=0) INTO **LSS23**

H1. e. Would you like to work again if there is a suitable job for you?

Yes   1   No   0

COMPUTE **LSS24**=H1e

Income

I3. Do you think that you have enough money to cover your daily expenses?
Would you say that you have...

Quite a bit more than what you need	5
A little more than what you need	4
Just enough	3
Not quite as much as what you need	2
Much less than what you need	1

RECODE I3 (3,4=3)(5=4)
COMPUTE **LSS25**=3-I3

I4. How much do you worry about being able to manage unexpected financial
strains in the future. Would you say that you worry about it...

A great deal	Somewhat	Not too much	Not at all
3	2	1	0

COMPUTE **LSS26**=I4

Ethnic/Regional issue

E1. Have you ever been discriminated because of ...

a. your place of birth?	Yes	1	No	0
b. your language or dialect?	Yes	1	No	0

E8. Now I would like to talk about things that happen to Asian Americans because of racial discrimination and prejudice. Have you ever felt ill-treated because you are a Chinese?

Yes   1   No   0

COMPUTE **LSS27**=SUM(E1a,E1b,E8)

Living Circumstances

Changes and events

E3. Have you moved to a new residence <u>during the past 3 years</u>?
Yes   1   No   0

E10. c. If you had a chance, would you immigrate again?
Yes   1   No   0

RECODE E10c (1=0)(0=1)
COMPUTE **LSS28**=SUM(E3,E10c)

E5. Were you robbed or was your home burglarized <u>in the past 3 years</u>?

Yes   1   No   0

COMPUTE **LSS29**=E5

E6. Have you lost anyone close to you through death in the past 3 years?
a. Who was it that died?

	Yes	No
1) Spouse	1	0
2) Child	1	0
3) Child-in-law	1	0
4) Grandchild	1	0
5) Sibling	1	0
6) Other relatives	1	0
7) Friend	1	0

COMPUTE **LSS30**=E6a1
COMPUTE **LSS31**=E6a2
RECODE E6a3 E6a4 E6a5 (1=2)
COMPUTE **LSS32**=SUM(E6a3 to E6a7)

E7. Have you lost contact with anyone close to you for any reason other than death in the past 3 years?

a. Who have you lost contact with?

	Yes	No
1) Spouse	1	0
2) Child	1	0
3) Child-in-law	1	0
4) Grandchild	1	0
5) Sibling	1	0
6) Other relatives	1	0
7) Friend	1	0

COMPUTE **LSS33**=E7a1
COMPUTE **LSS34**=E7a2
RECODE E7a3 E7a4 E7a5 (1=2)
COMPUTE **LSS35**=SUM(E7a3 to E7a7)

Home conditions

G3. Do you rent your place of residence?   Yes 1   No [Ask a] 0

a. Please specify   Self own residence   1
                     Offsprings own residence   2
                     Others   3
IF (G3=1) G3a=3
COMPUTE **LSS36**=G3a-1

G4. a. Is there a bathroom in your home?   Yes 1   No   0
    b. Is there a toilet in your home?   Yes 1   No   0
RECODE G4a G4b (1=0)(0=1)
COMPUTE **LSS37**=SUM(G4a,G4b)

G5. Is your home well lit? That is, you can see the staircase, furniture clearly day and night.

Yes 1   No 0

RECODE G5 (1=0)(0=1) INTO **LSS38**

G1. Do you feel safe in your home at night?

Yes, very much so 3   Yes, relative so 2   No 1

G2. Do you feel safe in your neighborhood during the day?

Yes, very much so 3   Yes, relative so 2   No 1

RECODE G1 G2 (3=0)(2=1)(1=2)
COMPUTE **LSS39**=SUM(G1,G2)

C16. How quickly can you get to the nearest hospital/clinic?

Minutes: ___

COMPUTE **LSS40**=C16/60

Work Stress

H1. At this time, do you consider yourself...[CHOOSE ONLY ONE RESPONSE CATEGORY]

Completely retired   1
Partially retired (still work some)   2
Employed full-time (not retired)   3
Unemployed   4
Never employed   5

RECODE H1 (3=3)(2=2)(1,4,5=0) INTO **LSS41**

Developmental (Aging) Stress

J3. Has becoming old effected your position in the family?

Greatly increased your status   1
Somewhat increased your status   2
No effect on your status   3
Somewhat decreased your status   4
Greatly decreased your status   5

    A. [UNDER WHAT CONDITION, WHEN ASKED]
       a. R is alone   1
       b. Children or family present   2
       c. Other   3

IF (J3A=3) J3=J3+0.5
IF (J3A=2) J3=J3+1
COMPUTE **LSS42**=J3-3

J4. Do you think young people today have more respect, about the same, or less respect for the elderly as when you were growing up?

More respect   3
About the same   2
Less respect   1

COMPUTE **LSS43**=2-J4

F2. Do you agree with the following statements?

	Agree	Disagree
1) I am just as happy as when I was younger	1	0
4) The things I do are as interesting to me as they ever were	1	0
5) Compare to other people of my age, I make a good appearance	1	0

RECODE F21 F24 F25 (1=0)(0=1)
COMPUTE **LSS44**=SUM(F21,F24,F25)

289

3a. Modified CES-D (17 Items)

I would like to ask you some questions about how you might have felt recently, that is, in the PAST WEEK.

During the past week:

	Rarely or none (<1 day)	Some or a little (1-2 days)	Occas-ionally (3-4 days)	Most/all the time (5-7days)
1) You were bothered by things that usually don't bother you	0	1	2	3
2) You did not feel like eating	0	1	2	3
3) You felt that you would not shake off the blues even with help from your family/friends	0	1	2	3
4) You had trouble keeping your mind on what you are doing	0	1	2	3
5) You felt depressed	0	1	2	3
6) You felt everything you did was an effort	0	1	2	3
7) You thought your life had been a failure	0	1	2	3
8) You felt fearful	0	1	2	3
9) Your sleep was restless	0	1	2	3
10) You were happy	0	1	2	3
11) You talked less than usual	0	1	2	3
12) You felt lonely	0	1	2	3
13) People were unfriendly	0	1	2	3
14) You enjoyed life	0	1	2	3
15) You felt sad	0	1	2	3
16) You felt that people dislike you	0	1	2	3
17) You could not get going	0	1	2	3

3b. Items used for the Depression Scale (DS) development

Mood disturbance

During the past week:	Rarely or none (<1 day)	Some or a little (1-2 days)	Occas-ionally (3-4 days)	Most/all the time (5-7days)
F105) You felt depressed	0	1	2	3
F103) You felt that you would not shake off the blues even with help from your family /friends	0	1	2	3
F115) You felt sad	0	1	2	3
F108) You felt fearful	0	1	2	3
F110) You were happy	0	1	2	3

COMPUTE **DS1**=F105
COMPUTE **DS2**=F103
COMPUTE **DS3**=F115
COMPUTE **DS4**=F108
RECODE F110 (0=3)(3=0)(1=2)(2=1) INTO **DS5**

Loss of interest

F2. Do you agree with the following statements?

	Agree	Disagree
F23) Most of the things I do are boring or monotonous	1	0

COMPUTE **DS6**=F23

During the past week:	Rarely or none (<1 day)	Some or a little (1-2 days)	Occas-ionally (3-4 days)	Most/all the time (5-7days)
F114) You enjoyed life	0	1	2	3

RECODE F114 (0=3)(3=0)(1=2)(2=1) INTO **DS7**

Psychomotor disturbance/decreased energy

During the past week:	Rarely or none (<1 day)	Some or a little (1-2 days)	Occas-ionally (3-4 days)	Most/all the time (5-7days)
F101) You were bothered by things that usually don't bother you	0	1	2	3

COMPUTE **DS8**=F101

C4. a. IN THE PAST YEAR, have you had any of the following symptoms continually?
    b. [For every YES, ask] How often did you have these conditions?
(daily=DL=4, several times a week=SW=3, several times a month=SM=2, once a month=OM=1, less than monthly=LM=0)

	a. Have?		b. How often?				
	Yes	No	DL	SW	SM	OM	LM
8) Bothered by nervousness	1	0	4	3	2	1	0

RECODE C4b8 (4=5)(3=4)(2=3)(1=2)(0=1)
IF (C4a8=0) C4b8=0
COMPUTE **DS9**=C4b8

During the past week:	Rarely or none (<1 day)	Some or a little (1-2 days)	Occas- ionally (3-4 days)	Most/all the time (5-7days)
F106) You felt everything you did was an effort	0	1	2	3
F117) You could not get going	0	1	2	3
F111) You talked less than usual	0	1	2	3

COMPUTE **DS10**=F106
COMPUTE **DS11**=F117
COMPUTE **DS12**=F111

C4. a. IN THE PAST YEAR, have you had any of the following symptoms continually?

b. [For every YES, ask] How often did you have these conditions?
(daily=DL=4, several times a week=SW=3, several times a month=SM=2, once a month=OM=1, less than monthly=LM=0)

	a. Have?		b. How often?				
	Yes	No	DL	SW	SM	OM	LM
11) Stiffness/swelling of joints	1	0	4	3	2	1	0
2) Tiredness/fatigue	1	0	4	3	2	1	0
9) Completely worn out at the end of the day	1	0	4	3	2	1	0

RECODE C4b11 C4b2 C4b9 (4=5)(3=4)(2=3)(1=2)(0=1)
IF (C4a11=0) C4b11=0, ...
COMPUTE **DS13**=C4b11
COMPUTE **DS14**=C4b2
COMPUTE **DS15**=C4b9

Sleep disturbance

During the past week:	Rarely or none (<1 day)	Some or a little (1-2 days)	Occas- ionally (3-4 days)	Most/all the time (5-7days)
F109) Your sleep was restless	0	1	2	3

COMPUTE **DS16**=F109

C4. a. <u>IN THE PAST YEAR</u>, have you had any of the following symptoms continually?

b. [For every YES, ask] How often did you have these conditions?
(daily=DL=4, several times a week=SW=3, several times a month=SM=2, once a month=OM=1, less than monthly=LM=0)

	a. Have? Yes No	b. How often? DL SW SM OM LM
10) Problems with sleep (hard to get to sleep, difficult to stay asleep, and waking up early)	1 0	4 3 2 1 0

RECODE C4b10 (4=5)(3=4)(2=3)(1=2)(0=1)
IF (C4a10=0) C4b10=0
COMPUTE **DS17**=C4b10

Decreased appetite/constipation

During the past week:	Rarely or none (<1 day)	Some or a little (1-2 days)	Occas- ionally (3-4 days)	Most/all the time (5-7days)
F102) You did not feel like eating	0	1	2	3

COMPUTE **DS18**=F102

C4. a. IN THE PAST YEAR, have you had any of the following symptoms continually?

b. [For every YES, ask] How often did you have these conditions?

(daily=DL=4, several times a week=SW=3, several times a month=SM=2, once a month=OM=1, less than monthly=LM=0)

	a. Have?		b. How often?				
	Yes	No	DL	SW	SM	OM	LM
1) Poor appetite	1	0	4	3	2	1	0
13) Constipation	1	0	4	3	2	1	0

RECODE C4b1 (4=5)(3=4)(2=3)(1=2)(0=1)
IF (C4a1=0) C4b1=0
COMPUTE **DS19**=C4b1
COMPUTE **DS20**=C4b13

Concentration problem

During the past week:	Rarely or none (<1 day)	Some or a little (1-2 days)	Occas- ionally (3-4 days)	Most/all the time (5-7days)
F104) You had trouble keeping your mind on what you are doing	0	1	2	3

COMPUTE **DS21**=F104

C4. a. IN THE PAST YEAR, have you had any of the following symptoms continually?

b. [For every YES, ask] How often did you have these conditions?

(daily=DL=4, several times a week=SW=3, several times a month=SM=2, once a month=OM=1, less than monthly=LM=0)

	a. Have?		b. How often?				
	Yes	No	DL	SW	SM	OM	LM
12) Unable to concentrate/losing memory	1	0	4	3	2	1	0

295

RECODE C4b12 (4=5)(3=4)(2=3)(1=2)(0=1)
IF (C4a12=0) C4b12=0
COMPUTE **DS22**=C4b12

Dissatisfaction

During the past week:	Rarely or none (<1 day)	Some or a little (1-2 days)	Occas-ionally (3-4 days)	Most/all the time (5-7days)
F107) You thought your life had been a failure	0	1	2	3

COMPUTE **DS23**=F107

F2. Do you agree with the following statements?

	Agree	Disagree
F22) My life could be happier than it is now	1	0
F27) As I look back on my life, I am fairly well satisfied	1	0
F28) I've got pretty much what I expected out of life	1	0

RECODE F27 F28 (0=1)(1=0)
COMPUTE **DS24**=SUM(F22,F27,F28)

Hopelessness

F2. Do you agree with the following statements?

	Agree	Disagree
F29) In spite of what people say, a lot of the average man is getting worse, not better	1	0
F26) I expect some interesting and pleasant things to happen to me in the future	1	0

RECODE F26 (0=1)(1=0)
COMPUTE **DS25**=SUM(F29,F26)

4a. Items used in personal coping proxy measure 1: Health Behaviors and Beliefs (HBB)

C17. Usually, when you are sick, how often do you...

	Very often	Sometimes	Not too often	Never
7) go to see a doctor right away	4	3	2	1
8) rather avoid going to the doctor for as long as possible	4	3	2	1
6) talk to a friend or family member	4	3	2	1

RECODE C177 C176 (4=3)(3=2)(2=1)(1=0) INTO **HBB1 HBB2**
RECODE C178 (4=-3)(3=-2)(2=-1)(1=0) INTO **HBB3**

C23. Please recall the last time you were sick enough to think about going to a doctor.

b. Did you go to a doctor for this condition?

      Yes 1   No 0

COMPUTE **HBB4**=C23b

C29. How often do you read articles or literature specifically to learn about protecting your health?

Regularly	Sometimes	Rarely or never
3	2	1

COMPUTE **HBB5**=C29

C30. How often do you watch or listen to programs on radio or TV in order to learn about protecting your health?

Regularly	Sometimes	Rarely or never
3	2	1

COMPUTE HBB6=C30

C31. How often do you exchange information or ideas with your friends about ways to keep your health at its best?

Regularly 3   Sometimes 2   Rarely or never 1

COMPUTE HBB7=C31

D3. How often do you exercise, e.g., Taichi, swimming, morning walk, jogging?

Never	0	Once a month at most	1
Several times a month	2	Once a week	3
Two or three times a week	4	Four times+ in a week	5

a. When you exercise, does it last 20 minutes or more every time?

Yes   1   No   0

b. How long have you been exercising regularly

Record number of years: ___

COMPUTE HBB8=D3
IF (D3=0 OR D3=1 OR D3=2 OR D3=3 OR D3a=0) D3b=0
COMPUTE HBB9=D3b

C19. How much do you trust...
  a. Western doctors? Would you say you trust Western doctors...
  b. Chinese doctors? Would you say you trust Chinese doctors...

A great deal	Somewhat	Not too much	Not much at all
4	3	2	1

COMPUTE **HBB10**=C19a
COMPUTE **HBB11**=C19b

4b. Items used in personal coping proxy measure 2: Attitudes Toward Social Support (ATSS)

Marriage

G10. If an old man loses his wife, do you think it is appropriate for him to remarry?

No 0   Yes 1   Depends 2   Other 3

G11. If an old woman loses her husband, do you think it is appropriate for her to remarry?

No 0   Yes 1   Depends 2   Other 3

RECODE G10 G11 (0=0)(2,3=1)(1=2) INTO **ATSS1 ATSS2**

Living arrangements

G8. When an old person/old couple gets older, should he/they live with a married son, stay on his/their own, or something else?

Live with married son	1
Live with married child (son or daughter)	2
Live with married daughter	3
Stay on his/their own	4
Not sure, depends	5
Something else	6

RECODE G8 (4=0)(5=1)(6=2)(1,2,3=3) INTO **ATSS3**

G9. If the old person/old couple has no son, should he/they go to live with a married daughter, move to an old age home, or something else?

Live with married daughter	1
Stay on his/their own	2
Move to old age home	3
Not sure, depends	4
Something else	5

RECODE G9 (2=0)(4=1)(5=2)(3=3)(1=4) INTO **ATSS4**

Caring arrangements

I6. We have talked about many things regarding the needs of the elderly. Who, do you think, should satisfy their needs in ...

a. financial well-being
b. satisfactory housing
c. transportation
d. health care
e. dealing with outside agencies, include filling out forms and handling money

Self/spouse	1
Children	2
Relatives	3
Friends/neighbors	4
Churches/religious organizations	5
Government, e.g., Social Welfare Department	6
Others	7

RECODE I6a TO I6e (1=0)(7=1)(5,6=2)(4=3)(2,3=4) INTO **ATSS5 TO ATSS9**

4c. Items used in personal coping proxy measure 3: Attitudes Toward Elderly (ATE)

J5. The following are some statements made about elderly people. Do you agree with it when people say...

	Strgly agree	Smwhat agree	Don't care	Smwhat disagree	Strongly disagree
a. Old people are burdens of family and society	1	2	3	4	5
b. Old people's experience and tradition are out-dated and worthless	1	2	3	4	5
c. They may still be able to do something useful	1	2	3	4	5
d. They have abundant experience and good tradition	1	2	3	4	5

RECODE J5c J5d (1=2)(5=-2)(2=1)(4=-1)(3=0) INTO **ATE1 ATE2**
RECODE J5a J5b (1=-2)(5=2)(2=-1)(4=1)(3=0) INTO **ATE3 ATE4**

Bibliography

Abramson, L.Y., & Alloy, L.B. (1990), 'Search for the "negative cognition" subtype of depression', in McCann, C.D., & Endler, N. (eds.), *Depression: New Directions in Theory, Research and Practice*, Wall & Emerson, Toronto.

Acosta-Cooper, Carmel Theresa (1989), *The Influence of Support Systems on the Subjective Well-Being of Mexican-American Elderly*, unpublished doctoral dissertation, Harvard University.

Alloway, Ruth, & Bebbington, Paul (1987), 'The buffer theory of social support - A review of the literature', *Psychological Medicine*, 17:91-108.

Alloy, L.B. (ed.) (1988), *Cognitive Processes in Depression*, Guilford Press, New York.

Alloy, L.B., Hartlage, S. & Abramson, L.Y. (1988), 'Testing the cognitive diathesis-stress theories of depression: Issues of research design, conceptualization, and assessment', in Alloy, L.B. (ed.), *Cognitive Processes in Depression*, Guilford Press, New York.

Altshuler, Lori L., et al. (1988), 'Who seeks mental health care in China? Diagnoses of Chinese outpatients according to DSM-III criteria and the Chinese classification system', *American Journal of Psychiatry*, 145(7):872-75.

American Psychiatric Association (1987), *Diagnostic and Statistical Manual of Mental Disorders*, 3rd Ed. (revised), American Psychiatric Association, Washington, D.C.

Babbie, Earl (1992), *The Practice of Social Research*, 6th Ed., Wadsworth Publishing Company, Belmont, CA.

Bandura, A. (1982), 'Self-efficacy mechanism in human agency', *American Psychologist*, 37:122-47.

Barrera, Manuel, Jr., & Ainlay, Sheila L. (1983), 'The structure of social support: A conceptual and empirical analysis', *Journal of Community Psychology*, 11:133-42.

Bech, Per (1992), 'Symptoms and assessment of depression', in Paykel, Eugene S. (ed.), *Handbook of Affective Disorders*, 2nd Ed., the Guilford Press, New York.

Beck, A.T. et al. (1961), 'An inventory for measuring depression', *Archives of General Psychiatry*, 4:53-63.

Becker, Joseph, & Kleinman, Arthur (eds.) (1991), *Psychosocial Aspects of Depression*, Lawrence Erlbaum Associates, Hillsdale, NJ.

Bentler, P.M. (1985), *Theory and Implementation of EQS: A Structural Equations Program*, BMDP Statistical Software, Los Angeles.

Bentler, P.M. (1989), *EQS: Structural Equations Program Manual*, BMDP Statistical Software, Los Angeles.

Blaik, R. (1980), *Perception of Social Support Satisfaction and Perception of Social Contact: Psychometric Instrument Development*, unpublished Ph.D. dissertation, University of North Carolina.

Blalock, H.M. (1962), 'Four-variable causal models and partial correlations', *American Journal of Sociology*, 68:182-94.

Bloom, Joan R. et al. (1991), 'Social supports and the social well-being of cancer survivors', *Advances in Medical Sociology*, 2:95-114.

Boudon, R. (1965), 'A method of linear causal analysis: dependence analysis', *American Sociological Review*, 30:365-74.

Brown, G.W., & Harris, T.O. (1978), *Social Origins of Depression: A Study of Psychiatric Disorder in Women*, Free Press, New York.

Brown, G.W., & Harris, T.O. (1989), 'Depression', in Brown, G.E., & Harris, T.O. (eds.), *Life Events and Psychiatric Illness,* the Guilford Press, New York.

Campbell, Angus (1974), 'Quality of life as a psychological phenomenon', in Strumpel, Burkhard (ed.), *Subjective Elements of Well-Being.* Organisation for Economic Co-Operation and Development, Paris.

Caplan, G. (1974). *Support Systems and Community Mental Health: Lectures on Concept Development*, Behavioral Publications, New York.

Cassel, J. (1974), 'Psychosocial Processes and "Stress": Theoretical Formulations', *International Journal of Health Services*, 4:471-82.

Cassel, J. (1976), 'The contribution of the social environment to host resistance', *American Journal of Epidemiology*, 104:107-23.

Caplan, G. (ed.) (1974), *Support Systems and Community Mental Health*, Basic Books, New York.

Chan, David W. (1991), 'Depressive symptoms and depressed mood among Chinese medical students in Hong Kong', *Comprehensive Psychiatry*, 32(2):170-80.

Chen, Shengzhang (1991), 'A research report of the health survey on the elderly in Guangzhou', paper presented at the Cross-National Conference on Asian and Asian-American Elderly Research, August, Los Angeles.

Chen, Sheying (1996), *Social Policy of the Economic State and Community Care in Chinese Culture: Aging, Family, Urban Change, and the Socialist Welfare Pluralism*, Avebury, Brookfield, Vermont/Aldershot, UK.

Chi, Iris, & Lee, Jik-Joen (1989), 'A health survey of the elderly in Hong Kong', Resource Paper Series No.14, Department of Social Work and Social Administration, University of Hong Kong.

Chi, Iris, & Boey, K.W. (1992), 'Validation of measuring instruments of mental health status of the elderly in Hong Kong', Resource Paper Series No.17, Department of Social Work and Social Administration, University of Hong Kong.

Chi, Iris, & Boey, K.W. (1994), 'A mental health and social support study of the old-old in Hong Kong', Resource Paper Series No.22, Department of Social Work and Social Administration, University of Hong Kong.

Chu, Godwin C. (1985), 'The emergence of the new Chinese culture', in Tseng, Wen-Shing, & Wu, David Y.H. (eds.) (1985), *Chinese Culture and Mental Health*, Academic Press, Orlando, Florida.

Cleary, Patrick J. (1980), 'A checklist for life event research', *Journal of Psychosomatic Research*, 24:199-207.

Cobb, S. (1976), 'Social support as a moderator of life stress', *Psychosomatic Medicine*, 38(5):300-14.

Cohen, S., & Edwards, J.R. (1989), 'Personality characteristics as moderators of the relationship between stress and disorder', in Neufeld, R.W.J. (ed.), *Advances in the Investigation of Psychological Stress*, John Wilky & Sons, New York.

305

Cohen, S., & G. McKay (1984), 'Social support, stress and the buffering hypothesis: A theoretical analysis', in Baum, A., Taylor, S.E. & Singer, J.E. (eds.), *Handbook of Psychology and Health*, Erlbaum, Hillsdale, N.J.

Cohen, S., & Wills, T.A. (1985), 'Stress, social support, and the buffering hypothesis', *Psychological Bulletin*, 98:310-57.

Coombs, C. H. (1964), *A Theory of Data*, Wiley, New York.

Costello, Charles G. (ed.) (1993), *Symptoms of Depression*, John Wiley & Sons, New York.

Culyer, A.J. (1981), 'Health and health indicators: Proceedings of a European workshop', a report to the British Social Science Research Council and the European Science Foundation, University of York.

DeVellis, Robert F. (1991), *Scale Development: Theory and Applications*, Sage Publications, Newbury Park, CA.

Davis, James A. (1985), *The Logic of Causal Order*, Sage University Paper Series on Quantitative Applications in the Social Sciences, 07-055. Sage, Newbury Park, CA.

Davison, Mark L. (1983), *Multidimensional Scaling*, John Wiley & Sons, New York.

Dean, Alfred (1986), 'Social support in epidemiological perspective', in Lin, N., Dean, A. & Ensel, W. *Social Support, Life Events, and Depression*, Academic Press, Orlando, FL.

Dobelstein, Andrew W., & Johnson, Ann B. (1985), *Serving Older Adults: Policy, Programs, and Professional Activities*, Prentice-Hall, Englewood Cliffs.

Dohrenwend, B.S., et al. (1984), 'Symptoms, hassles, social supports, and life events: Problems of confounded measures', *Journal of Abnormal Psychology*, 93:222-30.

Donald, Cathy A. and Ware, John E., Jr. (1984), 'The measurement of social support', *Research in Community and Mental Health*, 4:325-70.

Duncan, O.D. (1966), 'Path analysis: Sociological examples', *American Journal of Sociology*, 72:1-16.

Dunham, H. W. (1965), *Community and Schizophrenia: An Epidemiological Analysis*, Wayne State University Press, Detroit, Mich.

Eaton, William W. (1986), *The Sociology of Mental Disorders*, 2nd Ed., Praeger, New York.

Finch, Janet (1986), 'Age', in Burgess, Robert G. (ed.), *Key Variables in Social Investigation*, Routledge & Kegan Paul, London.

Frankenhaeuser, Marianne (1986), 'A psychobiological framework for research on human stress and coping', in Appley, H., & Trumbell, R. (eds.), *Dynamics of Stress*, Plenum Press, N.Y.

Freden, Lars (1982), *Psychosocial Aspects of Depression: No Way Out?* John Wiley & Sons, Chichester.

Freud, S. (1959), 'Mourning and Melancholia' (first published in 1917), *Collected Papers*, Vol.4, Basic Books, New York.

Ghiselli, Edwin E. (1964), *Theory of Psychological Measurement*, McGraw-Hill Book Company, New York.

Gordon, Milton M. (1964), *Assimilation in American Life*, Oxford University Press, New York.

Gore, Susan (1981), 'Stress-buffering functions of social supports: An appraisal and clarification of research models', in Dohrenwend, B.S., & Dohrenwend, B.P. (eds.), *Stressful Life Events and Their Contexts*, Prodist, New York. pp.202-22.

Gotlib, Ian H., & Hammen, Constance L. (1992), *Psychological Aspects of Depression: Toward a Cognitive-Interpersonal Integration*, J. Wiley, New York.

Gottlieb, Benjamin H. (1983), *Social Support Strategies: Guidelines for Mental Health Practice*, Sage Publications, Beverly Hills, CA.

Grob, G.N. (1983), *Mental Illness and American Society*, Princeton University Press, Princeton, NJ.

Grove, William M. & Andreasen, Nancy C. (1992), 'Concepts, diagnosis and classification', in Paykel, Eugene S. (ed.), *Handbook of Affective Disorders*, 2nd Ed., the Guilford Press, New York.

Guilford, J.P. (1978), 'When not to factor analyze', in Jackson, Douglas N., & Messick, Samuel (eds.), *Problems in Human Assessment*, Robert E. Krieger Publishing Company, Huntington, NY.

Gurland, B. (1976), 'The comparative frequency of depression in various adult age groups', *Journal of Gerontology*, 31:283-92.

Hammen, Constance (1984), 'Mood disorders (unipolar depression)', in Hersen, M. & Turner, S. (eds.), *Adult Psychopathology and Diagnosis*, Wiley, New York.

Hammen, Constance (1992), 'Cognitive, life stress, and interpersonal approaches to a developmental psychopathology model of depression', *Development and Psychopathology*, 4:189:206.

Hathaway, S.R., & McKinley, J.C. (1942), 'A multiphasic personality schedule (Minnesota): III. The measurement of symptomatic depression', *Journal of Psychology*, 14:73-84.

Healer, K. (1979). 'The effects of social support: Prevention and treatment implications', in Goldstein, A.P., & Kanter, F.H. (eds.), *Maximizing Treatment Gains: Transfer Enhancement in Psychotherapy*, Academic Press, New York.

Henderson, A.S. (1992), 'Social support and depression', in Veiel, Hans O.F. and Baumann, Urs (eds.), *The Meaning and Measurement of Social Support*, Hemisphere Publishing Corporation, New York.

Herzog, A. Regula, Rodgers, Willard L., & Woodworth, Joseph (1982), *Subjective Well-Being among Different Age Groups*, Institute for Social Research, the University of Michigan, Ann Arbor.

Hobfoll, Stevan E. (1988), *The Ecology of Stress*, Hemisphere, New York.

Holahan, Charles J., & Moos, Rudolf H. (1985), 'Life stress and health: Personality, coping, and family support in stress resistance', *Journal of Personality and Social Psychology*, 49(3):739-47.

Holmes, T.H. and Rahe, R.H. (1967), 'The Social Readjustment Rating Scale', *Journal of Psychosomatic Research*, 11:213-18.

Hooyman, Nancy R., & Kiyak, H. Asuman (1991), *Social Gerontology: A Multidisciplinary Perspective*, 2nd Ed., Allyn and Bacon, Boston.

Horst, Paul (1966), *Psychological Measurement and Prediction*, Wadsworth Publishing Company, Inc., Belmont, CA.

House, James S., & Kahn, Robert L. (1985), 'Measures and concepts of social support', in Cohen, S., & Syme, L. (eds.), *Social Support and Health*, Academic Press, New York.

Hsu, F. L. K. (1971), 'Psychosocial homeostasis and jen: Conceptual tools for advancing psychological anthropology', *American Anthropologist*, 73:23-33.

Hsu, (1985), In: Tseng, Wen-Shing, & Wu, David Y.H. (eds.), *Chinese Culture and Mental Health*, the Academic Press, Orlando.

Hwu H-G, Yeh E-K, Chang L-Y (1989), 'Prevalence of psychiatric disorders in Taiwan defined by the Chinese Diagnostic Interview Schedule', *Acta Psychiatrica Scandinavica*, 79:136-47.

Ikels, Charlotte (1989), 'Disability in China: Cultural issues in measurement and interpretation', paper presented at the Modern China Seminar, February, Harvard University.

Jacoby, William G. (1991), *Data Theory and Dimensional Analysis*, Sage University Paper Series on Quantitative Applications in the Social Sciences, 07-078, Sage, Newbury Park, CA.

Jalowiec, A., & Powers, M.J. (1981), 'Stress and Coping in Hypertensive and Emergency Room Patients', *Nursing Research*, 30:10-15.

James, L.R., Mulaik, S.A. & Brett, J.M. (1982), *Causal Analysis: Assumptions, Models, and Data*, Sage, Beverly Hills, CA.

Jöreskog, K.G., & Sörbom, D. (1989), *LISREL 7: A Guide to the Program and Applications*, 2nd Ed., SPSS Inc., Chicago.

Kahn, R. L. (1979), 'Aging and Social support', in Riley, M.W. (ed.), *Aging from Birth to Death: Interdisciplinary Perspectives*, Westview Press, Boulder, CO.

Kane, Rosalie A., & Kane, Robert L. (1981), *Assessing the Elderly: A Practical Guide to Measurement*, LexingtonBooks, Lexington, MA.

Kantor, Martin (1992), *The Human Dimension of Depression: A Practical Guide to Diagnosis, Understanding, and Treatment*, Praeger, New York.

Kendell, R.E. (1968), *The classification of depressive illness*, Oxford University Press, Oxford.

Kim, J. and Mueller, C.W. (1978), *Factor Analysis: Statistical Methods and Practical Issues*, Sage University Paper Series on Quantitative Applications in the Social Sciences, 07-014. Beverly Hills, CA.

Kitano, Harry H.L. (1969), *Japanese Americans: The Evolution of a Subculture*, Prentice-Hall, Englewood Cliffs, N.J.

Kleinman, A. (1982), 'Neurasthenia and depression: A study of somatization and culture in China', *Culture, Medicine and Psychiatry*, 6, 117-190.

Kleinman, A. (1986), *Social Origins of Distress and Disease: Depression, Neurasthenia, and Pain in Modern China*, Yale University Press, New Haven.

Klerman, Gerald L. (1987), 'The nature of depression: Mood, symptom, disorder', in Marsella, A.J., Hirschfeld, R.M.A. & Katz, M.M. (eds.), *The Measurement of Depression*. Guilford press, New York.

Klerman, G.L., & Weissman, M.M. (1989), 'Increasing rates of depression', *Journal of the American Medical Association*, 261:2229-35.

Kobasa, S. C., Maddi, S. R. & Kahn, S. (1982), 'Hardiness and health: a prospective study', *Journal of Personality and Social Psychology*, 42:168-177.

Kraepelin, E. (1921), *Manic-Depressive Insanity and Paranoia*, E & S. Livingstone, Edinburgh.

Krauthammer, C., & Klerman, G.L. (1979), 'The Epidemiology of Mania', in Shopsin, B. (ed.), *Manic Illness*, Raven Press, New York.

Kuo, Wen H. (1984), 'Prevalence of depression among Asian-Americans', *The Journal of Nervous and Mental Disease*, 172(8):449-57.

Larson, James S. (1993), 'The measurement of social well-being', *Social Indicators Research*, 28:285-96.

Lazarus, R.S. (1966), *Psychological Stress and the Coping Process*, McGraw-Hill, New York.

Lazarus, R.S., & Folkman, S. (1984), *Stress, Appraisal, and Coping*, Springer, New York.

Levine, Sol, & Scotch, Norman A. (1970), *Social Stress*, Aldine Publishing Company, Chicago.

Li, Pei-liang (1988), *Shehui Yanjiu de Tongji Fenxi* (Statistical Analysis in Social Research), *Juliu* Books Co., Taipei. (in Chinese)

Lieberman, M.A. (1986), 'Social supports - The consequence of psychologizing: A commentary', *Journal of Consulting and Clinical Psychology*, 54:461-65.

Lin, N. et al. (1979), 'Social support, stressful life-events and illness: A model and an empirical test', *Journal of Health and Social Behavior*, 20:108-19.

Lin (1985), in Tseng, Wen-Shing, & Wu, David Y.H. (eds.), *Chinese Culture and Mental Health*, the Academic Press, Orlando.

Lin, Nan (1986), 'Modeling the effects of social support', in Lin, N., Dean, A. & Ensel, W., *Social Support, Life Events, and Depression*, Orland Academic Press, Orlando, FL.

Lin, Nan (1989), 'Measuring depressive symptomatology in China', n.p. 177(3):121-31.

Lin, N., & Ensel, Walter M. (1989), 'Life stress and health: Stressors and resources', *American Sociological Review*, 54:382-99.

Lin, N., Dean, A. & Ensel, W. (1979), 'Constructing social support scales: A methodological note', paper presented at the Conference on Stress, Social Support, and Schizophrenia, September 24-25, Burlington, Vermont.

Lin, N., Dean, A. & Ensel, W. (1986) *Social Support, Life Events, and Depression*, Orland Academic Press, Orlando, FL.

Lubben, James E. (1983), 'Health and psychosocial assessment instruments for community based long term care: The California Multipurpose Senior Services Project experience', unpublished doctoral dissertation, University of California, Berkeley.

Lubben, James E. (1987), 'A short, reliable, and valid instrument for assessing the social networks of elderly persons: The Lubben Social Network Scale (LSNS)', paper presented at the 40th Annual Meeting of the Gerontological Society of America, November, Washington, D.C.

Lubben, James E. (1988), 'Assessing social networks among elderly populations', *Family & Community Health*, November, 11(3):42-52.

Lyman, Stanford M. (1974), *Chinese Americans*, Random House, New York.

MacCallum, R.C. (1974), 'Relations between factor analysis and multidimensional scaling', *Psychological Bulletin*, 81:505-16.

Macintyre, Sally (1986), 'Health and illness', in Burgess, Robert G. (ed.), *Key Variables in Social Investigation*, Routledge & Kegan Paul, London.

McDowell, Ian, & Newell, Claire (1987), *Measuring Health: A Guide to Rating Scales and Questionnaires*, Oxford University Press, New York.

McFarlane, Allan H., et al. (1981), 'Methodological issues in developing a scale to measure social support', *Schizophrenia Bulletin*, 7(1):90-100.

McGrath, J.E. (ed.) (1970), *Social and Psychological Factors in Stress*, Holt, Rinehart & Winston, New York.

McIver, John P., & Carmines, Edward G. (1981), *Unidimensional Scaling*, Sage University Paper Series on Quantitative Applications in the Social Sciences, 07-024, Sage, Beverly Hills, CA.

Michell, Joel (1990), *An Introduction to the Logic of Psychological Measurement*, Lawrence Erlbaum Associates, Hillsdale, NJ.

Monroe, Scott M., & Simons, Anne D. (1991), 'Diathesis-stress theories in the context of life stress research: Implications for the depressive disorders', *Psychological Bulletin*, 110(3):406-25.

Moos, Rudolph H., & Billings, Andrew G. (1982), 'Conceptualizing and measuring coping resources and processes', in Goldberger, Leo, & Breznitz, Shlomo (eds.), *Handbook of Stress: Theoretical and Clinical Aspects*, the Free Press, New York.

Morgan, D.H.J. (1986), 'Gender', in Burgess, Robert G. (ed.), *Key Variables in Social Investigation*, Routledge & Kegan Paul, London.

Morrison, Donald F. (1990), *Multivariate Statistical Methods*, 3rd Ed., McGraw-Hill, New York.

Murphy, Elaine (ed.) (1986), *Affective Disorders in the Elderly*, Churchill Livingstone, New York.

Murphy, Elaine, & Macdonald, Alastair (1992), 'Affective disorders in old age', in Paykel, Eugene S. (ed.), *Handbook of Affective Disorders*, 2nd ed., the Guilford Press New York.

Myers, J.K., Lindentrhal, J.J. and Pepper, M.P. (1975), 'Life events, social integration and psychiatric symptomatology', *Journal of Health and Social Behavior*, 16:21-27.

Myers, J.K., et al. (1984), 'Six month prevalence of psychiatric disorders in three communities', *Archives of General Psychiatry*, 41:959-67.

Nakane, Y. et al. (1988), 'Comparative study of affective disorders in three Asian Countries I. Differences in Diagnostic Classification', *Acta Psychiatr Scand*, 78:698-705.

Nakane, Y. et al. (1991), 'Comparative study of affective disorders in three Asian Countries II. Differences in Prevalence Rates and Symptom Presentation', *Acta Psychiatr Scand*, 84:313-19.

Norusis, Marija J. (1988), *SPSS-X Introductory Statistics Guide*, SPSS Inc., Chicago.

Nunnally, J.C. (1978), *Psychometric Theory*. New York: McGraw-Hill.

Paykel, Eugene S. (ed.) (1992), *Handbook of Affective Disorders*, 2nd Ed., the Guilford Press, New York.

Paykel, Eugene S., & Cooper, Zafra (1992), 'Life events and social stress', in Paykel, Eugene S. (ed.), *Handbook of Affective Disorders*, 2nd ed., the Guilford Press, New York.

Paykel, E.S., & Norton, K.R.W. (1986), 'Self-report and clinical interview in the assessment of depression', in Sartorius, N., & Ban, T.A. (eds.), *Assessment of Depression*, Springer, Berlin.

Pearlin, L.I.(1989), 'The sociological study of stress', *Journal of Health and Social Behavior*, 30(September):241-56.

Pearlin, Leonard I., & Aneshensel, Carol S. (1986), 'Coping and social supports: Their functions and applications', in Aiken, Linda H., & Mechanic, David (eds.), *Applications of Social Science to Clinical Medicine and Health Policy*, Rutgers University Press, New Brunswick, N.J.

Pedhazur, Elazar J. (1982), *Multiple regression in behavioral research: Explanation and prediction*, 2nd Ed., Holt, Rinehart & Winston, Fort Worth, Texas.

Pedhazur, Elazar J., & Schmelkin, Liora Pedhazur (1991), *Measurement, Design, and Analysis: An Integrated Approach*, Lawrence Erlbaum Associates, Hillsdale, NJ.

Perris, Carlo (1992), 'Bipolar-unipolar distinction', in Paykel, Eugene S. (ed.), *Handbook of Affective Disorders*, 2nd ed., the Guilford Press, New York.

Peterson, R.E. (1953), *Stress Concentration Design Factors*, New York.

Pinker, R. (1979), *The Idea of Welfare*, Heinemann, London.

Rabkin, Judith G., & Donald F. Klein (1987), 'The clinical measurement of depressive disorders', in Marsella, A.J., Hirschfeld, R.M.A. & Katz, M.M. (eds.), *The Measurement of Depression*, Guilford Press, New York.

Rende, R., & R. Plomin (1992), 'Diathesis-stress models of psychopathology: A quantitative genetic perspective', *Applied and Preventive Psychology*, 1:177-82.

Rook, Karen S. (1992), 'Detrimental aspects of social relationships: Taking stock of an emerging literature', in Veiel, Hans O.F., & Baumann, Urs (eds.), *The Meaning and Measurement of Social Support*, Hemisphere Publishing Corporation, New York.

Roth, M. (1977), 'The association of affective disorders and physical somatic disease and its bearing on certain problems of psychosomatic medicine, in Antonelli, F. (ed.), *Therapy in Psychosomatic Medicine*, Pozzi, Roma.

Roth, M., Gurney, C. & Mountjoy, C.Q. (1983), 'The Newcastle rating scales', *Acta Psychiatrica Scandinavica*, 68(suppl. 310):42-54.

Rotter, J.B. (1966), 'Generalized experiences for internal versus external control of reinforcement. *Psychological Monographs: General and Applied*, 80(1) (Whole No.609).

Rowe, John W. & Robert L. Kahn (1987), *Human Aging: Usual and Successful Science*, 237:143-49.

Sandler, Irwin N., & Barrera, Manuel Jr. (1984), 'Toward a multimethod approach to assessing the effects of social support', *American Journal of Community Psychology*, 12(1):37-52.

Sarason, I.G., & Sarason, B.P. (eds.) (1985), *Social Support: Theory, Research and Applications*, Martinus Nijhoff, Den Haag.

Saris, Willem, & Stronkhorst, Henk (1984), *Causal Modeling in Nonexperimental Research: An Introduction to the LISREL Approach*, Sociometric Research Foundation.

Schaefer, C., Conyne, J.C. & Lazarus, R.S. (1981), 'The health-related functions of social support', *Journal of Behavioral Medicine*, 4:381-406.

Schwarzer, Ralf, & Leppin, Anja (1992), 'Possible impact of social ties and support on morbidity and mortality', in Veiel, Hans O.F., & Baumann, Urs (eds.), *The Meaning and Measurement of Social Support*, Hemisphere Publishing Corporation, New York.

Scott, Janine (1992), 'Social and community approaches', in Paykel, Eugene S. (ed.), *Handbook of Affective Disorders*, 2nd ed., the Guilford Press, New York.

Selye, H. (1936), 'A syndrome produced by diverse nocuous agents', *Nature*, 138:32.

Selye, H. (1982), 'History and present status of the stress concept', in Goldberger, L., & Breznitz, B. (eds.), *Handbook of Stress*, the Free Press, New York.

Sewell, W.H. (1941), 'The development of a sociometric scale', *Sociometry*, 5:279-97.

Shively, W.P. (1980), *The Craft of Political Research: A Primer*, Prentice-Hall, Englewood Cliffs, NJ.

Shulman, K.I. (1989), 'Conceptual problems in the assessment of depression in old age', *Psychiatric Journal of the University of Ottawa*, 14:364-66.

Simon, H.A. (1954), 'Spurious correlation: A causal interpretation', *Journal of the American Statistical Association*, 49:467-79.

Skodol, Andrew E., et al. (1990), 'The nature of stress: Problems of measurement', in Noshpitz, Joseph D., & Coddington, R. Dean (eds.), *Stressors and the Adjustment Disorders*, John Wiley & Sons, New York.

Smith, Angela L., & Weissman, Myrna M. (1992), 'Epidemiology', in Paykel, Eugene S. (ed.), *Handbook of Affective Disorders*, 2nd ed., the Guilford Press, New York.

Soomer, Barbara, & Sommer, Robert (1991), *A Practical Guide to Behavioral Research: Tools and Techniques,* 3rd ed., Oxford University Press, New York.

Srole, L., & A.K. Fischer (1980), 'The midtown Manhattan longitudinal study versus the "paradise lost" doctrine', *Archives of General Psychiatry,* 37:209-21.

Stokes, Joseph P., & Wilson, Diane G. (1983), 'Social support, network structure, and the inventory of socially supportive behaviors', paper presented at the 91st Annual Convention of the American Psychological Association, August, Anaheim, CA.

Sue, Stanley, & Morishima, James K. (1982), *The Mental Health of Asian Americans: Contemporary Issues in Identifying and Treating Mental Problems,* Jossey-Bass Publishers, San Francisco.

Syme, S.L. (1982), 'Is Social Isolation a Risk Factor for Coronary Heart Disease?' Paper presented at the 9th Science Writers Forum of the American Heart Association, Charleston, SC.

Taylor, Robert B. (1969), *Cultural Ways: A Compact Introduction to Cultural Anthropology,* Allyn and Bacon, Boston, MA.

Taiwan Provincial Institute of Family Planning, & University of Michigan Population Studies Center & Institute of Gerontology (1989), '1989 survey of health and living status of the elderly in Taiwan: Questionnaire and survey design', Comparative Study of the Elderly in Four Asian Countries, Research Report No. 1.

Thoits, P.A. (1982), 'Conceptual, methodological, and theoretical problems in studying social support as a buffer against life stress', *Journal of Health and Social Behavior,* 23:145-59.

Timoshenko, S. & Young, D.H. (1962), *Elements of Strength of Materials,* 4th Ed., D.Van Nostrand Company, Princeton, NJ.

Torgerson, Warren S. (1958), *Theory and Methods of Scaling,* John Wiley & Sons, New York.

Tseng, Wen-Shing, & Wu, David Y.H. (eds.) (1985), *Chinese Culture and Mental Health,* Academic Press, Orlando.

Turner, R. Jay (1992), 'Measuring social support: issues of concept and method', in Veiel, Hans O.F. and Urs Baumann (eds.), *The Meaning and Measurement of Social Support,* Hemisphere Publishing Corporation, New York.

Van de Geer, John P. (1971), *Introduction to Multivariate Analysis for the Social Sciences*, W.H. Freeman and Company, San Francisco.

Vaux, Alan, et al. (1986), 'The Social Support Appraisals (SS-A) Scale: Studies of reliability and validity', *American Journal of Community Psychology*, 14(2):195-219.

Vaux, Alan, Burde, Philip & Stewart, Doreen (1986), 'Orientation towards utilizing support resources', *Journal of Community Psychology*, 14:159-70.

Vaux, Alan (1988), *Social Support: Theory, Research, and Intervention*, Praeger, N.Y.

Vaux, Alan (1992), 'Assessment of Social Support,' in Veiel, Hans O.F. and Baumann, Urs (eds.), *The Meaning and Measurement of Social Support*, Hemisphere Publishing Corporation, New York.

Veiel, Hans O.F. and Baumann, Urs (eds.) (1992), *The meaning and measurement of social support*, Hemisphere Publishing Corporation, New York.

Wallis, C. (1983), 'Stress: Can We Cope?' *Time Magazine*, June 8, 48-54.

Wallston, B.S., et al. (1983), 'Social support and physical health,' *Health Psychology*, 2:367-91.

Weissman, M.M. & Myers, J.K. (1978), 'Affective disorders in a US urban community: The use of research diagnostic criteria in an epidemiological survey', *Archives of General Psychiatry*, 35:1304-11.

Wellman, B. (1985), 'From social support to social network', in Sarason, I.G., & Sarason, B.P. (eds.), *Social Support: Theory, Research and Applications*, Martinus Nijhoff, Den Haag.

Welner, A., et al. (1979), 'Psychiatric disorders among professional women', *Archives of General Psychiatry*, 36:169-73.

Wilkening, Eugene A., & Ahrens, Nancey W. (1979), 'Social determinants of subjective well-being in northwestern Wisconsin', *Research Bulletin*, R2968, Research Division, College of Agricultural and Life Sciences, University of Wisconsin.

Woodruff, R.A., et al. (1971), 'Unipolar and bipolar primary affective disorder', *British Journal of Psychiatry*, 119:33-38.

World Health Organization (1958), *The First Ten Years of the World Health Organization*, World Health Organization, Geneva.

World Health Organization (1978), *Mental Disorders: Glossary and Guide to Their Classification in Accordance with the Ninth Revision of the International Classification of Diseases*, WHO, Geneva.

Wright, S. (1934), 'The method of path coefficients', *Annals of Mathematical Statistics*, V:161-215.

Ying, Yu-wen (1988), 'Depressive symptomatology among Chinese-Americans as measured by the CES-D', *Journal of Clinical Psychology*, 44(5):739-46.

Zung, W.W.K. (1965), 'A self-rating depression scale', *Archives of General Psychiatry*, 12:63-70.